SITE-SPECIFIC CANCER SERIES

Gynecologic Cancers

Edited by
Lois Almadrones-Cassidy, RN, MS, FNP, MPA

Oncology Nursing Society
Pittsburgh, Pennsylvania

ONS Publishing Division
Publisher: Leonard Mafrica, MBA, CAE
Director, Commercial Publishing: Barbara Sigler, RN, MNEd
Managing Editor: Lisa M. George, BA
Technical Content Editor: Angela D. Klimaszewski, RN, MSN
Staff Editor: Amy Nicoletti, BA
Copy Editor: Laura Pinchot, BA
Graphic Designer: Dany Sjoen

Site-Specific Cancer Series: Gynecologic Cancers

Library of Congress Control Number: 2009934463

ISBN: 978-1-890504-86-1

Publisher's Note

This book is published by the Oncology Nursing Society (ONS). ONS neither represents nor guarantees that the practices described herein will, if followed, ensure safe and effective patient care. The recommendations contained in this book reflect ONS's judgment regarding the state of general knowledge and practice in the field as of the date of publication. The recommendations may not be appropriate for use in all circumstances. Those who use this book should make their own determinations regarding specific safe and appropriate patient-care practices, taking into account the personnel, equipment, and practices available at the hospital or other facility at which they are located. The editors and publisher cannot be held responsible for any liability incurred as a consequence from the use or application of any of the contents of this book. Figures and tables are used as examples only. They are not meant to be all-inclusive, nor do they represent endorsement of any particular institution by ONS. Mention of specific products and opinions related to those products do not indicate or imply endorsement by ONS. Web sites mentioned are provided for information only; the hosts are responsible for their own content and availability. Unless otherwise indicated, dollar amounts reflect U.S. dollars.

ONS publications are originally published in English. Publishers wishing to translate ONS publications must contact the ONS Publishing Division about licensing arrangements. ONS publications cannot be translated without obtaining written permission from ONS. (Individual tables and figures that are reprinted or adapted require additional permission from the original source.) Because translations from English may not always be accurate or precise, ONS disclaims any responsibility for inaccuracies in words or meaning that may occur as a result of the translation. Readers relying on precise information should check the original English version.

Printed in the United States of America

ONS
Where Oncology Nurses Connect

Oncology Nursing Society
Integrity • Innovation • Stewardship • Advocacy • Excellence • Inclusiveness

Contributors

Editor

Lois Almadrones-Cassidy, RN, MS, FNP, MPA
Retired Clinical Nurse Specialist, Gynecologic Oncology
Memorial Sloan-Kettering Cancer Center
New York, New York
Chapter 1. Overview
Chapter 14. Long-Term Symptom Management

Authors

Paula J. Anastasia, RN, MN, AOCN®
Gynecology-Oncology Clinical Nurse Specialist
Cedars-Sinai Medical Center
Los Angeles, California
Chapter 7. Epithelial Ovarian Cancer, Fallopian Tube Carcinoma, and Primary Peritoneal Carcinoma

Kathleen Appollo, RN, BSN, OCN®
Clinical Research Nurse, Gynecologic Oncology
Memorial Sloan-Kettering Cancer Center
New York, New York
Chapter 14. Long-Term Symptom Management

Karen Bess, RN, MaEd, MSN
Affiliate Assistant Professor, Goldfarb School of Nursing
Barnes-Jewish College
St. Louis, Missouri
Chapter 10. Trophoblastic Disease

Frances Cartwright-Alcarese, PhD, RN, AOCN®
Director of Nursing, Oncology Services
New York University Langone Medical Center
New York, New York
Chapter 2. Anatomy, Physiology, and Pathophysiology

Jane Duffy-Weisser, MS, RN, ANP-BC
Adult Nurse Practitioner, Gynecologic Medical Oncology
Nurse Practitioner Coordinator for NP/Hospitalist Services
Memorial Sloan-Kettering Cancer Center
New York, New York
Chapter 11. Vulvar and Vaginal Cancers

Dorothy Dulko, PhD, RN, AOCNP®
Ambulatory Cancer Center and Advanced Practice Nursing Director
Department of Hematology Oncology
Dartmouth-Hitchcock Medical Center
Lebanon, New Hampshire
Chapter 9. Gynecologic Sarcomas

Kathleen Farley-Omerod, RN, MS, APN/CNS, AOCN®
Breast Health Advanced Practice Nurse
Central DuPage Hospital
Winfield, Illinois
Chapter 3. Prevention and Early Detection of Cancers of the Cervix, Ovaries, and Endometrium

Sheryl Redlin Frazier, RN, MSN, OCN®
Clinical Learning Consultant
Nursing Education and Development
Vanderbilt University Medical Center
Nashville, Tennessee
Chapter 6. Endometrial Cancer

Eileen Fusco, MSN, APRN-BC, AOCNP®
Nurse Practitioner, Radiation Medicine
North Shore-Long Island Jewish Health System
New Hyde Park, New York
Chapter 3. Prevention and Early Detection of Cancers of the Cervix, Ovaries, and Endometrium
Chapter 4. Preinvasive Disease of the Cervix, Vulva, and Vagina

Randy E. Gross, MS, RN, NP, WHNP-BC, ACNS-BC, AOCNP®
Nurse Practitioner, Gynecologic Medical Oncology Service
Memorial Sloan-Kettering Cancer Center
New York, New York
Chapter 14. Long-Term Symptom Management

Catherine Hydzik, RN, MS, AOCN®
Manager/Clinical Nurse Specialist
Memorial Sloan-Kettering Cancer Center at Sleepy Hollow
Sleepy Hollow, New York
Chapter 13. Acute Symptom Management

Virginia R. Martin, RN, MSN, AOCN®
Clinical Director, Ambulatory Care
Fox Chase Cancer Center
Philadelphia, Pennsylvania
Chapter 8. Nonepithelial Ovarian Cancer

Altagracia (Grace) I. Mota, RN, MSN, OCN®
Nursing Professional Development and Education Manager
Coordinator, Nurse Residency Program
Memorial Sloan-Kettering Cancer Center
New York, New York
Chapter 12. Pelvic Exenteration and Reconstruction

Kathleen A. O'Connor, RN, BSN
Clinical Nurse IV–Ambulatory Services
Memorial Sloan-Kettering Cancer Center
New York, New York
Chapter 13. Acute Symptom Management

Janette O'Sullivan, CNM, RN, MS
Midwife, Private Practice
Adjunct Lecturer, Nursing
Kingsborough Community College
Brooklyn, New York
Chapter 2. Anatomy, Physiology, and Pathophysiology

Sharon Schwartz, MSN, CRNP
Nurse Practitioner, Gynecologic Surgery
Fox Chase Cancer Center
Philadelphia, Pennsylvania
Chapter 5. Invasive Cervical Cancer

Blanca Vasquez-Clarfield, MA, RN
Nurse Leader, Women's Oncology Unit
Memorial Sloan-Kettering Cancer Center
New York, New York
Chapter 11. Vulvar and Vaginal Cancers

Nasrin Vaziri-Kermani, RN, CPSN
Ambulatory Office Practice Nurse
Office of Chief, Plastic and Reconstructive Surgery
Memorial Sloan-Kettering Cancer Center
New York, New York
Chapter 12. Pelvic Exenteration and Reconstruction

Terry L. Wood, PhD, RN
Clinical Assistant Professor
Southern Illinois University, Edwardsville
Edwardsville, Illinois
Chapter 10. Trophoblastic Disease

Disclosure

Editors and authors of books and guidelines provided by the Oncology Nursing Society are expected to disclose to the participants any significant financial interest or other relationships with the manufacturer(s) of any commercial products.

A vested interest may be considered to exist if a contributor is affiliated with or has a financial interest in commercial organizations that may have a direct or indirect interest in the subject matter. A "financial interest" may include, but is not limited to, being a shareholder in the organization; being an employee of the commercial organization; serving on an organization's speakers bureau; or receiving research from the organization. An "affiliation" may be holding a position on an advisory board or some other role of benefit to the commercial organization. Vested interest statements appear in the front matter for each publication.

Contributors are expected to disclose any unlabeled or investigational use of products discussed in their content. This information is acknowledged solely for the information of the readers.

The contributors provided the following disclosure and vested interest information:

Kathleen A. O'Connor, RN, BSN, Society of Gynecologic Nurse Oncologists, board member

Contents

Preface ix

Chapter 1. Overview 1
- Introduction 1
- References 2

Chapter 2. Anatomy, Physiology, and Pathophysiology 3
- Introduction 3
- Internal Female Reproductive Organs 3
- External Genitalia (Vulva) 9
- Lymphatic Drainage of the Female Genital Tract 10
- Breasts 11
- Sexual Function 11
- Sexually Transmitted Diseases 12
- Pelvic Inflammatory Disease 13
- Pelvic Pain 13
- Menstrual Issues/Differential Diagnosis 13
- Summary 14
- References 14

Chapter 3. Prevention and Early Detection of Cancers of the Cervix, Ovaries, and Endometrium 17
- Introduction 17
- Cervical Cancer 17
- Ovarian Cancer 23
- Endometrial Cancer 28
- Summary 31
- References 31

Chapter 4. Preinvasive Disease of the Cervix, Vulva, and Vagina 37
- Introduction 37
- Preinvasive Disease 37
- Evaluation of the Cervix 37
- Diagnostic Tests 38
- Vulvar Intraepithelial Neoplasia 39
- Vaginal Intraepithelial Neoplasia 40
- Risk Factors for Premalignant Vaginal and Vulvar Lesions 40
- Management of Preinvasive Disease 40
- Special Considerations 42
- Summary 43
- References 43

Chapter 5. Invasive Cervical Cancer 47
- Introduction 47
- Types of Cervical Cancer and Histology 47
- Signs, Symptoms, and Diagnosis of Cervical Cancer 47
- Cervical Cancer Staging 51
- Treatment 51
- Special Situations 57
- Palliative Care 57
- Future Directions 58
- Summary 58
- References 58

Chapter 6. Endometrial Cancer 63
- Introduction 63
- Etiology and Epidemiology 63
- Risk Factors 64
- Risk Reduction and Protective Effects 65
- Treatment 67
- Recurrent Disease 71
- Future Trends 71
- Summary 71
- References 71

Chapter 7. Epithelial Ovarian Cancer, Fallopian Tube Carcinoma, and Primary Peritoneal Carcinoma 75
- Introduction 75
- Epidemiology and Risk Factors 75
- Hereditary Epithelial Ovarian Cancer 76
- Screening, Presentation of Symptoms, and Diagnostic Testing 77
- Staging Surgery 79
- Pathology 80
- Immunomarkers 80
- Adjuvant Chemotherapy 80
- Consolidation and Maintenance Therapy 83
- Radiotherapy 83
- Surveillance 83
- Recurrent Disease 84
- Future Outlook 85
- Summary 86
- References 86

Chapter 8. Nonepithelial Ovarian Cancer 91
Introduction 91
Ovarian Germ Cell Tumors 91
Sex Cord Stromal Tumors 96
Rare Nonepithelial Ovarian Tumors 98
Summary 99
References 99

Chapter 9. Gynecologic Sarcomas 103
Introduction 103
Etiology and Epidemiology 103
Clinical Presentation and Diagnostic Evaluation 107
Staging 107
Treatment 107
Recurrent Disease 108
Summary 108
References 108

Chapter 10. Trophoblastic Disease 113
Introduction 113
Epidemiology of Trophoblastic Variants 113
Gestational Trophoblastic Disease 114
Gestational Trophoblastic Neoplasia 117
Placental Site Trophoblastic Tumor 121
Evidence-Based Practice 122
Psychosocial Impact of Trophoblastic Disease 122
Summary 123
References 123

Chapter 11. Vulvar and Vaginal Cancers 127
Vulvar Cancer 127
Vaginal Cancer 131
Summary 137
References 137

Chapter 12. Pelvic Exenteration and Reconstruction 139
Introduction 139
Exenterative Surgery 140
Nursing Care 144
Summary 147
References 148

Chapter 13. Acute Symptom Management 149
Introduction 149
Surgery 149
Chemotherapy 149
Radiation Therapy 158
Summary 158
References 158

Chapter 14. Long-Term Symptom Management 165
Introduction 165
Peripheral Neuropathy 165
Lower Extremity Lymphedema 168
Menopausal Management 172
Summary 178
References 178

Appendix: International Federation of Gynecology and Obstetrics Staging Classification for Gynecologic Cancer 183

Index 187

Preface

Nurses and other healthcare providers who care for women with gynecologic cancers practice in a unique subspecialty of oncology. It is unique for several reasons. First, a gynecologic oncologist's training includes four additional years of a surgical fellowship in a certified gynecologic oncology program after completion of an obstetrics and gynecologic residency. During this fellowship, a full year is spent performing laboratory and clinical research on some aspect of gynecologic cancer. During the other three years, the physician learns the unique surgical skills and techniques necessary to perform gynecologic surgery, as well as the medical oncologist's knowledge and skills of caring for women undergoing chemotherapy. Therefore, most gynecologic oncologists in the United States care for women with gynecologic cancer throughout the entire cancer experience from diagnosis, surgery, and chemotherapy to follow-up well-woman care.

The second unique aspect of gynecologic oncology is the organization formed by gynecologic oncologists, the Society of Gynecologic Oncologists (SGO), for the purpose of sharing knowledge with one another and other oncologists through publications and annual scientific meetings. SGO spawned the nursing group, the Society of Gynecologic Nurse Oncologists (SGNO), for nurses who practice this subspecialty and need the unique skills to deliver optimum care to women with gynecologic cancers throughout the trajectory of cancer care. Since 1983, SGNO has shared knowledge through publications and annual meetings and has become the premier resource for gynecologic oncology nursing.

The third unique aspect of gynecologic oncology is the Gynecologic Oncology Group, a national cooperative funded primarily by the National Cancer Institute expressly for the purpose of searching for better treatments for women with gynecologic cancers through scientifically designed clinical trials. All these aspects of gynecologic oncology translate into a dynamic subspecialty in which nurses may practice and also may find many professional opportunities.

This book is written by 20 of these unique gynecologic oncology nurse experts. Each was chosen for his or her expertise in a particular type of gynecologic oncology care. Each author shares knowledge gained by direct care of women with gynecologic cancer. Each desires to mentor other nurses in order to provide the best care for the courageous women who live with gynecologic cancers.

CHAPTER 1

Overview

Lois Almadrones-Cassidy, RN, MS, FNP, MPA

Introduction

Gynecologic cancers, specifically uterine corpus and ovarian, were among the 10 leading types of cancer diagnoses in females in the United States in 2008 (Jemal et al., 2008). Both of these cancers represent 9% of all new cases and deaths in the United States. The estimated total incidence of all types of new gynecologic cancers is 78,490 (11%), and estimated deaths total 28,490 (10.5%). Worldwide, this percentage is higher, with cervical cancer the second highest cancer killer after breast cancer (Yang, Bray, Parkin, Sellors, & Zhang, 2004). Trends in ovarian, uterine cervix, and uterine corpus survival rates in Caucasian women in the United States have significantly improved since 1975. However, survival rates have remained relatively stable in African American women (Jemal et al.).

Nurses who care for women with gynecologic cancer are challenged by the complexity of the multidisciplinary management approach. Experitse is needed in the management of not one cancer but in many cancers that affect the reproductive tract. Not only is knowledge about the biology of these cancers needed, but nurses also must know how to care for women who are undergoing surgery, chemotherapy, radiation therapy, or a combination of these modalities. This is made all the more challenging because good care must include the multifaceted psychosocial needs of the cancer survivor throughout the trajectory of her care. This kind of care touches the core of both nurses and women with cancer because it forces confrontation about "hot-button" issues related to sexuality, infertility, hereditary causes of cancer, and past and current sexual experiences. Ramondetta and Sills (2004) note that in our patients we see our mothers, our sisters, our friends, and ourselves. Spiritual issues arise because the genital tract is the source of recreating and sustaining life, and for some women, losing that ability can be personally diminishing of their life's purpose. Often, feelings of guilt, shame, and anger are present because the cancer, particularly cervical, is linked to sexual freedom and the ensuing increased probability of sexually transmitted disease. Being a part of assisting women to understand and cope with these complex issues as they and their families confront and manage the cancer experience is part of what makes gynecologic nursing care both challenging and rewarding.

The subspecialty of gynecologic oncology has evolved over the last three decades, and physicians are trained to specialize only in the multidisciplinary care of these women. This subspecialization has fostered nurses to become specialists also, and they are an integral part of the mutidisciplinary team. Undergirding the direct care of women with a gynecologic cancer is research into the biology of gynecologic cancers, the causes, best treatments for cure and control, and preventive strategies. This research is carried out by government-funded cooperative groups like the Gynecolgic Oncology Group, which work closely with community and international cooperative groups to carry out timely research trials that seek to improve the survival rates, find cures, and discover screening tests and preventive strategies that can be used worldwide.

Nurses who specialize in gynecologic oncology nursing are fortunate to have a subspecialty organization, the Society of Gynecologic Nurse Oncologists (SGNO). This organization has as its mission

> To provide current information regarding gynecologic oncology nursing practice and women's health issues; to foster education about gynecologic oncology nursing; to promote a means of communication, networking and support among gynecologic oncology nurses; and to promote the application of current information to all levels of gynecologic oncology practice. (SGNO, 2008)

This book seeks to give oncology nurses an overview of the current evidence-based information related to the major types of gynecologic cancers, causes, screening, and preventive strategies, as well as the current surgical, chemotherapeutic, and radiation treatments used to treat all stages of the cancer. However, the book begins with a thorough explanation of the anatomy and pathophysiology of the female reproductive tract that is essential for the optimal care of the patient with gynecologic cancer. Two chapters address management of acute and long-term side effects that greatly affect survivorship. The authors are all experts in the care of women with these malignancies.

References

Jemal, A., Siegel, R., Ward, E., Hao, Y., Xu, J., Murray, T., et al. (2008). Cancer statistics, 2008. *CA: A Cancer Journal for Clinicians, 58*(2), 71–96.

Ramondetta, L.M., & Sills, D. (2004). Spirituality in gynecological oncology: A review. *International Journal of Gynecological Cancer, 14*(2), 183–201.

Society of Gynecologic Nurse Oncologists. (2008). Society of Gynecologic Nurse Oncologists mission statement. *Journal of Gynecologic Oncology Nursing, 18*(1), 3.

Yang, B.H., Bray, F.I., Parkin, D.M., Sellors, J.W., & Zhang, Z.F. (2004). Cervical cancer as a priority for prevention in different world regions: An evaluation using years of life lost. *International Journal of Cancer, 109*(3), 418–424.

CHAPTER 2

Anatomy, Physiology, and Pathophysiology

Frances Cartwright-Alcarese, PhD, RN, AOCN®, and Janette O'Sullivan, CNM, RN, MS

Introduction

The management of most gynecologic malignancies requires multimodal therapy (National Comprehensive Cancer Network, 2009a, 2009b, 2009c). Consideration of the multiple anatomical structures and their function is critical to understand how treatment options affect physical and psychosocial aspects of care. Knowledge of the anatomy, physiology, and pathophysiology of the female genital tract is essential to provide optimal care of women with a gynecologic malignancy.

The female reproductive system includes the internal reproductive organs: the ovaries, fallopian tubes, uterus, cervix, and vagina. The *vulva* refers to the external genitalia and is composed of the mons pubis, the labia majora, the labia minora, the clitoris, and the vestibule where the urinary and vaginal openings and the ducts of the greater vestibular glands are located. The female reproductive tract includes several ducts that receive and transport the gametes, and accessory glands and organs that secrete fluids.

The content of this chapter is a synthesis of many authors who have provided expert reviews of these topics (Adams-Hillard, 2002; Aikins-Murphy, 1990; Barbieri, 2002; Bickley & Szilagyi, 2007; Botash, 2006; Cespedes, Cross, & McGuire, 1999; Cohen, 2006; Cunningham et al., 2005; DeCherney, 2002; Dondero & Lichtman, 1990; Godfrey, 2004; Gray, 2003; Grube & Giuliano, 2002; Hatcher & Namnoum, 2004; Hillard, 2002; Hurd, Amesse, & Randolph, 2002; Jackson & Lichtman, 1990; Jolin, 2002; Mashburn, 2006; Nelson & Stewart, 2004; Osuch, Bonham, & Morris, 1999; Peck, 1990; Policar, 2004; Scalone, 1990; Schillings & McClamrock, 2002; Soper, 2002; Sullivan, 1990; Varney, Kribes, & Gegor, 2004).

This chapter is organized by a discussion of the normal structure and function of the internal and external organs. Each topic is followed by a description of relevant "benign pathophysiology." Although the term *benign* is used to indicate noncancerous conditions, infections of the gynecologic tract and some disorders can have serious consequences and require immediate attention and treatment. The multisystem etiology of sexually transmitted diseases (STDs), menstrual disorders, and pelvic inflammatory disease (PID) lends itself to a separate discussion; therefore, each of these topics is described under their own heading.

Internal Female Reproductive Organs

The female reproductive organs are located within the bony pelvis, composed of the sacrum, coccyx, and innominate bones (see Figure 2-1).

Ovaries

The two ovaries (female gonads) are almond-shaped structures located near the lateral walls of the pelvic cavity, one on each side of the uterus. They are stabilized by a pair of supporting ligaments, the ovarian ligament and the broad ligament, or suspensory ligament. The ovary is attached to the broad ligament by the mesovarium. In women of reproductive age (puberty through menopause), each ovary is approximately 3–5 cm long, 2.5 cm wide, and 2 cm thick, varying in size depending on the phase of the menstrual cycle. The ovaries atrophy after menopause (Bickley & Szilagyi, 2007; Cunningham et al., 2005; Jackson & Lichtman, 1990).

Internally, the ovary contains follicles, each containing layers of cells enclosing an immature egg cell called an oocyte. The central part, called the medulla, is composed of connective tissue and contains a large number of small arteries, veins, and lymphatic vessels. The cortex is the outer layer that surrounds the medulla.

The ovaries are the primary female reproductive organs. From puberty to menopause (cessation of menstruation), they have two main functions: the production of female sex hormones and the development and release of ova (female gametes). Although primarily they produce the female sex hormones estrogen and progesterone, they also produce

Figure 2-1. Internal Female Genitalia and Other Pelvic Organs

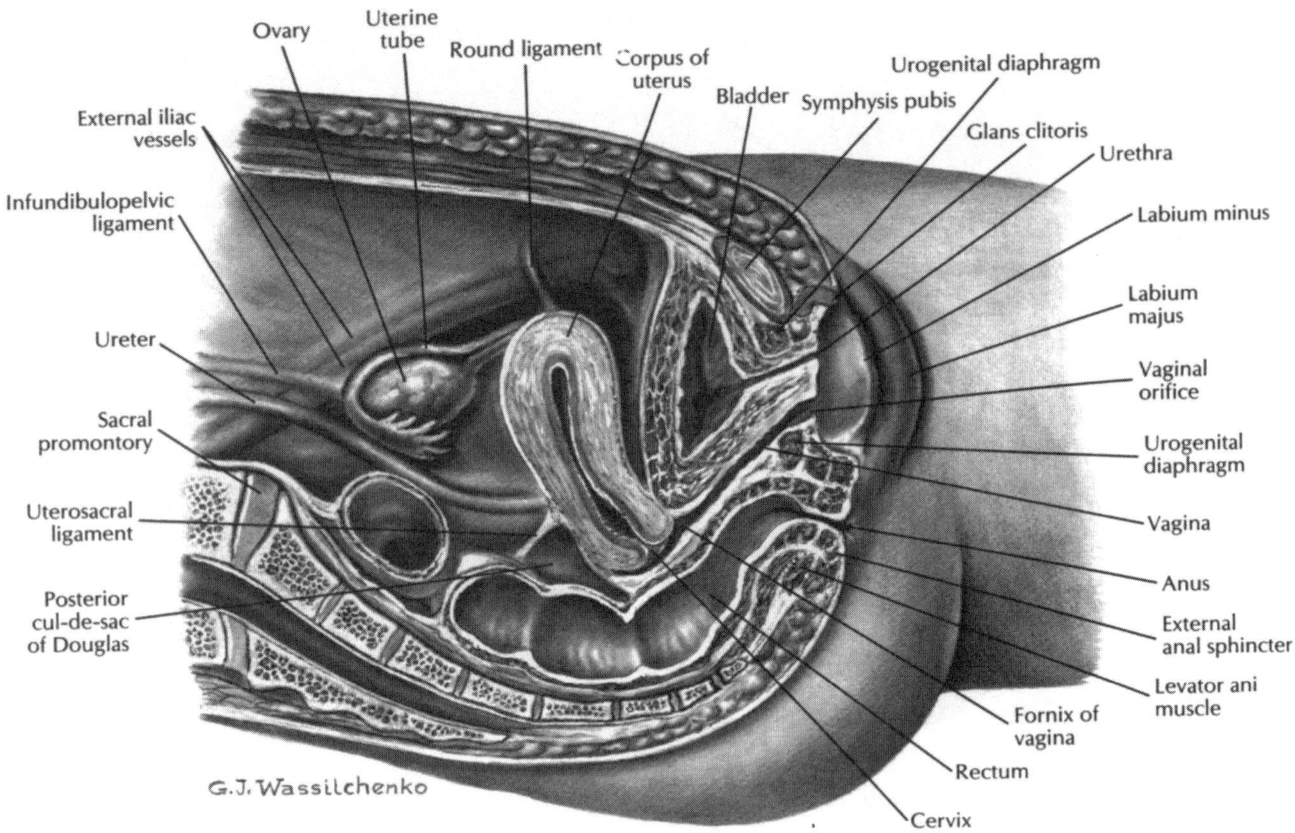

Note. From "Reproduction and Sexuality" (p. 110), by I.M Bobak in I.M. Bobak, M.D. Jensen, and D.L. Lowdermilk (Eds.), *Maternity and Gynecologic Care* (5th ed.), 1993, St. Louis, MO: Mosby. Copyright 1993 by Mosby. Reprinted with permission.

androgens and relaxin. Sex hormones are secreted by the following cells, which are present within the ovarian cortex: (a) cells of the stroma or tissue matrix, (b) two types of cells in the ovarian follicle (granulosa and theca cells), and (c) cells of the corpus luteum. These cells contain receptors for the gonadotropins, luteinizing hormone (LH) and follicle-stimulating hormone (FSH). Estrogen, primarily estradiol, is produced by cells in the developing ovarian follicle. Progesterone is produced by the cells of the corpus luteum, which is the structure that develops from the ruptured ovarian follicle after ovum release or ovulation. Androgens are produced within the ovarian follicle, adrenal glands, and adipose tissue.

Ova maturation and release is dependent on the interaction between the hypothalamus and the target cells. Gonadotropin-releasing hormone (GnRH) is synthesized in the hypothalamus and via the anterior pituitary produces FSH and LH. The level of hormone release varies depending on the phase of the menstrual cycle. Although the ovarian cycle can vary greatly from woman to woman, most authors indicate that it is approximately 28 days in duration (Cunningham et al., 2005; Hatcher & Namnoun, 2004; Scalone, 1990). As shown on Figure 2-2, the ovarian cycle consists of the physiologic and structural changes in the female reproductive tract as it responds to changes in the levels of ovarian hormones. The following four phases are named for these ovarian and endometrial changes: (a) the follicular/proliferative phase, (b) ovulation, (c) the luteal/secretory phase, and (d) menstruation. A brief description of each phase is described below. These events also are illustrated on the upper three sections of Figure 2-3.

The follicular/proliferative phase begins with release of GnRH by the hypothalamus, causing release of FSH and LH. Rising estradiol levels increase the FSH receptors on the destined or dominant follicle, resulting in even greater estradiol levels and a means of maintaining adequate FSH support for the dominant follicle when FSH release is inhibited. FSH promotes ovarian follicular growth by causing the granulosa cells that line each follicle to proliferate and produce estrogen. The dominant follicle enlarges as the layer of the surrounding granulosa cell grows and forms a new

Figure 2-2. Cross Section of Uterus, Fallopian Tube, and Ovary

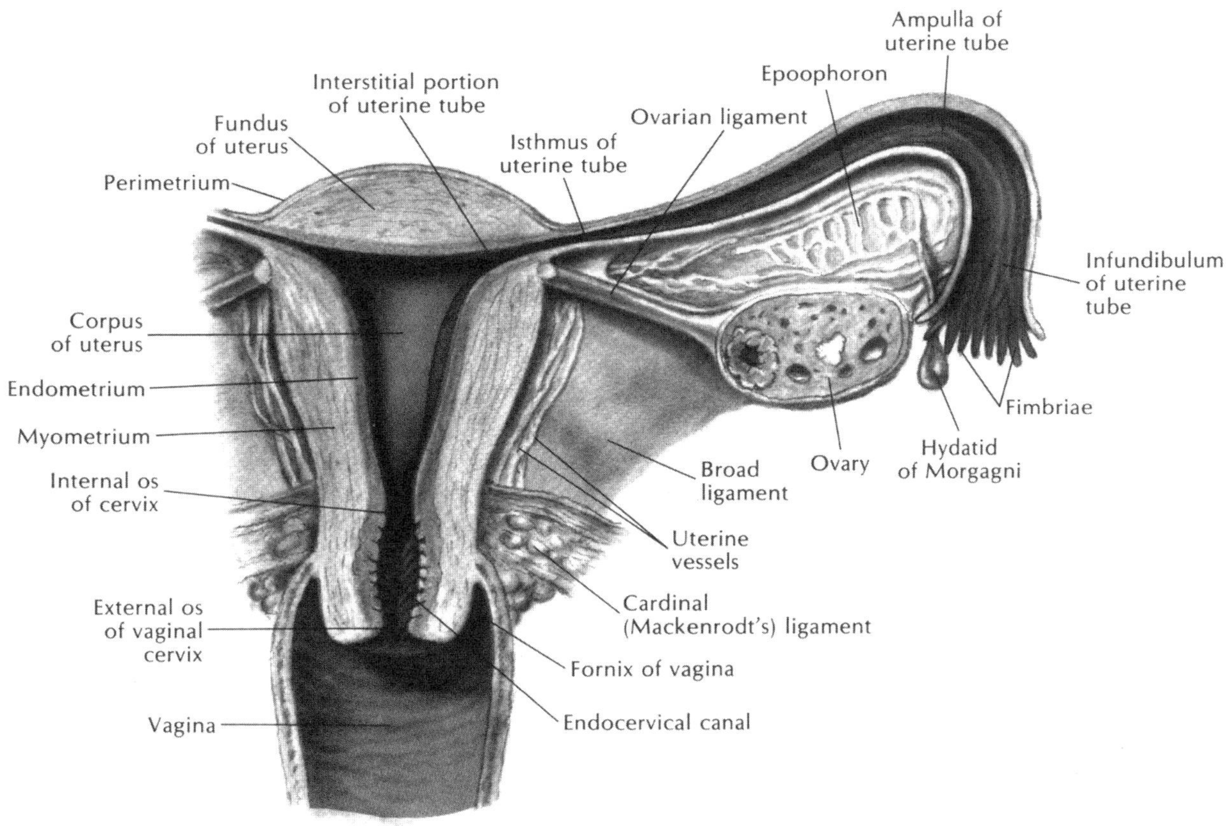

Note. From "Reproduction and Sexuality" (p. 110), by I.M Bobak in I.M. Bobak, M.D. Jensen, and D.L. Lowdermilk (Eds.), *Maternity and Gynecologic Care* (5th ed.), 1993, St. Louis, MO: Mosby. Copyright 1993 by Mosby. Reprinted with permission.

layer of cells, called the theca. The theca cells are adjacent to the granulosa cells. LH stimulates androgen production in the theca cells. The increase in FSH also stimulates conversion of androgen to estrogen. Estrogen production in the circulation and release of inhibin B by the granulosa cell inhibits the pituitary from producing FSH. Therefore, only the dominant follicle continues to grow. Toward the end of the follicular phase, the estrogen-rich environment causes increases in bioactive LH, resulting in luteinization of the granulosa cell layer of the follicle and progesterone production that is needed for ovulation.

Ovulation occurs from the surging levels of LH and is supported by the subsequent release of increased progesterone. Progesterone causes an increase in the elasticity of the follicular wall. The LH surge also results in high prostaglandin levels in the follicular fluid causing the follicle to rupture, marking the beginning of the luteal phase. The androgens convert estrogen-secreting granulosa cells to progesterone-secreting cells after ovulation.

The luteal/secretory phase is marked by a decrease in plasma estrogen caused by the LH surge and inhibition of GnRH and granulosa cell multiplication. The resulting decrease in plasma estrogen levels causes a decrease in LH levels and increased progesterone in the luteinized cells of the follicle. The function of the newly developed corpus luteum is to produce progesterone and estrogen to prepare the uterus for implantation. If this does not occur, the corpus luteum degenerates, causing a drop in estrogen and progesterone, which then stimulates secretion of GnRH and FSH, thus beginning the cycle again.

Menstruation is marked by the degeneration of the corpus luteum and endometrial vasodilation followed by vasoconstriction, resulting in interstitial hemorrhage and slough that results in menstrual flow. The amount and duration of blood flow varies greatly but averages 20–80 ml, lasting approximately 3–7 days. As menstruation occurs, estrogen and FSH levels transiently rise, which preserves a group of follicles for further development.

Between puberty and menopause, the ovarian cortex contains follicles and ova in various stages of development. Females are born with approximately 60,000 immature ovarian follicles. During a woman's lifetime, only about 400 ovarian follicles mature

Figure 2-3. Menstrual Cycle Events

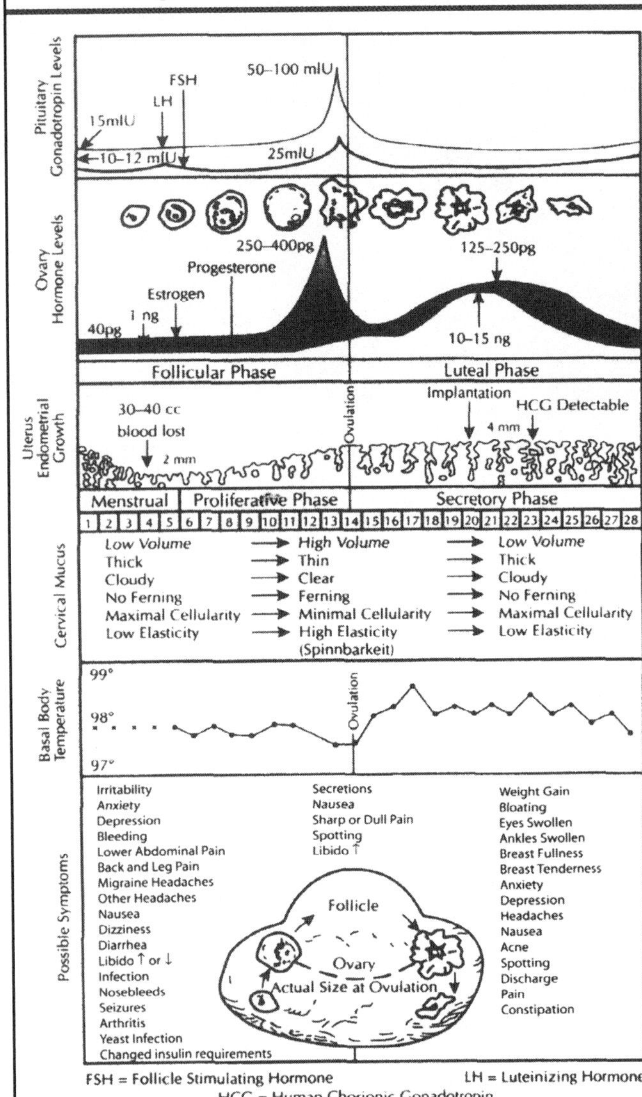

Note. From "The Menstrual Cycle" (p. 69), by R.A. Hatcher and A.B. Namnoum in R.A. Hatcher, J. Trussell, F. Stewart, A.L. Nelson, W. Cates, F. Guest, et al. (Eds.), *Contraceptive Technology* (18th ed.), 2004, New York: Ardent Media. Copyright 2004 by Ardent Media. Reprinted with permission.

completely and release an ovum. The number of ova decline during a woman's reproductive life. For example, Cunningham et al. (2005) cited a study conducted in 1952 that reported that a woman in her mid-30s has approximately 34,000 ova. The remaining follicles either fail to develop or degenerate without maturing completely.

Benign Pathophysiology of the Ovaries

Normally, the ovaries are somewhat tender and usually are palpable on pelvic examination in slender, relaxed women but are difficult or impossible to detect in others who are obese or unable to relax during the exam (Bickely & Szilagy, 2007). In perimenopausal and postmenopausal women, as ovarian function declines, the ovaries begin to atrophy, and they cannot be felt on bimanual examination (Bickley & Szilagyi; Cohen, 2006). Therefore, an ovary that can be palpated in a menopausal or postmenopausal woman should be considered an abnormality.

Benign ovarian tumors: Adams-Hillard (2002) describe the following categories of benign ovarian tumors: (a) functional, (b) inflammatory, (c) neoplastic, (d) epithelial, and (e) other. Functional includes follicular, corpus luteum, and theca lutein. *Inflammatory* includes tubo-ovarian abscess or complex. *Neoplastic* includes germ cell, benign cystic teratoma, other, and mixed. *Epithelial* includes serous cystadenoma, fibroma, cystadenofibroma, Brenner tumor, and mixed tumor. *Other* includes endometrioma.

Ovarian cysts: Ovarian cysts are growths arising from ovarian components and are usually benign (Adams-Hillard, 2002; Jackson & Lichtman, 1990; Snyder, 2005). Ovarian cysts include functional, para-ovarian, and paratubal cysts. They commonly arise from functional changes in the ovary such as from a Graafian follicle or from persistent corpus luteum. Dermoid cysts may develop from abnormal embryonic epithelium. They are found frequently during childbearing years; however, masses found in women older than age 50 are more often malignant.

Polycystic ovarian syndrome: Polycystic ovarian syndrome is a functional derangement of the hypothalamo-pituitary ovarian axis and is associated with anovulation. This is a result of high LH levels and low FSH levels resulting in an increased LH to FSH ratio. This is a complex syndrome with androgenic side effects, despite low serum total testosterone levels, as well as insulin resistance. Etiology is unknown. Women may present with amenorrhea, hirsutism, obesity, acne, and infertility.

Premature ovarian failure: Premature ovarian failure occurs as a result of the depletion of ovarian follicles from the ovary prior to the normal age of menopause, inducing premature menopause. Although the etiology is unclear, it is associated with chromosomal abnormalities such as Turner syndrome or autoimmune disease, or it may follow infections such as mumps. It may follow cancer treatment (e.g., systemic chemotherapy, pelvic irradiation). Anovulation secondary to polycystic ovary disease commonly occurs in obese women. Women who experience abrupt menopause report greater symptom distress than women who experience menopause naturally (Ganz, Greendale, Petersen, Kahn, & Bower, 2003; Knobf, 2006). Long-term symptom management associated with abrupt menopause, regardless of the cause, is an important quality-of-life issue.

Fallopian Tubes

The two fallopian tubes, oviducts or uterine tubes, each measure about 8–12.5 cm in length and 1 cm in width. They are located on each side of the uterus, just below the fundus, with an infundibulum, a fringed funnel-shaped end that curves up and over the two ovaries. The infundibulum has numerous irregular projections called fimbriae extending toward the ovary. The elongated segment of the fallopian tube proximal to the infundibulum is the ampulla. The ampulla leads to the isthmus, a short, narrow segment that opens into the uterine wall. The epithelium lining, the *ampulla*, has numerous sack-like grooves, and the exposed surface has hair-like appendages called *cilia*.

No structural connection exists between the fallopian tubes and the ovaries. The primary function of the fallopian tube is to propel the ovum via cilia and peristalsis from the space around the ovaries to the uterus. When the ovum is released from the ovarian follicle, it is swept into the fallopian tube by the wave-like action of the fimbriae. Here, the ovum may or may not encounter sperm, and it continues to travel through the fallopian tube to the uterus. Fertilization normally occurs in the ampulla of the fallopian tubes. If fertilized, the blastocyst implants itself in the endometrial layer of the uterine wall. If not fertilized, the ovum degenerates and leaves the uterus with the menstrual fluids.

Benign Pathophysiology of the Fallopian Tubes

Fallopian tube disorders include congenital malformations, infection, tubal pregnancy, and edematous fallopian tubes caused by PID. Disorders that affect the fallopian tubes can block the path of sperm and ovum and cause infertility.

Uterus

The uterus, or womb, is a hollow, flattened, pear-shaped, fibromuscular organ. Although it varies greatly in size, it is approximately 7.5 cm long and 6.5 cm wide, has muscular walls 1.5–3.0 cm thick, and is located medially within the anterior portion of the pelvic cavity resting in the lower pelvis. The uterus weighs approximately 30–60 grams and is surrounded by and held loosely in place by ligaments, peritoneal tissue folds, and the pressure of adjacent organs (especially the urinary bladder, sigmoid colon, and rectum). In most women, the uterus is anteverted (tipped forward) resting on the urinary bladder. It may also be retroverted (tipped backward), or less often, midposition (upright). All of these variations are considered normal.

The uterus is composed of two parts: the body or corpus, which is the superior, thick-walled portion, and the cervix, the lower portion that extends into the vagina. These two parts are joined together by the isthmus, which is the narrowed part of the corpus. The fundus is the convex upper portion of the uterus where the fallopian tubes are suspended. The diameter of the uterine cavity is widest at the fundus and narrowest at the isthmus.

The thick uterine wall has three layers. The superficial layer (*serosa*) is the outer serous tissue that covers the uterus and is continuous with the pelvic peritoneum. The middle layer, called the *myometrium*, is composed of a thick layer of smooth muscle, which is thickest at the fundus. The *endometrium*, the uterine lining, composed of a thick inner functional layer called the *stratum functionalis*, is the site of embryo implantation. Because the endometium is hormonally responsive, changes in its morphology fluctuate during the menstrual cycle (see Figure 2-3). When fertilization does not occur, the stratum functionalis of the endometrium sloughs off during menstruation. The deep layer, called the stratum basalis, provides tissue for regeneration of the stratum functionalis following menstruation. This layer's form and structure remains constant, regardless of hormonal fluctuations.

The functions of the uterus are to secure and protect the fertilized ovum, provide an optimal environment while it develops, and through the contractions of labor, facilitate birth. Uterine or endometrial events of the menstrual cycle are caused by ovarian hormones (see Figure 2-3).

Benign Pathophysiology of the Uterus

Uterine prolapse: Uterine prolapse is an abnormal position of the uterus in which the uterus protrudes downward. Uterine prolapse may be associated with rectocele, cystocele, or an enterocele. This may be caused by herniation of the uterus through the pelvic floor resulting in prolapse into the vagina or beyond the introitus (procidentia). This usually is caused by obstetric trauma and overstretching of musculofascial supports. Degrees of uterine prolapse are as follows.

- First degree: Cervix prolapses into vaginal canal.
- Second degree: Cervix prolapses at the introitus.
- Marked procidentia: The entire uterus protrudes outside vaginal cavity.

Endometriosis: Endometriosis is the abnormal proliferation of uterine endometrial tissue outside the uterus, also occurring outside of the pelvic cavity. An intact uterus is not needed to have endometriosis. Incidence peaks in women ages 25–45 but may occur at any age. Risk increases among siblings of women who have endometriosis and among women with shorter menstrual cycles and longer duration of flow. It is more common in white women than black women and in those with sedentary lifestyles and who are obese. Endometriosis may be caused by embryonic tissue remnants that differentiate as a result of hormonal stimulation and spread via lymphatic or venous channels. It may be caused by retrograde menstruation through fallopian tubes into the peritoneal cavity and may also be transferred via surgical instruments. Menstruation resulting in accumulated blood and inflammation and subsequent adhesions also may be associated with endometriosis.

Elevated estrogen levels increase endometriosis, whereas lower estrogen levels and increased progestins cause regression of endometriosis. Therefore, hormonal contraceptive and androgen use will decrease symptoms of endometriosis. D'Hooghe and Hill (2002), Lichtman and Smith (1990), and

Quinn (1993) provide a comprehensive overview of etiology, prevalence, diagnosis, clinical presentation, and treatment of endometriosis.

Cervix

The *cervix*, or opening of the uterus, is the narrow, lower portion that extends from the isthmus to the vagina. The *external os* of the cervix, a slit-like depression, opens into the vagina dividing it into the anterior, posterior, and lateral fornices. The upper portion of the cervix, the *internal os*, opens into the uterus and its lower opening, the external os, is the endocervical canal that opens into the vagina. The lining of the endocervical canal is continuous with that of the outer cervix and vagina but is composed of columnar epithelial cells. The point at which the columnar epithelium of the cervix meets the squamous epithelium of the vagina is the transformation zone or the squamocolumnar junction. The transformation zone is an area of continuous cell renewal and provides an ideal environment for many types of the cancer precursor human papillomavirus (HPV) to thrive and, thus, is a common site of cancer.

The cervix acts as a mechanical barrier to infectious microorganisms that may be present in the vagina. Depending on hormonal fluctuations in the menstrual cycle, cervical mucus can be thick and sticky, which acts as a barrier to both microorganisms and sperm. During ovulation, the mucus becomes thin, clear, and slippery, which aids the passage of sperm. The mucus plug, which forms in pregnancy from secretions created by the increased growth of cervical glands, minimizes entry of organisms. In addition, the downward flow of cervical secretions moves microorganisms away from the cervix and uterus. Among women of reproductive age, the pH of these secretions is resistant to most bacteria. The mucosal secretions contain enzymes and antibodies, predominantly immunoglobulin A, that keep defenses intact; however, these defenses do not always prevent infection.

Benign Pathophysiology of the Cervix

As mentioned previously, the transformation zone is the usual site of cervical carcinoma. Cancer of the cervix is addressed in Chapter 5 of this text. Infections include condyloma, gonorrhea, syphilis, herpes simplex virus (HSV) ulceration, chlamydial cervicitis, and other cervicitis. Other benign abnormalities include endocervical polyps, nabothian cysts, and columnar epithelial eversion.

Vagina

The vagina is a flexible, elastic opening, measuring about 9–10 cm in length with the capacity to greatly expand during sexual activity and childbirth. It extends from the cervix to the vulva. The upper part of the vagina surrounds the cervix. This pouch-like space, the shallow recess around the cervix, is called the *fornix*. The vagina is divided by the cervix into the posterior and anterior fornices and the lateral fornices. The posterior fornix is deeper than the anterior fornix because of the angle at which the cervix meets the vaginal canal.

Two layers comprise the vagina: a mucous layer and a muscularis layer. The mucous layer is composed of nonkeratinized, stratified squamous epithelium that is supported by a thick lamina propia continuous with the membrane that covers the lower part of the uterus. In women of reproductive age, the mucosal layer is arranged in transverse wrinkles or folds, called *rugae*. The rugae permit the muscosal layer to stretch during vaginal intercourse and childbirth.

The muscularis is composed of autonomically innervated smooth muscle fibers arranged into an outer longitudinal and inner circular layer. The second layer of the intermediate muscularis is lined by stratified squamous epithelium and a subdermal layer of fibrous connective tissue with a rich network of blood and lymphatic vessels and capillaries. The *adventitia*, the outer layer of the muscularis, is rich in collagen and elastic tissue, provides structural support to the vagina, and allows for expansion of the vagina during intercourse and childbirth.

The vagina is a site for sexual intercourse, provides a passage for menstrual fluids to leave the body, and is the passageway for the birth of the newborn. Because the vaginal wall does not contain glands, the mucus lining is reliant on secretions that drain into the vagina from the uterus or enter from the vestibule, the vaginal and urethral openings, the Bartholins glands and Skene glands. The smooth muscle of the vagina is active, especially during menstruation when it contracts periodically to expel the uterine/vaginal contents. These vaginal smooth muscle contractions normally go unnoticed, but they can be painful if spasms occur (dysmenorrheic pain).

The vaginal mucosa is colonized predominantly by *Lactobacillus acidiophilus*, a neutral bacterium that helps to maintain pH at acidic levels of 3.5–4.5. Between puberty and menopause, vulnerability to infection varies somewhat with cyclical changes in pH and epithelial thickness. Natural defenses are greatest when estrogen levels are high and the vagina contains a normal population of *Lactobacillus acidophilus*. Conditions that cause the vaginal pH to rise, such as low estrogen levels or destruction of *Lactobacillus acidophilus* by antibiotics, compromise the vaginal defenses against infection. After menopause, the pH rises to more alkaline levels and the epithelium thins resulting in an increased risk of infection. It may also contribute to dyspareunia.

Benign Pathophysiology of the Vagina

Adams-Hillard (2002) describes the following categories of benign conditions of the vagina:

- Embryonic origin
- Disorders of pelvic support
- Atypical vaginal prolapse

- Posterior vaginal prolapse
- Other.

Conditions of *embryonic origin* include mesonephric, paramesonephric, and urogential sinus cysts, adenosis related to diethylstilbestrol, vaginal septa, or duplications. Disorders of *pelvic support* include anterior vaginal prolapse, cystourethrocele, and cystocele. *Atypical vaginal prolapse* includes uterovaginal and vaginal vault prolapse. *Posterior vaginal prolapse* includes enterocele and rectocele. *Other* includes condyloma, urethral diverticula, fibroepithelial polyp, and vaginal endometriosis.

The morphology and physiology of the vagina and cervix at different phases of the life cycle can result in an environment that at times may be conducive to the growth of a variety of different organisms, causing infection.

Vaginal discharge/differential infection: Changes in the normal vaginal discharge may indicate vaginitis, trichomoniasis, bacterial vaginosis, candidiasis or monilia, HPV, HSV, chlamydia, gonorrhea, pediculosis, syphilis, PID, or genital malignancy.

Vaginitis in adult women is the most common reason for a gynecologic consultation (Botash, 2006). Vaginitis is inflammation of the vagina caused by infectious pathogens that may be associated with sexually transmitted organisms or overgrowth of other common organisms. Normal vaginal secretions as a result of estrogen secretion and acidity inhibit the growth of pathogens. Conditions such as diabetes mellitus, pregnancy, stress, sexual intercourse, and menopause alter the normal vaginal environment.

Vaginal fistula: A vaginal fistula is an abnormal, tortuous opening between the vagina and the rectum or between the vagina and urethra. Women from countries that have inadequate obstetric care and who experience very long labors are at risk for vaginal fistula. Other causes may include pelvic surgery such as a hysterectomy or vaginal reconstructive procedures, extensive malignant disease, and complications of cancer treatment such as radiation therapy.

External Genitalia (Vulva)

The majority of authors who discuss the anatomy and location of the gynecologic structure similarly detail the external genitalia; Aikins-Murphy (1990, p. 3) states it best: "The term *vulva* refers to the structures that are visible externally in the perineal region (the area limited anteriorly by the symphysis pubis, posteriorly by the buttocks, and laterally by the thighs." The structures of the vulva are shown on Figure 2-4 and illustrate how these structures protect body openings. In addition the vulva provides an important role in sexual functioning.

The *mons pubis* is a mound of adipose tissue beneath the skin, overlying the pubic symphysis, and is covered with coarse pubic hair. The labia minora, two elongated fatty folds of adipose tissue, extend from the mons pubis (anterior prominence) of the symphysis pubis and posteriorly with the perennial body (posterior commissure). The folds of the labia majora partially conceal and protect the labia minora and structures of the vestibule, including the vaginal and urethral openings and two pairs of glands, the paired greater vestibular (Bartholin) glands and the paraurethral (Skene) glands.

The *labia minora* are two smaller, hairless, pink, delicate, thinner folds of skin beneath the labia majora that fuse anteriorly to form the prepuce and the clitoris. In the posterior aspect, the labia minora meet at the perineum, the skin area between the anus and the vulva. The folds of the labia minora are well supplied with nerves, blood vessels, and sebaceous glands that supply nutrients for protection of the vestibule and provide lubrication during sexual response. Variation in the size and prominence of these structures is normal. In some women, the labia majora completely cover the labia minora, and in others they may not.

The *clitoris* is an erectile organ that lies anterior to the labia minora and is capped externally by a fibrous hood (glans) about 20–30 mm in length and width formed in part by the fusion of the upper folds of the labia minora. The body of the clitoris measures approximately 3 cm in length, is composed of two paired erectile chambers, and is a cylindrical, richly innervated structure. It consists of trabecular smooth muscle and trabecular connective tissue, which are supporting bundles of fibers that cross over the body of the clitoris. The dorsal and clitoral cavernosal arteries arise from the iliohypogastric pudendal bed.

The ducts of Skene glands (also called the lesser vestibular or paraurethral glands) open on either side of the urinary meatus. The ducts of Bartholin glands (greater vestibular glands or vulvogaginal glands) open on either side of the introitus. In response to sexual stimulation, Bartholin glands secrete mucus that lubricates the inner labial surfaces. Secretions from Skene ducts help to lubricate the inner labial surfaces and the urinary meatus.

The vulva is a common site of infection. Its moist, warm surface provides an ideal growth medium for many different microorganisms that may ascend to internal structures through the urethra, vagina, or glandular ducts. Because it is a site of sexual activity and an ideal environment for organisms to grow, it is a common site for STDs.

Benign Pathophysiology of the Vulva

Adams-Hillard (2002) described the following categories of benign conditions of the vulva: skin conditions, pigmented lesions, tumors and cysts, ulcers, and nonneoplastic epithelial disorders.

Skin conditions: The perineal area is susceptible to skin irritation and dermatologic disorders. Inflammation to the vulva also can be caused by mechanical or chemical irritation, including but not limited to tight-fitting or synthetic fabrics,

Figure 2-4. External Female Genitalia

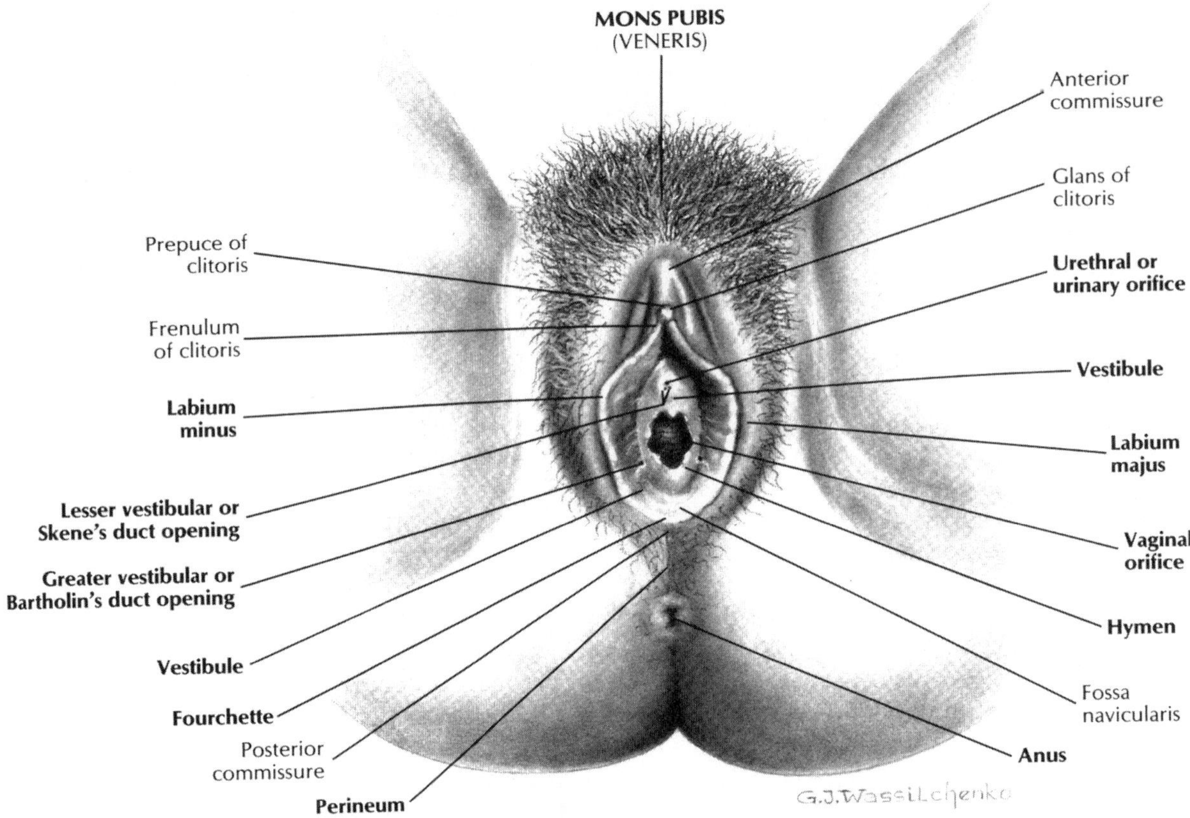

Note. From "Reproduction and Sexuality" (p. 105), by I.M Bobak in I.M. Bobak, M.D. Jensen, and D.L. Lowdermilk (Eds.), *Maternity and Gynecologic Care* (5th ed.), 1993, St. Louis, MO: Mosby. Copyright 1993 by Mosby. Reprinted with permission.

urine, feces, laundry detergents, vaginal deodorants, perfumed bubble bath, and chronic dermatologic conditions.

Vulvitis: Vulvitis, inflammation of the vulva, can be caused by infection from many organisms, including trichomonas, molluscum contagiosum, bacterial vaginosis, and a variety of fungi.

Bartholinitis: Bartholin cyst or abscess, also called bartholinitis, is an infection of the greater vestibular gland, causing cyst or abscess formation. The abscess or cyst may spontaneously rupture or enlarge and become painful. Most are sterile or abscess/cellulites caused by mixed vaginal flora but also may be caused by sexual transmission of gonorrhea, chlamydia or occasionally herpes.

Lymphatic Drainage of the Female Genital Tract

Gynecologic cancer spreads via direct extension into surrounding structures and via the lymphatic system to local, regional, and distant sites. Baggish (2006) and Gray (2003) provide a detailed description of the gynecologic lymphatic system that includes illustrations. The lymphatic secretions from both the ovaries and uterus drain into the pelvic nodes, into the inguinal lymph nodes, and along the ovarian lymphatics in the infundibulopelvic ligaments directly to the paraaortic nodes. Lymph from the middle third of the vagina can flow into either the inguinal nodes or the pelvic and abdominal lymph nodes. Lymph from the cervix and upper vagina drains along the uterine arteries and cardinal ligaments to the pelvic lymph nodes that include the external iliac, internal iliac (hypogastric), and obturator pelvic lymph nodes and continues to drain through the common iliac lymph nodes and paraortic nodes. Lymph from the lower third of the vagina and vulva drains to the external and internal inguinal nodes.

Approximately 15–20 lateral aortic nodes on each side of the aorta receive lymphatic drainage from the iliac lymph nodes, ovaries, and other pelvic viscera (apart from the alimentary tract), and it is this group of nodes that are sampled in the surgical staging of gynecologic cancer (Baggish, 2006).

Breasts

The breasts or mammary glands are modified sweat glands and function as apocrine glands in the production of milk. Each breast is located between the margin of the sternum and the midaxillary line on either side of the chest wall. They are surrounded by fascia, separating each breast from the chest muscles, the pectoralis major and the pectoralis minor. The breast can be divided into three components: glandular tissue, fibrous tissue, and adipose tissue. The glandular tissue is composed of 15–20 lobes containing milk-secreting apocrine glands (alveolar glands) drained by mammary ducts (alveolar ducts). The fibrous tissue is composed of suspensory ligaments, which connect to the skin and underlying fascia. The outermost adipose layer of the breast becomes more prominent with age. The *areola*, a pigmented circular area on the tip of each breast, has both sebaceous and sweat glands. The tubercles of Montgomery are sebaceous glands that lubricate the aerolae and secrete a milk-like substance during pregnancy and for breast feeding (Bickley & Szilagyi, 2007; Bobak, 1993; Lawrence & Lawrence, 2005).

The lymphatics of the breast drain into the infraclavicular nodes, into the chest or abdominal nodes, and to the opposite breast (see Figure 2-5). The pectoral nodes located inside the anterior axillary fold drain the chest wall and most of the breast. The subscapular group of nodes is located deep in the posterior axillary fold and drains the posterior chest wall. The lateral group of nodes is located along the upper humerus and drains most of the arm (Bickley & Szilagyi, 2007; Bobak, 1993; Gray, 2003).

Virtually all breasts are somewhat asymmetrical, but degree varies greatly among women. Hormonal cyclic changes result in variable fibrocystic physiologic nodularity in the breast as well as changes in breast size and sensitivity. Reports vary regarding when the breast has the fewest changes, but all range within approximately 4–10 days after the start of menstrual flow (Dondero & Lichtman, 1990; Grube & Giuliano, 2002; Lawrence & Lawrence, 2005; Osuch et al., 1999; Policar, 2004). Because these changes vary among women, a careful history, documentation of reports from women conducting monthly breast self-examination, and findings during timing of clinical breast examination may help to individualize the optimal time to conduct breast examination (Bickley & Szilagyi, 2007).

Benign Pathophysiology of the Breast

Dondero and Lichtman (1990), Fuss (2006), Grube and Giuliano (2002), and Osuch et al. (1999) provide an overview of benign breast diseases, clinical findings, differential diagnosis, and management. These diseases can be categorized into breast masses and breast cysts.

The breast undergoes changes in response to the menstrual cycle and hormonal changes from adolescence through adulthood, including childbearing, and through menopause and postmenopause. As a result, the breast may have different fibrocystic physiologic nodularity resulting in a change in breast shape, size, or texture. Breast masses include cysts, which are fluid-filled sacks and may be cyclic, as opposed to fibroadenomas, which present as a benign breast mass that may or may not be painful, and multiple papilloma, a rare breast mass that is associated with an increased risk of invasive cancer. Fibroadenoma, the most common benign tumor of the breast, occurs more often in women younger than age 35 and is usually painless. Obstruction of a breast duct called a galactocele may be enlarged and tender. A breast abscess resulting from infection is usually associated with redness, tenderness, and inflammation. A woman with an abscess that does not respond immediately to antibiotics needs to be evaluated for cancer, regardless of her age.

Benign breast disorders include cyclic pain versus continuous, fibrocystic changes, which may present as an asymptomatic mass but more commonly are painful or tender and may be accompanied by nipple discharge. Although there are many benign causes for nipple discharge, careful consideration and evaluation are needed when any nipple discharge is present in a nonlactating woman. Mastalgia, a condition that presents with breast engorgement, pain, and tenderness, is related to premenstrual symptoms.

The diagnosis and treatment of these disorders is beyond the scope of this chapter; however, the reader may refer to authors who provide a comprehensive discussion of these topics (Barbieri, 2002; Bickley & Szilagyi, 2007; Botash, 2006; Cespedes et al., 1999; D'Hooghe & Hill, 2002; Hatch & Berek, 2002; Hatcher & Namnoum, 2004; Hillard, 2002; Hurd et al., 2002; Jolin, 2002; Lichtman & Papera, 1990; Mashburn, 2006; Nelson, 2004; Nelson & Stewart, 2004; Schillings & McClamrock, 2002; Soper, 2002).

Sexual Function

Although gynecologic cancer and its treatment can have a profound effect on all aspects of a woman's sexuality, natural hormonal changes related to the menstrual cycle and menopause are usually accompanied by symptoms that may or may not cause distress (Nelson, 2004; Nelson & Stewart, 2004). A brief discussion of the female sexual physiology is provided here.

Although sexual arousal can occur at any time during the ovarian cycle, the androgen level increase that occurs during the follicular phase may contribute to enhanced sexual arousal. During sexual arousal the vaginal wall and the erectile tissues in the clitoris become congested with blood. The mucosal lining of the vagina, composed of a substantial network of blood vessels, lymphatics, and neural innervation, cause this congestion in the vaginal wall. This stimulates fluid flow to the surface of the mucosa, providing lubrication and enhancing sexual arousal. This secretion combined with the smooth,

Figure 2-5. Cross-Section of the Breast

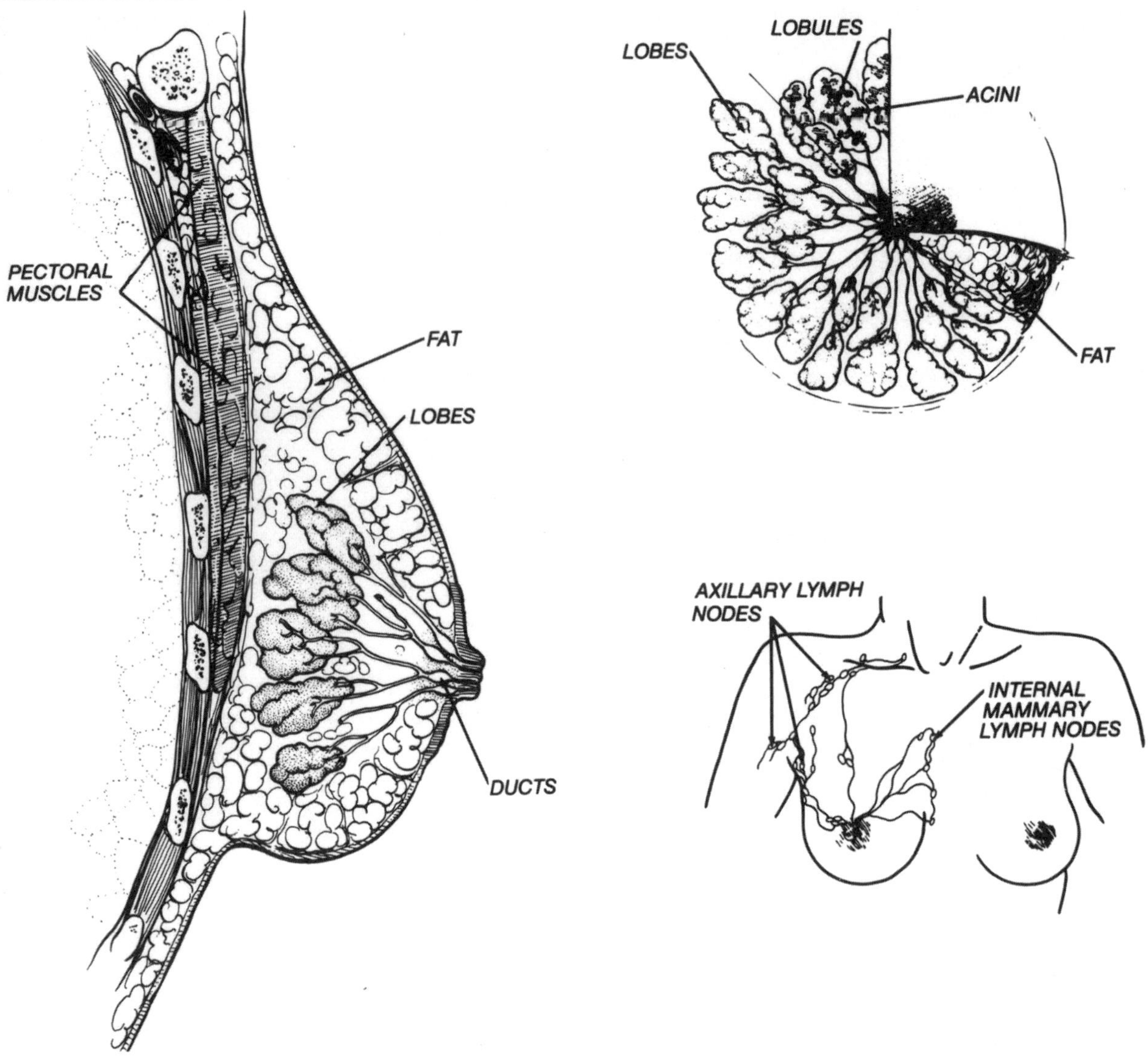

Note. Figure courtsey of the National Cancer Institute.

slippery cervical mucus, as well as the secretions from the sebaceous glands of the labia minora, all provide lubrication during sexual arousal and sexual intercourse. These secretions can be altered from normal cycle changes or from chemotherapy-induced menopause or radiation therapy to the gynecologic structures.

Sexually Transmitted Diseases

Lichtman and Duran (1990, p. 203) "advise all practitioners to stay abreast of new developments by reading up-to-date journals, attending conferences, and being particularly aware of recommendations of the [U.S.] Centers for Disease Control (CDC)." This remains relevant today. Despite the increased amount of knowledge regarding the prevention, diagnosis, and management of STDs during the last four decades, these diseases remain prevalent. The incidence of genital herpes, genital warts, and vaginal trichomoniasis has steadily increased during the decades from 1966–2007 (CDC, 2008). According to CDC reports titled *Trends in Reportable Sexually Transmitted Diseases in the United States, 2007: National Surveillance Data for Chlamydia, Gonorrhea, and Syphilis* (CDC, 2009) and *Sexually Transmitted Disease Surveillance 2007* (CDC, 2008), the number of new cases of chlamydia, gonorrhea, syphilis, vaginal trichomoniasis, other vaginitis, and PID reported each year remains alarmingly high. In addition, these estimates are falsely low because these infections are both underdiagnosed and underreported. A recent article in the *New York Times* citing as-yet unpublished data reported that 25% of all teenage girls in the United States are infected with one of the following four STDs: HPV, chlamydia, genital herpes, or trichomoniasis (Altman, 2008). Women who have undiagnosed and untreated STDs are at risk for infertility, ectopic pregnancy, PID, chronic pelvic pain, cervical cancer, genital warts, and other disorders. Add to these concerns the fact that more than one million Americans are living with HIV, 24%–27% of whom are unaware of their infection (CDC, 2009). It is essential that oncology healthcare professionals encourage women to see a healthcare practitioner who will provide screening for STDs, prevention strategies (which now include the option of vaccination against HPV in adolescent and young women), diagnosis, and treatment. In addition to the CDC Web site, Cates (2004), Cohen (2006), and Lichtman and Duran (1990) provide a comprehensive discussion of reproductive tract infections that includes risk, prevention strategies, assessment, diagnosis, and treatment. Treatment guidelines for STDs are also available (CDC, 2006).

Pelvic Inflammatory Disease

PID is an infection that may involve the fallopian tubes, ovaries, uterus, or peritoneum. The incidence of PID has been increasing with a high recurrence rate because of reinfections from polymicrobial organisms. Common polymicrobial causative agents include *Neisseria gonorrhoeae*, *Chlamydia trachomatis*, anaerobes, gram-negative bacteria, and streptococci.

A cervical infection can ascend through the endometrium into the fallopian tubes and possibly into the peritoneal cavity. Risk factors include multiple sexual partners; early onset of sexual activity; and procedures such as intrauterine device insertion, therapeutic abortion, cesarean section, and hysterosalpingogram.

Pelvic Pain

Pelvic pain may indicate conditions arising from relaxed pelvic muscles, PID, endometriosis, interstitial cystitis, ectopic pregnancy, miscarriage, or cervical or uterine cancer. In addition to these organic causes, women may experience pain associated with factors related to menstrual cycle and hormonal changes.

Menstrual Issues/Differential Diagnosis

As Lichtman and Papera (1990) stated in *Gynecology Well-Woman Care,* "Menstruation is a part of every woman's life whether it proceeds normally or not. It is crucial for women's health practitioners to understand the great varieties of normalcy in menstruation and to promptly recognize abnormalities" (p. xiv). Interventions should be individualized by considering a woman's specific needs and priorities (Dodd et al., 2001).

Dysmenorrhea

Dysmenorrhea, or painful menstruation, is a common gynecologic disorder. Causes include chlamydia, gonorrhea, ectopic pregnancy, tumor, cysts, or endometriosis. However, this is not an exhaustive list. Secondary dysmenorrhea can be caused by endometriosis, adenomyosis (presence of ectopic endometrial glands and stroma in the myometrium of the uterus), pelvic adhesions and infection, and pelvic congestion (engorgement and thrombosis of the pelvic veins). Other causes include cervical stenosis; when the menstrual flow is impeded at the level of the internal cervical os causing increased pressure and pelvic pain, and psychological stress.

Premenstrual Syndrome

Premenstrual syndrome (PMS) is a complex set of symptoms including but not limited to anxiety, irritability, appetite changes, headache, fatigue, back pain, abdominal bloating, lower extremity edema, weight gain, and breast tenderness and is associated with emotional distress. Symptoms occur 4–10 days prior to menstruation and dissipate when menstruation begins (Bobak, 1993; Nelson, 2004). Because all women can experience one or all of these symptoms at varying levels of severity ranging from mild to very severe, the condition "premenstrual syndrome" is relevant when physical, psychological, social, or spiritual aspects of a woman's life are negatively affected.

Irregular Uterine Bleeding

Irregular bleeding may indicate infection of the vagina or cervix; malignancy of the vulva, vagina, cervix, or uterus; benign tumor of the uterus or ovarian cyst; pregnancy; or endometriosis. Dysfunctional uterine bleeding (DUB) is abnormal uterine bleeding that has no organic cause, such as tumor, infection, or pregnancy. Rather, it may be caused by immature hypothalamic stimulation in adolescents, impaired follicular formation or rupture, or corpus luteum dysfunction. Ovarian changes in perimenopausal women are a frequent cause of DUB. Other causes include temporary estrogen withdrawal at ovulation, psychological stress, malnutrition, and changes in exercise. Hypothyroidism can cause menorrhagia.

Amenorrhea

Amenorrhea is absence of menstrual flow caused by pregnancy, lactation, menopause, or corpus luteal ovarian cysts.

Excessive exercise or inadequate nutrition with decreased body fat stores is a significant cause of amenorrhea in young women. Ovarian, adrenal, or pituitary tumors and thyroid disease (hyperthyroidism) are hormonal causes of amenorrhea. Amenorrhea may be a result of depression, severe psychological trauma, physical trauma, or radiation therapy to the pelvis. Medications such as phenothiazines, chemotherapy, and hormonal contraceptives may also induce amenorrhea.

Menopause

Menopause is defined as the cessation of menstruation for a period of 12 months or greater. Women who have had surgical removal of their ovaries or who have menopausal subclinical levels of estradiol are menopausal (Bickley & Szilagyi, 2007; Cohen, 2006; Nelson & Stewart, 2004). Women in menopause report vasomotor changes, including hot flashes, sleep disruption, memory loss, and vaginal dryness from atrophy of the vaginal mucosa. Additionally, women are at increased risk for osteoporosis because of bone loss. These symptoms can be exacerbated in women who experience abrupt menopause related to systemic cancer treatments (Ganz et al., 2003; Knobf, 2006). Acute and chronic symptoms of cancer treatments are addressed in subsequent chapters of this text.

Summary

Understanding the well woman undergoing cancer screening is important, as well as women with a cancer diagnosis during treatment, recovery, and ongoing survivorship who experience benign pathology of the gynecologic tract. Nurses who are caring for women with a gynecologic cancer are in a pivotal position to provide effective screening for benign gynecologic disorders that require prompt attention. Survivors of gynecologic cancer need ongoing support to address symptoms as well as strategies to maintain or adopt a healthy lifestyle. Women with a gynecologic cancer will experience symptoms related to the cancer diagnosis and treatment and perhaps symptoms related to the menstrual cycle and hormonal changes relevant to her stage in the life span.

Understanding the perception of symptom experience related to these benign disorders will add to an appreciation of how these disorders may complicate the cancer diagnosis and treatment and their impact on distress, quality of life, and other outcomes. Guided by this information, nurses can work with women to identify which aspects of symptom experience are of most concern and cause the greatest distress (Armstrong, 2003; Goodell & Nail, 2005). By screening for these benign disorders, resources can then be directed toward the cause of distress, symptom management, and education to promote optimal health during this challenging time in a woman's life.

Special thanks to Kathleen Lutz, MSN, WHNP, for her review of this chapter.

References

Adams-Hillard, P.J. (2002). Benign diseases of the female reproductive tract: Symptoms and signs. In J.S. Berek (Ed.), *Novak's gynecology* (13th ed., pp. 351–420). Philadelphia: Lippincott Williams & Wilkins.

Aikins Murphy, P. (1990). Anatomy and physiology of the female reproductive system. In R. Lichtman & S. Papera (Eds.), *Gynecology well-woman care* (pp. 3–17). East Norwalk, CT: Appleton and Lange.

Altman, K. (2008, March 12). Sex infections found in quarter of teenage girls. *The New York Times*, p. 1.

Armstrong, T.S. (2003). Symptom experience: A concept analysis. *Oncology Nursing Forum, 30*(4), 601–606.

Baggish, M.S. (2006). Introduction to pelvic anatomy. In M.S. Baggish & M.M. Karram (Eds.), *Atlas of pelvic anatomy and gynecologic surgery* (2nd ed., pp. 5–60). Philadelphia: Elsevier.

Barbieri, R.L. (2002). *Endometriosis: Diagnosis. ACP Medicine Online.* Retrieved December 16, 2007, from http://www.medscape.com/viewarticle/534289

Bickley, L.S., & Szilagyi, P.G. (2007). *Bates' guide to physical examination and history taking* (9th ed.). Philadelphia: Lippincott Williams & Wilkins.

Bobak, I. (1993). Reproduction and sexuality. In I.M. Bobak, M. Jensen, & D.L. Lowdermilk (Eds.), *Maternity and gynecologic care* (5th ed., pp. 102–153). St. Louis, MO: Mosby.

Botash, A.S. (2006, July). *Vaginitis*. Retrieved January 1, 2008, from http://www.emedicine.com/emerg/TOPIC631.HTM

Cates, W. (2004). Reproductive tract infections. In R.A. Hatcher, J. Trussell, F. Stewart, A.L. Nelson, W. Cates, F. Guest, et al. (Eds.), *Contraceptive technology* (18th ed., pp. 191–220). New York: Ardent Media.

Cespedes, R.D., Cross, C.A., & McGuire, E.J. (1999). Pelvic prolapse: Diagnosing and treating uterine and vaginal vault prolapse. *Medscape General Medicine, 1*(3), 1–8. Retrieved February 11, 2009, from http://www.medscape.com/viewarticle/408889

Cohen, C.K. (2006). Gynecologic disorders. In S.M. Nettina (Ed.), *Lippincott manual of nursing practice* (8th ed., pp. 807–853). Philadelphia: Lippincott Williams & Wilkins.

Cunningham, F.G., Leveno, K.J., Bloom, S.L., Hauth, J.C., Gilstrap, L.C., & Wenstrom, K.D. (Eds.). (2005). *Williams obstetrics* (22nd ed.). New York: McGraw-Hill.

DeCherney, A.H. (2002). *Dysmenorrhea: Secondary dysmenorrheal. ACP Medicine Online.* Retrieved December 16, 2007, from http://www.medscape.com/viewarticle /534247

D'Hooghe, T.M., & Hill, J.A. (2002). Endometriosis. In J.S. Berek (Ed.), *Novak's gynecology* (13th ed., pp. 931–972). Philadelphia: Lippincott Williams & Wilkins.

Dodd, M., Janson, S., Facione, N., Faucett, J., Froelicher, E.S., Humphreys, J., et al. (2001). Advancing the science of symptom management. *Journal of Advanced Nursing, 33*(5), 668–676.

Dondero, T., & Lichtman, R. (1990). The breasts. In R. Lichtman & S. Papera (Eds.), *Gynecology well-woman care* (pp. 141–171). East Norwalk, CT: Appleton and Lange.

Fuss, E.P. (2006). Breast conditions. In S.M. Nettina (Ed.), *Lippincott manual of nursing practice* (8th ed., pp. 854–872). Philadelphia: Lippincott Williams & Wilkins.

Ganz, P.A., Greendale, G.A., Petersen, L., Kahn, B., & Bower, J.E. (2003). Breast cancer in younger women: Reproductive and late health effects of treatment. *Journal of Clinical Oncology, 21*(22), 4184–4193.

Godfrey, J.R. (2004). Toward optimal health: The experts discuss abnormal uterine bleeding. *Journal of Women's Health, 13*(3), 259–264.

Goodell, T.T., & Nail, L.M. (2005). Operationalizing symptom distress in adults with cancer: A literature synthesis. *Oncology Nursing Forum, 32*(2), E42–E47. Retrieved February 11, 2009, from http://ons.metapress.com/content/3017235611mq3840/fulltext.pdf

Gray, H. (2003). The female organs of generation. In P. Pick & R. Howden (Eds.), *Gray's anatomy* (16th ed., pp. 1025–1040). Ann Arbor, MI: Ann Arbor Media Group.

Grube, B.J., & Giuliano, A.E. (2002). Benign breast disease. In J.S. Berek (Ed.), *Novak's gynecology* (13th ed., pp. 543–567). Philadelphia: Lippincott Williams & Wilkins.

Hatch, K.D., & Berek, J.S. (2002). Intraepithelial disease of the cervix, vagina, and vulva. In J.S. Berek (Ed.), *Novak's gynecology* (13th ed., pp. 471–506). Philadelphia: Lippincott Williams & Wilkins.

Hatcher, R.A., & Namnoum, A.B. (2004). The menstrual cycle. In R.A. Hatcher, J. Trussell, F. Stewart, A.L. Nelson, W. Cates, F. Guest, et al. (Eds.), *Contraceptive technology* (18th ed., pp. 63–72). New York: Ardent Media.

Hillard, P.J.A. (2002). Benign diseases of the female reproductive tract: Symptoms and signs. In J.S. Berek (Ed.), *Novak's gynecology* (13th ed., pp. 351–420). Philadelphia: Lippincott Williams & Wilkins.

Hurd, W.W., Amesse, L.S., & Randolph, J.F., Jr. (2002). Menopause. In J.S. Berek (Ed.), *Novak's gynecology* (13th ed., pp. 1109–1142). Philadelphia: Lippincott Williams & Wilkins.

Jackson, V., & Lichtman, R. (1990). The ovaries. In R. Lichtman & S. Papera (Eds.), *Gynecology well-woman care* (pp. 283–294). East Norwalk, CT: Appleton and Lange.

Jolin, J.A. (2002). Pelvic pain and dysmenorrhea. In J.S. Berek (Ed.), *Novak's gynecology* (13th ed., pp. 421–452). Philadelphia: Lippincott Williams & Wilkins.

Knobf, T. (2006). Reproductive and hormonal sequelae of chemotherapy in women. *American Journal of Nursing, 106*(Suppl. 3), 60–65.

Lawrence, R.A., & Lawrence, R.M. (Eds.). (2005). *Breastfeeding: A guide for the medical profession*. Philadelphia: Mosby.

Lichtman, R., & Duran, P. (1990). Sexually transmitted diseases. In R. Lichtman & S. Papera (Eds.), *Gynecology well-woman care* (pp. 203–248). East Norwalk, CT: Appleton and Lange.

Lichtman, R., & Papera, S. (Eds.). (1990). Introduction. In R. Lichtman, & S. Papera (Eds.), *Gynecology well-woman care* (pp. iii–xvi). East Norwalk, CT: Appleton and Lange.

Lichtman, R., & Smith, S.M. (1990). Multiorgan disorders. In R. Lichtman & S. Papera (Eds.), *Gynecology well-woman care* (pp. 309–330). East Norwalk, CT: Appleton and Lange.

Mashburn, J. (2006). Etiology, diagnosis, and management of vaginitis. *Journal of Midwifery and Women's Health, 51*(6), 423–430.

National Comprehensive Cancer Network. (2009a). *NCCN Clinical Practice Guidelines in Oncology™: Cervical cancer* [v.1.2009]. Retrieved March 11, 2009, from http://www.nccn.org/professionals/physician_gls/PDF/cervical.pdf

National Comprehensive Cancer Network. (2009b). *NCCN Clinical Practice Guidelines in Oncology™: Ovarian cancer* [v.1.2009]. Retrieved March 11, 2009, from http://www.nccn.org/professionals/physician_gls/PDF/ovarian.pdf

National Comprehensive Cancer Network. (2009c). *NCCN Clinical Practice Guidelines in Oncology™: Uterine neoplasms* [v.2.2009]. Retrieved March 11, 2009, from http://www.nccn.org/professionals/physician_gls/PDF/uterine.pdf

Nelson, A.L. (2004). Menstrual problems and common gynecologic concerns. In R.A. Hatcher, J. Trussell, F. Stewart, A.L. Nelson, W. Cates, F. Guest, et al. (Eds.), *Contraceptive technology* (18th ed., pp. 109–151). New York: Ardent Media.

Nelson, A.L., & Stewart, F.H. (2004). Menopause. In R.A. Hatcher, J. Trussell, F. Stewart, A.L. Nelson, W. Cates, F. Guest, et al. (Eds.), *Contraceptive technology* (18th ed., pp. 73–108). New York: Ardent Media.

Osuch, J.R., Bonham, V.L., & Morris, L.L. (1999). Primary care guide to managing a breast mass: Step-by-step workup. *Medscape General Medicine, 1*(3), 1–29. Retrieved February 11, 2009, from http://www.medscape.com/viewarticle/443381

Peck, D. (1990). Premenstrual syndrome. In R. Lichtman & S. Papera (Eds.), *Gynecology well-woman care* (pp. 333–344). East Norwalk, CT: Appleton and Lange.

Policar, M.S. (2004). Female genital tract screening. In R.A. Hatcher, J. Trussell, F. Stewart, A.L. Nelson, W. Cates, F. Guest, et al. (Eds.), *Contraceptive technology* (18th ed., pp. 37–61). New York: Ardent Media.

Quinn, E.B. (1993). Health promotion and screening. In I.M. Bobak & M. Duncan-Jensen (Eds.), *Maternity and gynecologic care: The nurse and the family* (5th ed., pp. 1245–1275). St. Louis, MO: Mosby.

Scalone, M.R.C. (1990). Natural family planning and fertility awareness. In R.L. Lichtman & S. Papera (Eds.), *Gynecology well-woman care* (pp. 59–70). East Norwalk, CT: Appleton and Lange.

Schillings, W.J., & McClamrock, H. (2002). Amenorrhea. In J.S. Berek (Ed.), *Novak's gynecology* (13th ed., pp. 843–870). Philadelphia: Lippincott Williams & Wilkins.

Snyder, U. (2005). *Medscape ob/gyn and women's health*. Retrieved January 3, 2008, from http://www.medscape.com/viewarticle/496841_print

Soper, D.E. (2002). Genitourinary infections and sexually transmitted diseases. In J.S. Berek (Ed.), *Novak's gynecology* (13th ed., pp. 453–470). Philadelphia: Lippincott Williams & Wilkins.

Sullivan, N. (1990). Dysmenorreha. In R. Lichtman & S. Papera (Eds.), *Gynecology well-woman care* (pp. 345–353). East Norwalk, CT: Appleton and Lange.

U.S. Centers for Disease Control and Prevention. (2006). Sexually transmitted diseases treatment guidelines, 2006. *Morbidity and Mortality Weekly Report, 55*(RR-11), 1–94.

U.S. Centers for Disease Control and Prevention. (2008, December). *Sexually transmitted disease surveillance, 2007*. Atlanta, GA: Author.

U.S. Centers for Disease Control and Prevention. (2009, January). *Trends in reportable sexually transmitted diseases in the United States, 2007: National surveillance data for chlamydia, gonorrhea, and syphilis.* Retrieved March 17, 2009, from http://www.cdc.gov/std/stats07trends.pdf

Varney, H., Kribes, J., & Gegor, L. (2004). *Varney's midwifery* (4th ed.). Sudbury, MA: Jones and Bartlett.

CHAPTER 3

Prevention and Early Detection of Cancers of the Cervix, Ovaries, and Endometrium

Kathleen Farley-Omerod, RN, MS, APN/CNS, AOCN®, and
Eileen Fusco, MSN, APRN-BC, AOCNP®

Introduction

Women who encounter a diagnosis of gynecologic cancer experience a severe threat to their physical, spiritual, psychological, and social well-being. Oncology nurses are in a unique position to provide care for women undergoing evaluation for gynecologic cancer and provide information about the nature, cause, prevention, predictability, and prognosis to all women.

Cervical Cancer

The incidence of cervical cancer in the United States has steadily declined in both Caucasian and African American women and is among the lowest in the world (American Cancer Society [ACS], 2007). The death rate for cervical cancer in the United States declined by 74% between 1955 and 1992, in large part because of the effectiveness of Pap smear screening. The widespread availability of and improvements in technology that combine cytologic, histologic, and DNA technology maximize screening efforts.

Pathophysiology

An understanding of the pathophysiology of cervical cancer, cervical intraepithelial neoplasia (CIN), its association with the squamo-columnar junction (SCJ), and the transformation zone of the cervix is necessary to understand the rationale for cervical Pap smears and prevention and screening strategies.

The cervix is the lower one-third of the uterus and is tubular in shape. It extends downward into the upper portion of the vagina. The cervix surrounds the opening called the *cervical orifice* or *os*, through which the uterus communicates with the vagina. The cervix contains three types of tissue. The two main cell types are columnar epithelium and squamous epithelium, and their distribution is established embryonically. The endocervical canal is lined with columnar epithelium, and the exocervix is composed of squamous epithelium. The meeting point of the endocervix and the exocervix is called the SCJ. This area is responsive to hormonal stimulation and exogenous factors. The SCJ, normally located in the endocervical canal, comes out of the endocervical canal during puberty or reverts to a position on the cervix. This endocervical tissue in a new position on the cervix is exposed to all things that enter through the vagina. A new SCJ is generated continually just above this area by the process of metaplasia. This area of constant repair (squamous metaplasia) between the old and the new junctions is called the transformation zone. After menopause, the uterus and cervix become smaller because of muscular atrophy (Netter, 2006), and this junction may lie in the canal. The process of metaplasia is less after menopause, as well. More than 90% of the squamous intraepithelial neoplasia occurs within the transformation zone (Addis, Hatch, & Berek, 2007; Herbst, 2001).

Risk Factors

The association of cervical cancer and its precursor lesions is substantially linked to persistent infection with oncogenic human papillomavirus (HPV). (See next section in this chapter for epidemiology of HPV.) HPV is sexually transmitted; therefore, all sexually active women are at risk. However, cofactors have been identified that increase the risk for certain women. These cofactors include early age at first intercourse and lifetime number of sexual partners. The sexual behavior of the male partner also has been found to affect a woman's risk of cervical cancer (Zunzunegui, Kink, Coria, & Charlet, 1986). Some studies suggest that partners of women with cervical cancer had more sexual partners, intercourse at an early age, and a greater history of venereal disease than partners of women without cervical cancer (Giuliano et al., 2001). Another study suggests that women married to men who previously had wives with cervical cancer are also at greater risk for developing cervical cancer (Holowaty, Miller, Rohan, & To, 1999).

Active and passive cigarette smoking have been implicated as risk factors for cervical cancer, especially squamous cell carcinoma (Trimble et al., 2005). Cotinine and nicotine exert mutagenic activity in the cervical mucus of smokers. Cigarette smoking produces a local immunosuppression in cervical epithelium, which may increase the likelihood of developing HPV neoplasia (Barton et al., 1988). Women who report having smoked cigarettes regularly have a 50% higher risk of cervical cancer compared with women who are nonsmokers. Women who smoke 40 or more cigarettes per day and those who smoked for 40 years or more have a significant twofold excess risk (Brinton et al., 1986). Among HPV-infected women, current and former smokers have approximately two to three times the incidence of high-grade CIN or invasive cancer. Passive smoking also is associated with increased risk, albeit to a lesser extent (Ho, Kadish, et al., 1998).

Increased risk of cervical neoplasia has been noted with any use of combined oral contraceptives, with the greatest increase in women who use them for five years or more (World Health Organization Collaborative Study of Neoplasia and Steroid Contraceptives, 1993). The mechanism of action of oral contraceptives on the cervical epithelium is unclear. Among women with HPV, those who use combined oral contraceptives for 5–9 years have approximately three times the incidence of invasive cancer, and those who use them for 10 years or longer have approximately four times the risk (Miller, Blumenthal, & Blanchard, 2004; Moreno et al., 2002). In contrast, women who use barrier methods, such as diaphragm, vaginal spermicide, or condom, are at a lower cervical cancer risk than women who use hormonal contraceptives (Manhart & Koutsky, 2002).

Women who are iatrogenically immunosuppressed because of medical conditions (e.g., bone marrow or organ transplant) have a greater incidence of cervical and other cancers of the reproductive tract and anus (anogenital). Women who undergo renal transplants are shown to have an incidence of cervical cancer five times higher than that of age-matched controls (Penn, 2000). The progression of HPV infection to the development of cervical neoplasia in women who are HIV-positive correlates to the degree of immunosuppression (Schafer, Friedman, Meilke, Schwartlander, & Koch, 1991).

Jemal et al. (2008) reported a higher incidence of cervical cancer among African American and Hispanic women. This disparity may be because of differences in increased exposure to risk factors and diminished access to high-quality regular screening, timely diagnosis, and treatment.

See Figure 3-1 for factors that contribute to the development of cervical cancer; note that many are modifiable behaviors such as smoking.

Figure 3-1. Factors Contributing to Cervical Cancer

- Multiple sexual partners
- Presence of sexually transmitted disease
- Early onset of sexual activity
- Lack of cervical cancer screening
- Cigarette smoking
- Immune suppression (e.g., HIV, pregnancy)
- Long-term oral contraception use

Note. Based on information from Koutsky, 1997; U.S. Centers for Disease Control and Prevention, 2007.

Epidemiology of the Human Papillomavirus

Papillomaviruses are double-stranded DNA tumor viruses. They infect epithelial cells of the skin and mucous membranes preferentially. This may produce warts at the site of epithelial proliferation. Genital HPV has been shown to be present in the squamous cells and the glandular epithelium of the cervix. Primary infection with HPV causes no symptoms and resolves unnoticed. More than 100 types of HPV exist, and 40 distinct types infect the genital tract. At least 14 high-risk or oncogenic types have been associated with significant progression over time to invasive cervical cancer. Most of these types are related to either HPV type 16 (e.g., 31, 33, 35, 52, 58) or HPV type 18 (e.g., 39, 45, 59, 68) (Bosch et al., 1995).

Walboomers et al. (1997) reanalyzed the data from Bosch et al. (1995) and used different techniques to measure for the presence of HPV. After excluding inadequate specimens, they concluded that HPV prevalence in cervical carcinoma was 99.7%. Data from Schiffman et al. (1993) and Bosch et al. (1995) support this.

Bosch, Lorincz, Munoz, Meijer, and Shah (2002) provided information for the first time that established a definitive causal relationship between an infection with HPV and the development of cervical cancer (see Figure 3-2). Bosch's review of the literature met the criteria traditionally set forth in research such as temporal relationship, consistency, specificity, biologic plausibility, and coherence.

These pivotal research findings set the stage for combining the already widely used screening Pap test and HPV testing in established and developing screening programs. Establishing the causal factor as HPV infection clearly made the case for the development of a vaccine to prevent HPV infection.

Figure 3-2. Cervical Cancer and Human Papillomavirus (HPV) Association

1. A strong relationship exists between the presence of HPV DNA and development of cervical cancer.
2. HPV infections precede the development of cervical cancer by a substantial number of years.
3. The risk of cervical cancer may be related to persistent viral load.
4. This model is analogous to other virus-induced carcinomas.

Note. Based on information from Bosch et al., 2002.

A meta-analysis published in 2003 by Clifford, Smith, Plummer, Muñoz, and Franceschi sought to clarify regional distribution of HPV by type. They reviewed 85 studies published on invasive cervical cancer that discussed prevalence of HPV type. A total of 10,058 cases were reviewed that used only polymerase chain reaction (PCR) in the analysis. The analysis included variables such as geographic region, histologic type of invasive cervical carcinoma, and type of PCR testing. Mean age was not considered to be significantly related to overall HPV prevalence. Cases chosen were distributed regionally among Asia, Europe, Africa, North America, South America, Central America, and Australia. They extracted data on squamous cell carcinoma (SCC) and adenosquamous carcinoma (ADC). The analysis identified that HPV prevalence was about 80%. HPV DNA was detected in 87% of the SCC cases and 77% of the ADC cases, and this was statistically significant. Interestingly, when the combination of cervical biopsy and cytology was reviewed, HPV prevalence was significantly higher at 92.5%. The most common types of HPV identified were HPV 16 and 18. HPV 16 was identified in more than 50% of the SCC cases, compared to 31% of ADC cases, and that was statistically significant. Conversely, HPV 18 was more common in ADC cases than SCC. More than two-thirds of the cases surveyed were associated with HPV 16 or 18. Compared to HPV 16, HPV 18 has been described to be associated with increased oncogenic potential, more rapid transition to invasive cervical cancer, and poorer prognosis.

Castellsagué et al. (2006) did an analysis of eight case-controlled studies of adenosquamous carcinomas and adenocarcinomas that arose in the cervix. His data confirmed the association between the development of cervical cancer and HPV infection. Again, HPV types 16 and 18 were the most commonly detected.

In a prospective study, Ho, Bierman, Beardsley, Chang, and Burk (1998) focused on persistence and progression. They confirmed that many cases of CIN regress spontaneously but that persistence of HPV coincided with persistence of CIN.

Woodman et al. (2001) described the natural history of HPV infection in the United Kingdom and its relationship to the occurrence of CIN. In an attempt to focus on a population that was not already infected with the virus, young women between the ages of 15 and 19 years of age who were being seen for contraception were recruited. On study entry, participants completed detailed risk factor profiles that included information about social, sexual, and behavioral issues. Cervical sampling was performed during initial examination and serum and cytology samples were obtained for future reference. There was continuity in the examiners of the cytologic and histologic samples. The final cohort was made up of 1,075 women who had negative cytology and histology on study entry. The median age was 18 years. The median number of sexual partners was two, and years of sexual activity was one. The cumulative risk of obtaining HPV infection at five years was 44%, and the most common type was HPV 16. The median duration of the first HPV-positive episode was 13–17 months.

During three years of follow-up, 246 women had abnormal Pap smears, a cumulative risk of 28%, and median duration of the episode of eight months. High-grade CIN was diagnosed in 28 women, and 22 were diagnosed within 12 months. Positive cytology samples in 98 of these 246 women were tested for HPV and were negative. The majority of the cytologic abnormalities were associated with the detection of HPV, but concordance did not always occur. Another important point identified was that after the detection of HPV, the risk was great for a cytologic abnormality, but it quickly declined after six months. Recurrence of HPV-associated abnormalities were usually associated with the detection of new HPV types.

Winer et al. (2005) confirmed the transient nature with more frequent screening using HPV DNA testing and cytology. One difference between the data that Winer presented and that presented by Woodman (2001) and Moscicki, Schiffman, Kjaer, and Villa (2006) is that high-grade squamous intraepithelial lesions (HSIL) appeared earlier than anticipated, and their detection may have been as a result of the study schema of screening every four months rather than six months. In one study, only 9% of college-aged females remained HPV positive when assessed at two years (Ho, Bierman, et al., 1998).

These three previous studies confirmed the usual transient nature and usual short duration of an HPV infection as the immune system clears the infection over time.

Hildesheim et al. (1994) described persistent HPV infections and some potential outcomes. Women with persistent positive HPV cervical lavage sampling were more likely to be associated with high-risk types of HPV. Persistence also decreased with time between sampling in a reliable way in the group of women who were younger than 24 years of age.

In 1996, Chua and Hjerpe analyzed 88 archived Pap smears to determine if a relationship existed between persistent HPV infection and the development of cervical cancer. These smears were taken 1.5–7 years before the diagnosis of an HPV-containing invasive cervical cancer was made. They were able to demonstrate that in the majority of cancers diagnosed using PCR technology, persistent HPV infection could be demonstrated years before the cancer diagnosis. In those cases that did not demonstrate HPV preceding cancer development, the use of stored samples may have affected their ability to detect HPV and may have been a limitation of this study. The demonstration of a persistent infection with HPV was a sensitive indicator of patients at risk for developing cervical cancer in the future, although the presence of HPV did not always correlate with the cytology sample. However, used together, they provide helpful information and improved screening as is suggested by the Bethesda System (see Chapter 4).

In a meta-analysis done by Melnikow et al. (1998), Chua and Hjerpe's (1996) finding that high-grade lesions were more likely to be persistent and to progress to cancer were confirmed. This analysis also confirmed spontaneous regression of atypical squamous cells of undetermined significance and low-grade squamous intraepithelial lesion (LSIL) lesions without treatment.

The sexual transmission of HPV occurs orally or via vaginal or anal intercourse. It is very easy to transmit HPV, and infections are not limited to the cervix. It can be transmitted skin to skin from areas not covered by condoms during sexual activity (Koutsky & Kiviat, 1999). Infection is common after the first few years of sexual activity (Winer et al., 2003). The absence of visible warts cannot be used as an assessment of a partner's potential infection with HPV. Most genital warts are caused by HPV types 6 and 11. Warts, or condyloma acuminatum, may not be observable on the cervix and may be flat or not observable to the eye. Sexually transmitted high-risk HPV 16, 18, 31, 33, 39, 45, 51, 52, 56, 58, 59, 68, and 69 have been linked to cervical cancer in women (Walboomers et al., 1999). Table 3-1 provides a comprehensive list of HPV types and associated types of lesions.

Prevention

HPV Vaccination

Cervical cancer represents only a small portion of the impact of infection with HPV. More than a half a million new cases of genital warts are diagnosed annually in the United States. They are benign but often recur within six months of treatment. There are 1.5 million cases of low-grade CIN diagnosed, and 0.5 million cases of high-grade CIN diagnosed annually (Saslow et al., 2002).

These figures, in addition to the recent epidemiologic studies that have clearly established HPV as the causal factor in invasive cervical cancer, plainly identify the burden of HPV infection. With that identification, HPV has been the target of vaccine development.

Table 3-1. Human Papillomavirus (HPV) Types Associated With Genital Lesions

Type of Lesion	Types of HPV
Condyloma	6, 11, 16, 30, 40, 41, 42, 44, 45, 54, 55, 61
CIN, VIN, VAIN	6, 11, 16, 18, 30, 31, 33, 35, 39, 40, 45, 51, 52, 55, 59, 61, 62, 64, 66–70
Cervical cancer	16, 18, 31, 33, 35, 39, 45, 51, 52, 54, 55, 56, 58, 59, 66, 68

CIN—cervical intraepithelial neoplasia; VAIN—vaginal intraepithelial neoplasia; VIN—vulvar intraepithelial neoplasia

Note. Based on information from Muñoz, 2003.

Human papillomavirus quadrivalent vaccine (Gardasil®, Merck), the first vaccine to prevent HPV-related precancerous lesions and cervical cancer, was approved by the U.S. Food and Drug Administration (FDA) in June 2006. It has been shown to be effective against HPV types 6 and 11, which are associated with condyloma and LSIL, as well as HPV 16 and 18, which are associated with cervical changes more likely to progress to cervical cancer (Siddiqui & Perry, 2005). Recently, two large randomized trials confirmed a greater than 95% reduction in the incidence of HPV-related disease caused by HPV types 6, 11, 16, and 18 (FUTURE II Study Group, 2007; Villa et al., 2006). The Federal Advisory Committee on Immunization Practices has recommended that the vaccine be given to females aged 11–12 before they become sexually active. They also recommend administering catch-up vaccinations in women who are 19–26 years old (Atkinson et al., 2002; Markowitz et al., 2007). In 2007, the American Cancer Society published guidelines specifically addressing HPV vaccines (see Figure 3-3).

Figure 3-3. American Cancer Society Recommendations for Human Papillomavirus (HPV) Vaccination

- Routine use of the HPV vaccination in girls 9–12 years old.
- Catch-up vaccinations for the age group 13–18 are recommended.
- Vaccination currently is not recommended for women older than 26 years of age.
- Vaccination currently is not recommended for men.
- Cervical cancer screening should continue as per the established American Cancer Society guidelines.

Note. Based on information from Saslow et al., 2002.

Education

Using data from the 2000 National Health Interview Survey, Coughlin, Breslau, Thompson, and Benard (2005) analyzed the results related to women older than 18 years. Their objective was to determine the proportion of women who had not received a provider recommendation to get a Pap test with a focus on those women who were uninsured and in certain racial subgroups. Their discussion summary focused on three linked variables: (a) predisposing factors that were linked to the individual, (b) factors that were enabling, and (c) an external reinforcing associated with the system itself or the practitioner. Approximately 10% of the patients responded that they did not think they needed a Pap test or the practitioner did not order it. These two factors may contribute to the under-use of Pap screening by women who are at risk.

Multiple studies have identified that women's informational needs are not being met (Anhang, Goodman, & Goldie,

2004; Gilbert, Alexander, Grosshans & Jolley, 2003; Mays et al., 2000). Health education regarding the effects of HPV infection, safer sex strategies, condom use, and information about HPV vaccines may reduce the burden of HPV-related infections (Winer et al., 2006).

Controversies and Challenges

The successful screening programs in North America and Europe were all based on cytology screening alone. The addition of the ability to screen for specific types of HPV that place a woman at high risk for cervical cancer shows that now the focus must shift from the woman to the virus in order to identify the oncogenic potential in each woman.

Despite the advent of a new vaccine, it may or may not help women who are already infected with HPV. Some oncogenic HPV types are not included in the vaccine, and the length or duration of protection is unknown. A gap in the knowledge exists surrounding whether natural HPV infection confers a reduced risk of subsequent infection. Some evidence suggests that the production of antibodies provides cross-protection against other types of HPV (Smith et al., 2007). Screening of vaccinated and unvaccinated women should continue. Adequate screening in populations of people without access to care continues to be a problem, and vaccinating this underserved population is almost impossible.

One of the challenges practitioners face is the waxing and waning of infections versus the reemergence of disease. It is not clear if this is because of multiple types of viruses or persistence or reappearance of a previous infection. Screening efforts should include educational information about the natural history of the infection and the significance of the coincidence with the abnormal Pap smear (Woodman et al., 2001).

One of the challenges clinicians still face is the barriers to cervical cancer screening. They vary across the world, from country to country, and even within countries themselves with diverse populations and socioeconomic status. Barriers to screening are lack of knowledge, poverty, lack of access to healthcare systems and new technologies, and personal healthcare behaviors (Miller et al., 1996).

In a prospective design study by Walsh (2006), the impact of knowledge and perceived barriers and risk on attendance at a screening clinic were examined. Participants were sent questionnaires and letters inviting them to a free clinic visit that included a cervical Pap smear test. The questionnaires covered information concerning previous experiences with screening, knowledge, perception of risk, and barriers, as well as socioeconomic information. Of the 3,000 participants, 41% returned their questionnaires. Less than half the women that responded identified the fact that the Pap smear could prevent cancer. Many thought it was used to detect infection. Only 17% of the women contacted accepted the invitation and had an examination performed. Previous unpleasant experiences and poor perception of risk also were barriers to attendance.

A study published in 2005 by Brewster et al. attempted to overcome some of the previously listed barriers. In a randomized clinical trial (RCT) of 3,521 women, an attempt was made to educate and simplify the screening process by using a single visit approach. Women were provided with results of Pap tests on the day of the procedure with explanations of the importance of follow-up. In the group of women who were randomized to the single visit approach, if the Pap was significant for an abnormal cytology, with either HSIL or atypical gland cells of undetermined significance, an excision procedure was performed at the time of visit. Despite the intensive efforts to educate and treat the patients in a timely fashion, only 36% of the women returned for follow-up screening the following year.

Denny et al. (2005) also published an article about a screen-and-treat approach to cervical cancer prevention in South Africa. The RCT had advantages for the low-resource setting, as it was not reliant on cytology-based screening and colposcopy services. Using nurses as examiners, HPV screening and direct visualization was completed in one visit. This study did result in high rates of follow-up.

These three studies highlight the continued difficulty practitioners face worldwide. The unique availability of the cervix to visual inspection and cytologic and histologic sampling has led to improved overall cure rates of cervical cancer nationally and worldwide. Cervical cancer serves as a model of a cancer that has an identifiable precursor lesion, CIN, a slow progression to cancer, a minimally invasive screening test that is inexpensive and readily available, and an identified causal factor that is modifiable.

The identification of the causative factor, the burden of HPV disease, and the understanding of the natural history of the disease has presented an opportunity for practitioners to provide patient education. Cervical cancer is not a sexually transmitted disease. The cancer is not transmitted, only the virus is. This is a challenge for healthcare providers. Healthcare professionals need to clearly communicate to female patients that their sexual practices as well as their sexual partners' practices place them at risk for acquisition of HPV. As sexual activity onset occurs during adolescence, generally with the risk taking associated with that age group, the challenge is to educate both mothers and daughters. It involves an exchange of private information from patients to ascertain risk factors. It involves an intimate exam that very often is difficult for women, and it involves diagnostic techniques that are invasive and frightening.

Oncology nurses are in a unique situation as they can be effective in all the educational areas needed by women. Newly acquired scientific information about HPV and a new vaccine provide a unique opportunity for nurses to educate women confidently and accurately about how to keep themselves healthy. It is also an opportunity to eradicate cervical cancer across the globe.

Screening

Precancerous lesions, such as those that develop in cervical dysplasia, are ideal for screening and are asymptomatic (Kramer, 2004). The most widely used screening test for cervical dysplasia is the Pap smear, and the defined targets are sexually active females. The use of Pap tests for cervical cancer screening has reduced the incidence of cervical cancer by 79% and the mortality by 70% since 1950 (Ries, Eisner, & Kosary, 2004). Cervical cytology for screening is based on the premises that cervical cancer develops gradually and that cancer precursors are identifiable. Once identified, a successful treatment can be offered to reduce the progression to invasive cancer. Problems with sensitivity and specificity were identified in a literature review published by the Agency for Healthcare Research and Quality (AHRQ) (Fahey, Irwig, & Macaskill, 1995). Their conclusion was that sensitivity of conventional cytology tests for detecting precancerous changes was 51%. Bolick and Hellman, reporting for the AHRQ in 1998, stated that the use of liquid-based Pap test improved the sensitivity to 80%. Liquid-based Pap tests intended as a replacement for the conventional smears received FDA approval in 1996 for cervical cancer screening. They have been shown to be superior in several meta-analyses (Chacho, Mattie, & Schwartz, 2003). Studies show a more uniform cellular distribution, better preserved morphology, and a cleaner background was observed in the ThinPrep® (Hologic, Inc.) slides during the screening process than in Pap tests that were not liquid based. The traditional collection of cells that were placed on glass slides and air dried did not eliminate mucous, blood, or extraneous cells. These are eliminated by ThinPrep. The Pap is taken in the usual way (see the technique description that follows), and the cells are placed in a jar containing the preservative. A suspension is prepared and placed on a slide in a thin, well-distributed layer of cells. With this distribution, it is less likely to be obscured by extraneous cells or debris.

An additional benefit of ThinPrep technology is that the remaining fluid may be used for additional testing, including tests for HPV. This would not require another visit and may assist in the management of cervical screening results (Stoler, 2002). Reflexive DNA testing for HPV has been approved by the FDA for use as a screening test in combination with the Pap test in women older than 30 years of age. It also is being used clinically in those women who have previous cervical abnormalities.

In April of 2003, the FDA approved the Hybrid Capture 2® (Digene Corporation) test to be used conjunctively with a liquid-based Pap test. Cells are taken from the cervix in the usual way. The test assesses the sample for the presence of genetic material of HPV.

Pap Smear Collection

Ideally, a woman scheduled for a cervical cytology exam should not be menstruating, use douche, have intercourse, use tampons, or use intravaginal medication for at least 24 hours before the examination.

To collect the cells needed to make a Pap smear, the clinician begins by inserting a speculum into the vagina (see Figure 3-4). The speculum, lubricated only with water or a water-based lubricant, is placed carefully to expose the cervix. The clinician rotates an Ayer spatula 360° to gently scrape the entire circumference of the external cervical area (see Figure 3-5) to harvest cells from the area of the transformation zone. Meticulous technique in obtaining a Pap smear is essential in reducing false-negative results. An additional sample may be taken from the vaginal pool or the posterior vaginal fornix, but it is important to obtain an adequate sample from the endocervical canal. This is best done with an endocervical brush (see Figure 3-6). An adequate history also must accompany the smear, including information such as the date of the last menstrual period, hormonal medications, and prior genital tract neoplasia and treatment.

In certain populations, such as postmenopausal women, it is especially important to obtain a good endocervical sample. Obtaining endocervical cells can be challenging as the transformation zone migrates up the cervix because of the loss of estrogen. The healthcare provider may need to reposition the woman to obtain an adequate sample. A variety of specula should be available in the event of a stenotic os. Stenosis may occur as part of the aging process. Stenosis also may occur after radiation therapy to the vagina, cervix, or uterus.

From 2002 to 2003, several new screening guidelines were published by ACS (Saslow 2002), the American Col-

Figure 3-4. Pelvic Examination

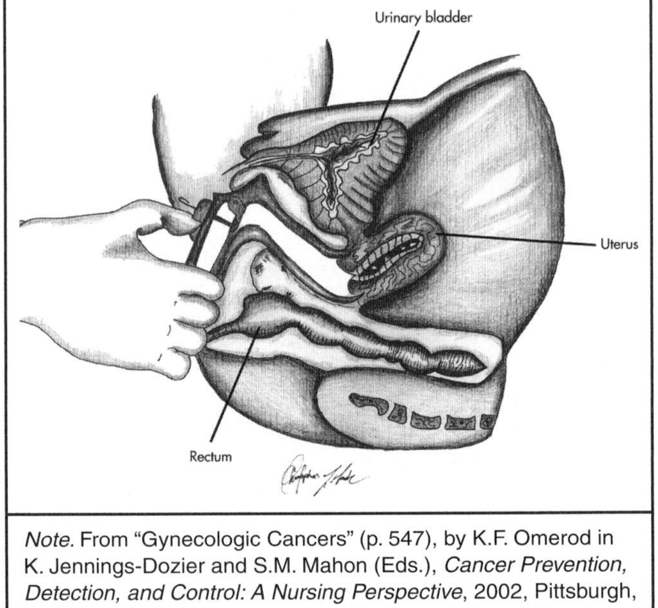

Note. From "Gynecologic Cancers" (p. 547), by K.F. Omerod in K. Jennings-Dozier and S.M. Mahon (Eds.), *Cancer Prevention, Detection, and Control: A Nursing Perspective*, 2002, Pittsburgh, PA: Oncology Nursing Society. Copyright 2002 by Oncology Nursing Society. Reprinted with permission.

lege of Obstetricians and Gynecologists (ACOG, 2003), and the U.S. Preventive Services Task Force (USPSTF, 2003). In summary,

1. All three organizations agree that screening should begin coincident with the onset of sexual activity, when the risk of transient HPV infection is the highest and the risk of cervical cancer is low.

Figure 3-5. Pap Smear

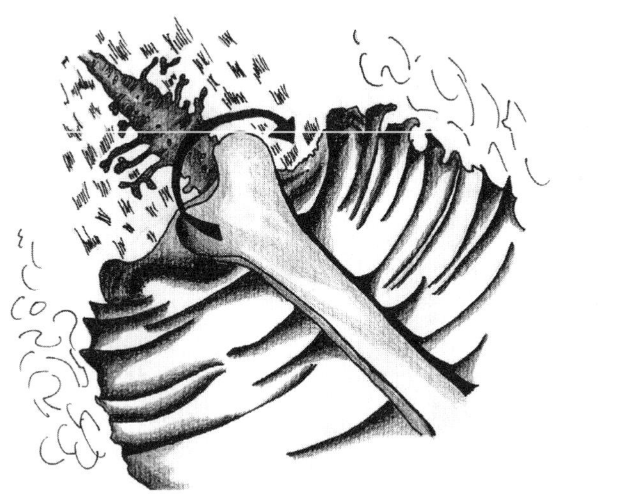

Note. From "Gynecologic Cancers" (p. 547), by K.F. Omerod in K. Jennings-Dozier and S.M. Mahon (Eds.), *Cancer Prevention, Detection, and Control: A Nursing Perspective*, 2002, Pittsburgh, PA: Oncology Nursing Society. Copyright 2002 by Oncology Nursing Society. Reprinted with permission.

Figure 3-6. Endocervical Pap Smear

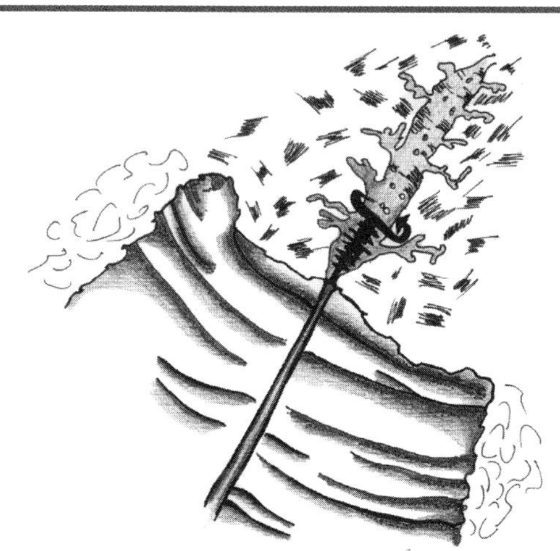

Note. From "Gynecologic Cancers" (p. 548), by K.F. Omerod in K. Jennings-Dozier and S.M. Mahon (Eds.), *Cancer Prevention, Detection, and Control: A Nursing Perspective*, 2002, Pittsburgh, PA: Oncology Nursing Society. Copyright 2002 by Oncology Nursing Society. Reprinted with permission.

2. ACS and USPSTF recommend stopping screening at age 65 or 70, if screening has been negative for three consecutive years.
3. Screening interval recommendations vary, but in women older than 30 years with a negative cytology result and a positive HPV high-risk type should have both tests repeated in 6–12 months.
4. All three guidelines recommend against routine cervical screening for women after a hysterectomy unless the surgery was performed for a gynecologic cancer.

A study by Solomon, Breen, and McNeel (2007) was published in an attempt to determine the impact of these new screening guidelines. Based on population projections, in the year 2010, 75 million Pap tests will be performed. If the guidelines are implemented, this number will be reduced by half.

Ovarian Cancer

At present, only 25% of ovarian cancers are detected in stage I because of the absence of specific symptoms and lack of effective screening. Early detection of ovarian cancer may significantly improve the overall survival rate of women with ovarian cancer if the cancers are clonal, are unifocal, and arise in the ovary rather than in the peritoneum; metastatic disease results from progression of clinically detectable stage I lesions, and cancers remain localized for a sufficient interval to permit cost-effective screening (Badgwell & Bast, 2007). To affect change in the morbidity and mortality associated with ovarian cancer, it is necessary to identify those women at increased risk, ensure prompt treatment, and improve treatment to prevent invasion and metastasis.

Risk Factors

The specific causes of ovarian cancer are still unknown. All women are at risk. Ovarian cancer occurs 50% more frequently in Caucasian women than African American women followed by Asian Americans. Native Americans have the lowest incidence. Age, hereditary, genetic, environmental, chemical, and hormonal factors have been identified as potentially causative (ACS, 2008a; Ozols, Rubin, Thomas, & Robboy, 2005) (see Figure 3-7).

Figure 3-7. Risk Factors for Developing Ovarian Cancer

- Increasing age
- Personal history of breast cancer
- Family history of ovarian or breast cancer
- Mutation of the *BRCA1* or *BRCA2* genes
- Presence of hereditary nonpolyposis colorectal cancer mutation
- Nulliparity
- Obesity

Note. Based on information from American Cancer Society, 2008a; O'Rourke & Mahon, 2003.

Age

Like breast cancer, ovarian cancer risk increases at the age of 40 years, and the incidence peaks in the eighth decade. The risk in the general population is 1.8% by age 70 years (ACS, 2008a). The mean age for developing ovarian cancer in the United States is 58 years (National Cancer Institute, 2008b). Incessant ovulation over time is one theory that may help to explain age as a significant factor in the risk of developing ovarian cancer (Terry et al., 2007).

Hereditary and Genetic Risk Factors

In general, ovarian cancer often occurs as a sporadic genetic mutation rather than hereditary cancer syndrome. The precise molecular events that cause ovarian cancer to develop have not been determined. Only 3%–9% of ovarian cancers are caused by a hereditary cancer syndrome (Kehoe & Kauff, 2007). However, family history of ovarian cancer is among the strongest risk factors for the disease. Women with second-degree (e.g., grandmother, aunt) relatives who have had ovarian cancer have a 4% increased risk, whereas women with two or more first-degree (e.g., mother, sister, daughter) relatives have a 7% increased risk (Piver, 2002).

Familial clusters of ovarian cancer suggest a genetic component. Researchers have conducted several case-controlled studies (Bast et al., 2007; Chen et al., 2006; Kehoe & Kauff, 2007; Satagopan et al., 2002) estimating the magnitude of genetic contribution. These studies demonstrate relative risks of 3.6%–2.9% associated with ovarian cancer in first- and second-degree relatives, respectively. Women with a positive family history of ovarian cancer often are diagnosed in their 40s or earlier. The risk also increases if other family members have premenopausal ovarian cancer or a history of breast, endometrial, colon, rectal, or pancreatic cancers in either female or male relatives.

A predisposing cancer gene, such as *BRCA1* and *BRCA2*, accounts for approximately 5%–10% of all ovarian cancer. More than 50% of women with *BRCA1* mutations who develop ovarian cancer are younger than 50 years of age. The lifetime risk of ovarian cancer conferred by a *BRCA1* or *BRCA2* mutation has been estimated to be 40%–50%, and the risk for carriers of a *BRCA2* mutation has been estimated to be 20%–30% (Lancaster et al., 2007; Thompson & Eaton 2001). Both *BRCA* proteins regulate gene transcription, expression, and the recognition or repair of certain forms of DNA damage, particularly double-strand breaks.

In North America, the incidence of ovarian cancer is higher among Ashkenazi Jewish women than non-Jewish women. Three common mutations are reported in this population: two in *BRCA1* (18delAG and 5382insC) and one in *BRCA2* (6174delT). The combined frequency of these three mutations in the Ashkenazi population is approximately 2%. These mutations may account for 30%–60% of all early-onset breast or ovarian cancer in this ethnic population (Antoniou et al., 2003; Chen et al., 2006; Moleshi et al., 2000; Satagopan et al., 2002).

Three recognized ovarian cancer syndromes have been identified: *site-specific familial,* in which two or more first-degree relatives or a first- and second-degree relative have or had ovarian cancer; *breast-ovarian,* in which breast and ovarian cancers occur among first- and second-degree relatives; and *hereditary nonpolyposis colorectal cancer* (HNPCC) or *Lynch syndrome II,* in which a family history of colorectal, endometrial, ovarian, pancreatic, or other types of cancer exist in male or female relatives (Figure 3-8). Hereditary ovarian cancers are usually associated with a *BRCA1* or *BRCA2* mutation and cause almost 90% of ovarian cancers (Martin, 2007; Piver, 2002).

Figure 3-8. Hereditary Syndromes in Ovarian Cancer

Hereditary Breast-Ovarian Syndrome
- Most common
- Three family members with early-onset (e.g., younger than 60 years of age) breast or ovarian cancer with at least one member with ovarian cancer
- *BRCA1:* 20%–44% risk
- *BRCA2:* 10%–27% risk

Site-Specific Ovarian Cancer
- Three or more family members with ovarian cancer at any age and no relatives with breast cancer diagnosed younger than age 50
- Ovarian cancer: 4%–7% risk
- Breast cancer: 4%–5% risk

Hereditary Nonpolyposis Colorectal Cancer
- Three or more first-degree relatives with colon or endometrial cancer with at least two individuals diagnosed with colon cancer at the age of 50 or younger

Note. Based on information from Martin, 2007; Piver, 2002.

Environmental Factors

Studies on diets high in meat and animal fat, dairy foods, and alcohol consumption as risk factors for ovarian cancer have been conflicting. Industrialized nations have the highest rates of ovarian cancer, which suggests that certain dietary factors may be associated with an increased risk. A diet high in fat may increase risk, and a diet high in fiber may decrease risk. Two studies suggest the increased risk and protective effect seen with certain dietary factors were minimal (Koralek et al., 2006; Kushi et al., 2006).

Researchers examined the relationship between obesity and ovarian cancer. A twofold increase in premenopausal ovarian cancer risk was associated with a body mass index (BMI) of 25 kg/m^2 or higher versus women with a BMI less than 20 kg/m^2 (Bertone, 2002; Fairfield et al., 2002; Tworoger, Gertig, Gates, Hecht, & Hawkinson, 2008). Certain endogenous levels of hormones, specifically estrogen, may affect the risk of developing ovarian cancer (Lukanova et al., 2002). In another study, an inverse relationship between increasing body weight and the risk for ovarian cancer was found (Schouten et al., 2008). The effect may be associated with an increased number of anovulatory cycles associated with a higher BMI. Further studies are required to determine the relationship between obesity and ovarian cancer.

Hazardous Chemicals

Exposure of the ovaries to industrial byproducts, triazine herbicides, and radiation has not been proven to be a risk factor. Migration of chemicals to the peritoneal cavity via the vagina and reproductive organs may account for exposure to carcinogens. Tests of talc and asbestos exposure as causes of ovarian cancer lack statistical significance (Mills, Riordan, Cress, & Young, 2004; Wong, Hempling, Piver, Natarajan, & Mertlin, 1999).

Hormonal Factors

Menopausal hormone replacement therapy (HRT) increases the risk of developing ovarian cancer (Lacey et al., 2006). Women who used estrogen replacement therapy (ERT) and those who used HRT for more than 10 years were at significantly increased risk for developing ovarian cancer. Additional studies determining the relationship between HRT and ovarian cancer are inconsistent. A nearly threefold increased risk was found in women who used infertility drugs with a substantially greater risk in those who failed to conceive; however, this was not a consistent finding, and most of these neoplasms were borderline tumors (Vine, Ness, Calingaert, Schildkraut, & Berchuck, 2001).

Prevention Strategies

Although the exact etiology of ovarian cancer is unknown, current epidemiologic and genetic data suggest several prevention strategies. These strategies include oral contraceptive use, pregnancy and breast-feeding, diet modifications, and risk-reducing salpingo-oophorectomy (RRSO) (Martin & Cherry, 2006; Rebbeck et al., 2002).

The risk of ovarian cancer is correlated with the length of time a woman has ovulated. Pregnancy, lactation, tubal ligation, oral contraceptives, and early menopause suppress ovulatory cycles and seem to decrease risk. The cascade of epithelial events prompted by ovulation include minor trauma; bathing of the surrounding tissue with estrogen-rich follicular fluid; and increased proliferation of epithelium, particularly near the point of ovulation, with resulting development of inclusions into the ovarian parenchyma (Ozols et al., 2005). Some or all of these events may lie in the causal path to ovarian cancer. This theory is consistent with most of the endocrine-related risk factors except for the risks associated with infertility.

Oral Contraceptives

Oral contraceptives decrease the risk of ovarian cancer in younger women by approximately 50%. Collaborative Group on Epidemiological Studies of Ovarian Cancer (2008) reviewed 45 studies that included 23,257 women with ovarian cancer and 87,303 without the disease. They concluded the longer a woman is taking oral contraceptives, the greater protection, and the protection persists for many years after stopping. Taking oral contraceptives for 15 years or more reduces a woman's risk by 58%; 10–14 years reduces risk by 44%; and 5–9 years reduces risk by 36%. Women with a *BRCA* mutation who have used oral contraceptives for a total of five years may decrease their risk of developing ovarian cancer by at least 30% (Narod et al., 2002; National Comprehensive Cancer Network [NCCN], 2009b; Whittemore et al., 2004). In a study evaluating the impact of progestin and estrogen potency on ovarian cancer risk, oral contraceptives with higher progestin dosages were associated with a greater reduction in ovarian cancer risk separate from the dose of estrogen (Schildkraut, Calingaert, Marchbanks, Moorman, & Rodriguez, 2002).

Pregnancy and Breast-Feeding

Two epidemiologic studies to evaluate risk factors for epithelial ovarian cancer indicate a higher incidence in nulliparous or low parity women. Women who have been pregnant and have breast-fed for at least three months have a lower chance of developing ovarian cancer than women without a history of breast-feeding. The longer a woman breast-feeds, the more she reduces her ovarian cancer risk. Breast-feeding for extended periods, as in 18 months over the course of a lifetime, confers the most benefit (Danforth et al., 2007).

Diet

All women should be counseled regarding the beneficial effects of a low-fat, high-vitamin-A diet on ovarian cancer prevention, especially because the benefits of such a diet on the prevention of other cancers are well established (Fairfield et al., 2004; Prentice et al., 2007). Eating foods containing kaempferol, a plant flavonoid, may provide protection from ovarian cancer. Gates (2007) reported a 30% decrease in the incidence of ovarian cancer among women with the highest intake of kaempferol consumed in broccoli and non-herbal tea compared to women with the lowest kaempferol intake. Nurses need to educate women regarding the benefits of lifestyle modifications that include low-fat, high-fiber diets, adequate vegetable and fruit intake, regular exercise, limiting alcohol intake, regular exercise, and avoidance of carcinogens such as cigarettes.

Salpingo-Oophorectomy

Tubal ligation or hysterectomy may decrease the risk of developing ovarian cancer but not to the magnitude associated with oral contraceptives. Women older than the age of 40 who are about to undergo a hysterectomy for a noncancerous condition involving the uterus, such as uterine fibroids, may decide to have an oophorectomy during the procedure to lessen the risk of ovarian cancer (Finch et al., 2006; Tworoger, Fairfield, Coldtiz, Rosner, & Hankinson, 2007). A woman deciding to have an elective oophorectomy at the time of hysterectomy for benign disease should be counseled based on age, parity, risk factors, menstrual status, and family and personal history. Nurses are in a key position to assist women with this highly individual decision-making process by providing information and counseling regarding the potential benefits and consequences of oophorectomy (Omerod, 2002).

RRSO for has become an important component of the management options in women with hereditary breast-ovarian cancer syndrome. For these women, the National Institutes of Health (NIH) Consensus Development Conference on Ovarian Cancer ("Ovarian Cancer," 1994) recommended use of oral contraceptives before childbearing and prophylactic oophorectomy after childbearing, preferably by age 35. Those women with a *BRCA1* or *BRCA2* mutation or with two or more first-degree relatives with ovarian cancer who have completed childbearing should be counseled and considered candidates for RRSO. Such women must consider the long-term physiologic and psychological effects of oophorectomy, including the use of HRP and management of menopausal symptoms (NCCN, 2009b) (see Chapter 14). Prevention and screening for cardiovascular disease and osteoporosis also are considerations. The risk of developing peritoneal carcinomatosis following RRSO is approximately 4% (Casey et al., 2005; Kauff et al., 2008). These reports suggest the peritoneum shares the same embryologic origin and undergoes malignant transformation simultaneously as the ovary or the primary cancer.

Early Detection of Ovarian Cancer

Currently, no procedure can reliably detect ovarian cancer in its early stages. Available potential screening techniques have included pelvic examination (ovarian palpation), ultrasound examinations, CA-125 and other tumor markers, and combined modality approaches. The objective of cancer screening is to find the disease in a precancerous stage prior to malignant transformation or at an early, highly curable stage.

Ovarian cancer has been considered a "silent disease" without any early warning symptoms. Although early symptoms are experienced by 78% of women, they often occur as a cluster of symptoms. These symptoms are not diagnostic on their own yet indicate that a woman should see a gynecologist so that further testing can be done. The Gynecologic Cancer Foundation consensus statement (see Figure 3-9) targets the most important early warning signs, including bloating, pelvic or abdominal pain, early satiety, and urinary symptoms including urgency or frequency. Women who have these target symptoms almost daily for more than a few weeks should see their primary care physician or gynecologist and undergo a recto-pelvic exam and/or a transvaginal ultrasound (TVUS) that could potentially diagnose ovarian cancer in the earliest stages of disease (Goff et al., 2007; NCCN, 2009a; "Ovarian Cancer," 1994).

Figure 3-9. Early Signs and Symptoms of Ovarian Cancer

- Bloating, a feeling of fullness, gas
- Frequent or urgent urination
- Nausea, indigestion, constipation, diarrhea
- Menstrual disorders, pain during intercourse
- Fatigue, backaches

Note. Based on information from Goff et al., 2007; NCCN, 2009b.

Routine screening for women at average risk is not recommended as no sufficiently accurate screening test is currently available. Pelvic examination only occasionally detects ovarian cancer, generally when the disease is advanced. However, the combination of a thorough pelvic exam, transvaginal ultrasound, and a blood test for the tumor marker CA-125 may be helpful in diagnosis but is not useful for routine screening (ACS, 2008c). A screening test for ovarian cancer must have a specificity of 99.6% to achieve a 10% positive predictive value; a test for women older than age 45 and women with a *BRCA1* mutation must have a specificity of 90% to achieve a 10% positive predictive value (Badgwell & Bast, 2007; Bast et al., 2007).

Pelvic Examinations

In a large retrospective study of more than 1,700 women with ovarian cancer, only 5% reported having no symptoms of the disease prior to diagnosis. More than 70% of women reported having symptoms, including lower abdominal discomfort or pain, dyspepsia, early satiety, abdominal distention or bloating, change in bowel habits, urinary frequency or incontinence, weight loss, and vaginal bleeding (Goff, Mandel, Melancon, & Muntz, 2004; Martin, 2007). Detecting an asymptomatic pelvic mass through routine bimanual pelvic examination may identify an ovarian carcinoma before abdominal dissemination occurs (see Figure 3-10). No data report the frequency with which annual recto-pelvic examination detects ovarian cancer in asymptomatic women.

Ultrasonography

The use of TVUS with color Doppler as a more specific alternative to abdominal ultrasonography may result in an increased resolution capable of detecting minimal morphologic changes in the ovary. TVUS may detect intra-ovarian vascular changes and the ability to track ovarian neovascularization, as detected by impeded blood flow, to help clinicians to dis-

Figure 3-10. Bimanual Pelvic Examination

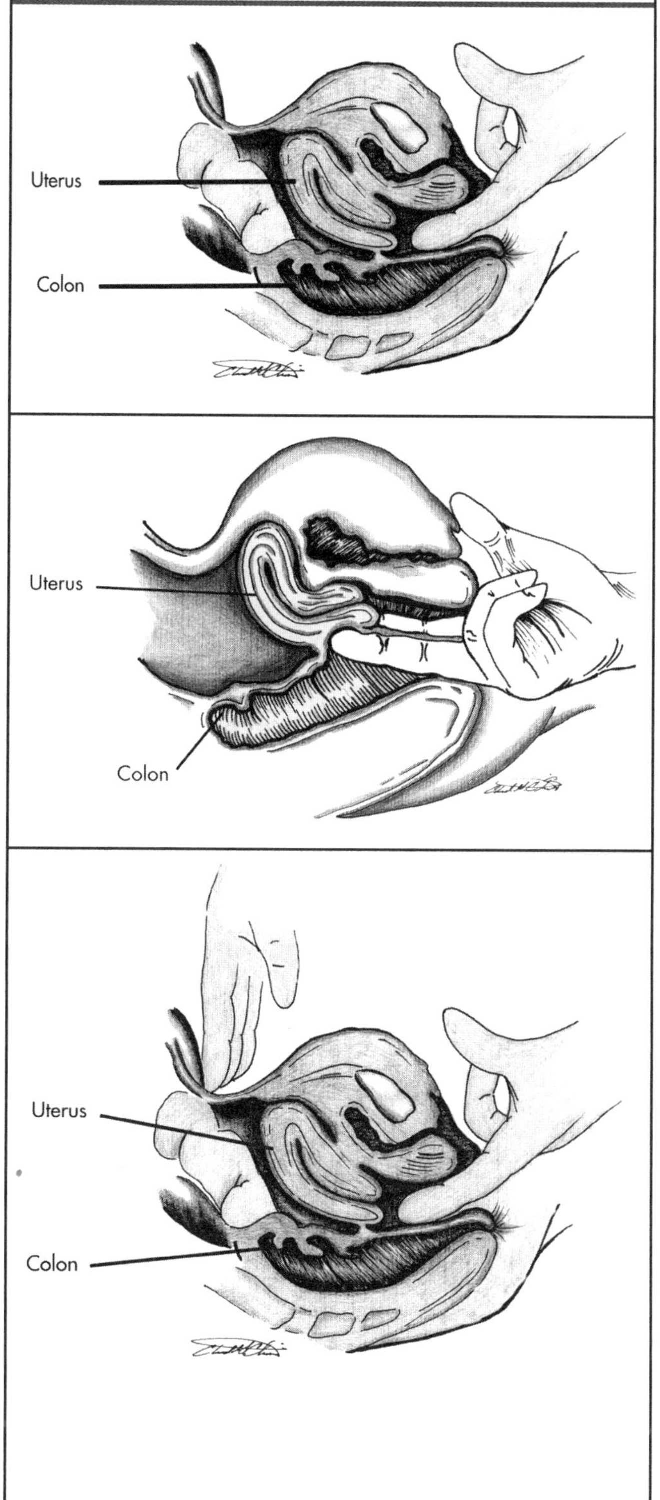

Note. From "Gynecologic Cancers" (p. 557), by K.F. Omerod in K. Jennings-Dozier and S.M. Mahon (Eds.), *Cancer Prevention, Detection, and Control: A Nursing Perspective*, 2002, Pittsburgh, PA: Oncology Nursing Society. Copyright 2002 by Oncology Nursing Society. Reprinted with permission.

criminate benign from malignant ovarian tumors. However, the results from two large trials demonstrated the limited value of TVUS as an independent modality for the detection of early-stage epithelial ovarian cancer in asymptomatic women who are at increased risk for disease (Fishman et al., 2005; van Nagell et al., 2007).

CA-125

CA-125, a protein associated with the surface of ovarian cancer cells, is expressed in 80% of nonmucinous epithelial ovarian cancer. Overall, more than 80% of women with advanced ovarian cancer will have an elevated CA-125 level (greater than 35 u/ml) (Lamb, Garcia, Goff, Paley, & Swisher, 2006). Nevertheless, the test is not useful in detecting early-stage disease because it is elevated only 50% of the time, particularly in premenopausal women. Noncancerous conditions (e.g., pregnancy, endometriosis, uterine fibroids, liver disease, benign ovarian cysts) also may cause an elevation in CA-125. Currently, the most beneficial use of CA-125 is to sequentially track a woman's response to cancer therapy (Badgwell & Bast, 2007; Bast et al., 2007).

Multimodal Screening

Preliminary studies using serial serum CA-125 levels, pelvic examinations, and TVUS have demonstrated that ovarian cancer can be detected in asymptomatic women. However, these procedures are associated with a significant false positive rate such that an unacceptably large number of negative laparotomies would result if each "positive" screening test resulted in surgical exploration aimed at diagnosing early ovarian cancer. A review of the NCI Prostate, Lung, Colorectal, and Ovarian Cancer Screening in 28,816 women from 1993 to 2001 showed 34 women (0.1%) had abnormal results in both TVUS and CA-125. Among women with abnormal test results, 29 tumors were detected, 20 of which were invasive cancers. The predictive value for an ovarian cancer screening test is around 10%. The predictive values for an abnormal CA-125 test is 3.7%, an abnormal TVUS is 1%, and if both tests were abnormal, 23.5%. The combined screening modality had a fairly high predictive value; only 9 of the 29 tumors (31%) were associated with abnormalities in both tests. Based on these considerations, NCI does not recommend ovarian cancer screening for women without risk factors (Buys et al., 2005).

Compared to women with a *BRCA* mutation who undergo prophylactic surgery, women with mutation who do not undergo surgery may be at significantly increased risk for the development of ovarian cancer (40%) as well as breast cancer (60%) by age 70. Therefore, these women require more intensive clinical surveillance (Robson, 2002). In addition, women with family histories consistent with a genetic predisposition to hereditary cancers require more intensive evaluations when presenting with abdominal/pelvic symptoms even if the symptoms are vague.

Women at increased risk should have at least annual screening that includes a comprehensive gynecologic examination (i.e., a pelvic exam that includes a rectovaginal exam), a test for serum marker CA-125 and TVUS or transabdominal ultrasound (Fields & Chevlen, 2006; Hensley, Casteil, & Robson, 2000; NCCN, 2009b; "Ovarian Cancer," 1994).

Research Initiatives

Little is known about the etiology of ovarian cancer at the molecular and genetic level. Developing molecular profiles of the changes relevant to tumor progression for sporadic ovarian cancer currently are being developed. This information may reveal early genomic or biologic changes to facilitate detection of early-stage epithelial ovarian cancer and may identify markers indicative of premalignant changes (Omerod, 2002).

To affect change in the morbidity and mortality associated with ovarian cancer, it is necessary to identify those individuals at increased risk and clinically apply the understanding of the biochemical and molecular biology of ovarian carcinogenesis. Ovarian carcinogenesis, invasion, and metastasis require a complex cascade of interrelated genetic, molecular, and biochemical events that regulate aberrations affecting cell cycle control, apoptosis, adhesion, angiogenesis, transmembrane signaling DNA repair, and genomic stability (Bast et al., 2007, Brewer et al., 2005; Mor et al., 2005; Omerod, 2002).

Research Developments in Screening Women at High Risk

Proteomic screening is one of the more sensitive and specific screening tests expected to be used for the early detection of ovarian cancer in the future. Proteomics documents the consequences of the genetic change, including protein mutation, rearrangement, loss, and amplification or silencing of genes (Boyce & Kohn, 2005). Clinical trials currently under way will validate and standardize proteomic testing (Bast et al., 2007; Brewer et al., 2005; Daly & Ozols, 2002; Martin, 2007; Ozols et al., 2003).

NCI currently is sponsoring five screening trials for women at high risk for ovarian cancer. Four are in progress in the United States and one in the United Kingdom. All studies evaluate CA-125 and TVUS using an algorithm that calculates cancer risk and will critically test the ability of the combination of both screening tests to improve survival in ovarian cancer (Bast et al., 2007; NCI, 2008b).

Endometrial Cancer

Cancer of the endometrium is the most common invasive gynecologic cancer and the fourth most frequently diagnosed cancer among American women today. Endometrial cancer is predominantly a disease of postmenopausal women, with an average age at diagnosis of 61 years (ACS, 2008b). However, 25% of cases occur in premenopausal women and 5% occur in women younger than 40 years (Duska et al., 2001; Parslov et al., 2000; Schmeler et al., 2005).

Major differences exist between black and white women in stages of endometrial cancer at detection and subsequent survival. Although the incidence of endometrial cancer is lower among black women, mortality rates are higher. NCI initiated a Black/White Cancer Survival Study and concluded that higher-grade and more aggressive histologies appear to be related to excess risk of advanced-stage disease for black women. It is difficult to disentangle the effects that biology and socioeconomic status may have on the lower survival rates of black women with endometrial cancer (Barrett et al., 1995).

Evidence from a Gynecologic Oncology Group study suggests that lower income is associated with advanced-stage disease, lower probability of undergoing a hysterectomy, and lower survival rates (Maxwell et al., 2006). Further research is necessary to understand why black women tend to be diagnosed with more aggressive disease and have a higher probability of dying than white women, despite their lower incidence of endometrial cancer.

Risk Factors

About 70% of all women diagnosed with endometrial cancer are postmenopausal (Sonoda & Barakat, 2006). Most studies support about a twofold risk associated with natural menopause after the age of 52 than before the age of 49 (Purdie, 2003). The effect of late age at menopause on risk may reflect prolonged exposure of the uterus to estrogen stimulation in the presence of anovulatory (progesterone deficient) cycles.

The two major types of endometrial cancer are type I and type II. Type I carcinomas are the most common type and are associated with unopposed estrogen, occur in young postmenopausal women, and often are diagnosed at a low-grade stage. Type II carcinomas are usually diagnosed in older women, are unrelated to estrogenic stimulation, and are associated with a poorer prognosis. Most identified risk factors are associated with type I carcinomas, whereas older age is the only identified risk factor for type II. Identified risk factors for type I carcinomas include obesity, unopposed estrogen use, early menarche, late menopause, polycystic ovarian syndrome, tamoxifen therapy, diabetes, hypertension, and a history of atypical hyperplasia (Barakat, Grigsby, Sabbatini, & Zaino, 2005; Purdie, 2003; Zhou, Dowdy, Podratz, & Jiang, 2007).

Obesity

Obesity is a well-recognized factor for endometrial cancer, with as much as 25% of the disease possibly explained by this factor (Purdie, 2003; Zhou et al., 2007). Very heavy women appear to have disproportionately high risks. Women weighing 200 pounds or more have a seven-fold excess risk compared with women weighing less than 125 pounds (Bakkum-Gamez, Gonzolez-Bosquet, Laack, Mariani, & Dowdy, 2008). Obesity appears to affect both premenopausal and postmenopausal endometrial cancer. Abnormalities in endogenous estrogen production or peripheral conversion of adrenally derived androstenedione in fat combined with a lack of progesterone effect on the endometrial lining associated with obesity may account for this increased risk.

Diet

Epidemiologic studies have evaluated the etiologic role of dietary factors. Geographic differences in disease rates (e.g., high rates in Western and low rates in Eastern societies) suggest that nutrition has a role, especially the high content of animal fat in Western diets (Madison, Schottenfeld, James, Schwartz, & Gruber, 2004). A correlation may exist between total fat intake and endometrial cancer incidence. Higher levels of plasma estrone, estradiol, and prolactin are found among women consuming a high-fat or omnivorous diet rather than a low-fat or vegetarian diet.

Hormonal and Reproductive Factors

Hormonal and reproductive factors play an important role in the development of endometrial cancer. Endogenous estrogen production associated with polycystic ovary syndrome has been identified as a risk factor. Endometrial proliferation associated with this syndrome may be reversed with clomiphene citrate, with progesterone, or by wedge resection of the ovary (Parazzini, La Vecchia, Bocciolone, & Franceschi, 1991; Zhou et al., 2007).

Nulliparity is a recognized risk factor for endometrial cancer and the risk decreases with increasing parity. Evidence from the Iowa Women's Health Study supports the association of endometrial cancer with early age at menarche, late age at natural menopause, and total length of ovulation span (Folsom et al., 1995). However, infertility and ages at first and last pregnancy may be unrelated to risk after adjustment for gravidity. Results suggest that a miscarriage late in reproductive life followed by a lack of a subsequent full-term pregnancy may be a marker for progesterone deficiency and supports the "unopposed" estrogen hypothesis for the etiology of endometrial cancer.

The relationship between exogenous hormones and risk of endometrial cancer has received considerable attention. The data suggests that any use of unopposed ERT is associated with a 2- to 12-fold elevation in risk of endometrial cancer (ACS, 2008b). In most investigations, the increased risk was not observed unless estrogen was used for at least two to three years, and longer use generally was associated with higher risk (Cooper & Stegmann, 2005).

The associations of risk with HRT are strongest among women who are thin, nondiabetic, and normotensive (Grady, Gebretsadik, Kerlikowske, Ernster, & Petitti, 1995; Lacey et al., 2006). These findings suggest that estrogen metabolism differs in these groups of women or that risk is already high enough in obese, hypertensive, or diabetic women that exposure of exogenous estrogens has only a small additional effect.

Further evidence for the role of exogenous hormones in the pathogenesis of endometrial cancer is derived from studies that evaluated the effects of oral contraceptives. These studies demonstrated significantly higher risks in users of sequential oral contraceptives (i.e., oral contraceptives containing a high dose of estrogen and a weak progestin) and significantly lower risks of endometrial cancer in women using estrogen-progestin combination pills (Pike & Ross, 2000).

A number of clinical trials and population-based case control studies have indicated an increased risk of endometrial cancer among women with breast cancer given adjuvant tamoxifen therapy. This finding is consistent with tamoxifen's estrogenic effects on the endometrium (American College of Obstetricians and Gynecologists Committee on Gynecologic Practice, 2006; van Leeuwen et al., 1994). The National Surgical Adjuvant Breast and Bowel Project B-14 trial revealed data regarding the rates of endometrial and other cancers. The reported relative risk is 7.5% (Fisher et al., 1994). Although other agents for hormonal manipulation in the treatment of breast cancer have been developed, tamoxifen continues to be an effective treatment for breast cancer despite an associated risk for endometrial cancer.

Raloxifene is a second-generation selective estrogen receptor modulator approved for prophylaxis against postmenopausal osteoporosis. Unlike tamoxifen, it does not have an estrogenic effect on the uterus. Women enrolled in STAR (Study of Tamoxifen and Raloxifene) were evaluated for the development of endometrial cancer. The women in the raloxifene group developed 36% fewer uterine cancers during the trial: 36 of 4,732 women in the tamoxifen group developed uterine cancers compared to 23 of the 4,712 women in the raloxifene group (NCI, 2008a). Results from the MORE (Multiple Outcomes of Raloxifene) randomized trial indicated that raloxifene reduced the risk of estrogen receptor–positive breast cancer but was not associated with an increased risk of developing endometrial cancer after 40 months of follow-up (Dickler & Norton, 2001; Grady et al., 2004).

Genetic Factors

A hereditary pattern, referred to as the Lynch syndrome II, is associated with endometrial cancer. Lynch syndrome II features a significant genetic association between hereditary nonpolyposis colorectal cancer and the development of endometrial carcinoma. Other cancers noted in the same families include carcinoma of the ovary, urologic system, stomach, small bowel, pancreas, and breast. Healthcare providers caring for women with endometrial cancer must obtain a complete family history to determine the possibility of a Lynch syndrome II phenomenon (Chen, Yang, Little, Cheung, & Caughey, 2007). Mutations in the *MLH1* gene or *MSH2* gene can increase the risk of developing endometrial cancer by as much as 60% (Bandera, 2005; Vasen et al., 2001). Genetic testing for the *MLH1* and *MSH2* genes is available commercially and is recommended for women meeting specific criteria as outlined in the NCI Bethesda guidelines (Strate & Syngal, 2005; Vasen et al., 2007). Women with a personal or family history of colorectal, endometrial, or ovarian cancer, particularly when the diagnosis is made in people younger than 50 years or in people with multiple primary cancers, should undergo genetic counseling and testing (American Society of Clinical Oncology, 2003; Lindor et al., 2006; Smith et al., 2001). Women with a known mutation should have annual screenings for colorectal cancer and consider prophylactic hysterectomy including removal of ovaries when childbearing is complete after age 35 (NCCN, 2009a).

Endometrial Hyperplasia

Endometrial hyperplasia is defined as an overgrowth of the endometrial lining of the uterus as a result of prolonged estrogenic stimulation of the endometrium. Endometrial hyperplasia may present clinically as abnormal bleeding with excessive blood loss and may be associated with anovulation and infertility or result from unopposed estrogen use (Ronnett, Seidman, Zaino, Ellenson, & Kurman, 2005).

Endometrial hyperplasia is considered a precursor state to endometrial cancer. The term *endometrial hyperplasia* refers to the histopathologic state of the endometrial glands and stroma. The histopathologic classification accepted by the International Society of Gynecologic Pathologists consists of three categories: simple (cystic without atypia), complex (adenomatous without atypia), and atypical (simple cystic with atypia or complex adenomatous with atypia) (Ronnett et al., 2005).

Endometrial hyperplasia with cellular atypia is considered to be premalignant, whereas those without atypia are benign. However, the endometrium continues to be predisposed to the development of cancer in the absence of cytologic atypia based on the underlying pathophysiologic state (Bakkum-Gamez et al., 2008). The progression of hyperplasia to cancer in women with simple hyperplasia is 1% and for women with complex hyperplasia is 3%. The progression rate to cancer is much higher when atypia accompanies hyperplasia. The rate rises to 8% with simple atypical hyperplasia and 29% with complex atypical hyperplasia (Barakat et al., 2005).

Women with atypical hyperplasia may be treated by periodic use of progestin or hysterectomy depending on age and reproductive desires. Hysterectomy is the preferred treatment in women with complex atypical hyperplasia. This approach not only cures the usual presenting symptoms of abnormal bleeding but also confers prophylaxis against the almost 30% risk of later developing endometrial cancer (Sonoda & Barakat, 2006). Those women treated with progestins should have a dilatation and curettage (D&C) performed before treatment to rule out the occasional occult carcinoma not detected by biopsy. A progestin should be administered daily and endometrial biopsies performed in three- to four-month intervals to assess treatment results. The addition of progestins to the regimens of women treated with exogenous estrogens usually prevents endometrial hyperplasia and subsequent development of cancer (Grady et al., 1995).

Another preventive measure in women who are perimenopausal with fluctuating levels of estrogen and amenorrheic or hypermenorrheic or in any woman with a suspected condition of unopposed endogenous estrogen production is periodic treatment with a progestin to create scheduled withdrawal bleeding to prevent hyperplasia. A progesterone challenge may be helpful in defining this group of women. This test involves challenging any nonpregnant amenorrheic woman with progesterone to see if withdrawal bleeding occurs (Pike & Ross, 2000). If bleeding does occur, endometrial sampling may be performed to confirm a diagnosis. Appropriate treatment and follow-up can then be established.

Screening Methods

No good screening test for endometrial cancer is available. The pelvic exam enables the clinician to detect only an abnormally sized uterus. The current recommendation for screening for endometrial cancer from ACS and ACOG is an annual pelvic exam and cervical cytology screening. Sampling of the endometrium is neither cost-effective nor indicated in the general population and is not required before or during HRT in asymptomatic women.

ACS (2008b) recommends that women with or at risk for HNPCC undergo annual screening with endometrial biopsy and TVUS beginning at age 35. NCI (2008a) recommends these women begin screening with endometrial biopsy and TVUS at age 25. The population of women includes those known to be carriers of an HNPCC gene mutation, women with a substantial risk for carrying the mutation, and women with a suspected autosomal dominant predisposition to colon cancer (Smith, Cokkinides, & Eyre, 2003; Tiffen & Mahon 2006; Vasen et al., 2007).

Most women with early and localized endometrial cancer present with abnormal uterine bleeding. About 90% of women diagnosed with endometrial cancer have abnormal uterine bleeding as a presenting symptom (ACS, 2008b), including changes in the frequency, duration, amount of bleeding, and bleeding between menstrual cycles (Albers, Hull, & Wesley, 2004). A thorough medical history, including an abdominal/pelvic examination, should be performed by a gynecologist. The commonly used diagnostic tests include TVUS and endometrial biopsy.

TVUS is performed to measure endometrial thickness and localize lesions to be sampled during biopsy. An endometrium thicker than 16 mm is a predictor of abnormal endometrial pathology in premenopausal women with a sensitivity of 67%, specificity of 75%, and a positive predictive value of 14%. In postmenopausal women, an endometrium thicker than 5 mm has a sensitivity of at least 82% and a specificity of 60% as a predictor of abnormal endometrial pathology (Thurmond et al., 2000). An endometrium of less than 5 mm is determined to rule out the diagnosis of endometrial cancer in postmenopausal women (Medverd & Dubinsky, 2002; Tiffen & Mahon, 2006).

Endometrial biopsy is performed when it is necessary to sample the endometrial tissue for pathologic evaluation. Endometrial biopsy has a high sensitivity, has minimal side effects, and can be performed in an office setting (NCI, 2008a).

Endometrial sampling is a favorable alternative to more invasive procedures such as fractional D&C when screening asymptomatic women. Several methods (e.g., Pipelle®, CooperSurgical, Inc.; Tao Brush™, Cook Medical; Uterine Explora® curette, CooperSurgical, Inc.) of endometrial sampling have been evaluated with regard to their ability to accurately identify abnormal endometrial pathology including endometrial cancer. These studies have been conducted among symptomatic populations and are difficult to assess with respect to their use in the asymptomatic population as widespread screening tools (Dubinsky, 2004). Histopathologic reports from D&C or hysterectomy remain the standard to which these sampling methods should be compared. No studies have evaluated the use of endometrial sampling as routine screening in reducing endometrial cancer mortality.

Prevention of Endometrial Cancer

The use of combination oral contraceptives is associated with a decreased risk of developing endometrial cancer. The highest protective effect was produced by preparations with the lowest estrogen and the highest progesterone content. The benefit ranges from a 50% reduction associated with 4 years of use up to 72% reduction in risk with 12 or more years of use (NCI, 2008a).

Women who are physically active have a 30%–40% reduced risk of endometrial cancer (Littman, Voigt, Beresford, & Weiss, 2001; Moradi et al., 2000), with the greatest reduction in risk among those who are most active. The possible association between physical activity and endometrial cancer is based on a limited number of studies, some of which indicate that inactive women have higher rates of endometrial cancer compared to physically active women. Changes in body mass and alterations in level and metabolism of sex hormones, such as estrogen, are the major biologic mechanisms thought to explain the association between physical activity and endometrial cancer (Friedenreich & Orenstein, 2002).

Researchers are studying the *PTEN* tumor suppressor gene to establish whether it has clinical cancer predicative value for endometrial cancer. *PTEN* is altered very early in endometrial carcinogenesis and displays decreased protein expression in 75% of premalignant and malignant endometrial lesions (Bischoff & Simpson, 2000; Hecht & Mutter, 2006). The goal is to develop a strategy for early detection and chemoprevention of endometrial cancer.

Summary

The issues of genetic counseling and cancer risk assessment for women who are at increased risk for ovarian cancer are of great importance (Mahon, 2000). Oncology nurses trained as genetic counselors can provide cancer genetic counseling and calculate cancer risk while providing education and emotional support (O'Rourke & Mahon, 2003). These nurses are uniquely positioned to influence the health promotion of women at risk for ovarian cancer and make individually tailored assessment plans based on social, educational, and economic status, particularly for women considering prophylactic surgery. In addition, these nurses can mobilize strategies from other aspects of oncology nursing care such as support groups, educational seminars, and peer or individual counseling that may be beneficial in reducing the negative impact of receiving genetic information and cancer risk assessment. Nurses can enhance the understanding of the meanings and perceived consequences for women at risk for ovarian cancer (Omerod, 2002).

Nurses can promote and educate women about risk-reduction strategies that include annual pelvic examination, sequencing progesterone with ERT, use of oral contraceptives for birth control, regular medical check-ups for control of medical conditions (e.g., diabetes, hypertension), and modifying the diet for weight control or weight loss. Any woman with abnormal uterine bleeding, bloating, pelvic or abdominal pain, early satiety, and urinary urgency or frequency should be encouraged to seek timely gynecologic evaluation. Educating women to take responsibility for their health and well-being is vital in reducing the morbidity and mortality associated with gynecologic cancer. Women who have detailed information can assume more responsibility for their health and, as a result, enhance their quality of life (Omerod, 2002).

References

Addis, I.B., Hatch, K.D., & Berek, J. (2007). Intraepithelial disease of the cervix, vagina, and vulva. In J.S. Berek (Ed.), *Berek and Novak's gynecology* (14th ed., pp. 561–600). Philadelphia: Lippincott Williams & Wilkins.

Albers, J.R., Hull, S.K., & Wesley, R.M. (2004). Abnormal uterine bleeding. *American Family Physician, 69*(8), 1915–1926.

American Cancer Society. (2007). *Cancer facts and figures, 2007.* Atlanta, GA: Author.

American Cancer Society. (2008a). *Cancer facts and figures, 2008.* Atlanta, GA: Author.

American Cancer Society. (2008b). *Endometrial (uterine) cancer.* Atlanta, GA: Author.

American Cancer Society. (2008c). *Ovarian cancer.* Atlanta, GA: Author.

American College of Obstetricians and Gynecologists. (2003). ACOG practice bulletin. Cervical cytology screening. Number 45, August 2003. *International Journal of Gynecology and Obstetrics, 83*(2), 237–247.

American College of Obstetricians and Gynecologists Committee on Gynecologic Practice. (2006). ACOG Committee opinion no. 336: Tamoxifen and uterine cancer. *Obstetrics and Gynecology, 107*(6), 1475–1478.

American Society of Clinical Oncology. (2003). American Society of Clinical Oncology policy statement update: Genetic testing for cancer susceptibility. *Journal of Clinical Oncology, 21*(12), 2397–2406.

Anhang, R., Goodman, A., & Goldie, S. (2004). HPV communications: Review of existing research and recommendations for patient education. *CA: A Cancer Journal for Clinicians, 54*(5), 248–259.

Antoniou, A., Pharoah, P.D., Narod, S., Risch, H.A., Eyfjord, J.E., Hopper, J.L., et al. (2003). Average risks of breast and ovarian cancer associated with *BRCA1* or *BRCA2* mutations detected in case series unselected for family history: A combined analysis of 22 studies. *American Journal of Human Genetics, 72*(5), 1117–1130.

Atkinson, W.L., Pickering, L.K., Schwartz, B., Weniger, B.G., Iskander, J.K., Watson, J.C., et al. (2002). General recommendations on immunization. Recommendations of the Advisory Committee on Immunization Practices (ACIP) and the American Academy of Family Physicians (AAFP). *Morbidity and Mortality Weekly Report: Recommendation and Reports, 51*(RR-2), 1–35.

Badgwell, D., & Bast, R.C., Jr. (2007). Early detection of ovarian cancer. *Disease Markers, 239*(5–6), 397–410.

Bakkum-Gamez, J.N., Gonzalez-Bosquet, J., Laack, N.N., Mariani, A., & Dowdy, S.C. (2008). Current issues in the management of endometrial cancer. *Mayo Clinic Proceedings, 83*(1), 97–112.

Bandera, C. (2005). Endometrial cancer in the hereditary nonpolyposis colorectal cancer syndrome. In G. Coukos & S.C. Rubin (Eds.), *Cancer of the uterus* (pp. 35–51). New York: Marcel Dekker.

Barakat, R.R., Grigsby, P.W., Sabbatini, P., & Zaino, R. (2005). Corpus: Epithelial tumors. In W.J. Hoskins, C.A. Perez, & R.C. Young (Eds.), *Principles and practice of gynecologic oncology* (4th ed., pp. 823–872). Philadelphia: Lippincott Williams & Wilkins.

Barrett, R.J., II, Harlan, L.C., Wesley, M.N., Hill, H.A., Chen, V.W., Clayton, L.A., et al. (1995). Endometrial cancer: Stage at diagnosis and associated factors in black and white patients. *American Journal of Obstetrics and Gynecology, 173*(2), 414–422.

Barton, S.E., Maddox, P.H., Jenkins, D., Edwards, R., Cuzick, J., & Singer, A. (1988). Effect of cigarette smoking on cervical epithelial immunity: A mechanism for neoplastic change? *Lancet, 332*(8612), 652–654.

Bast, R.C., Jr., Brewer, M., Zou, C., Hernandez, M.A., Daley, M., Ozols, R., et al. (2007). Prevention and early detection of ovarian cancer: Mission impossible? *Recent Results in Cancer Research, 174,* 91–100.

Bertone, E.R., Rosner, B.A., Hunter, D.J., Stampfer, M.J., Speizer, F.E., Colditz, G.A., et al. (2002). Dietary fat intake and ovarian cancer in a cohort of US women. *American Journal of Epidemiology, 156*(1), 22–31.

Bischoff, F.Z., & Simpson, J.L. (2000). Heritability and molecular genetic studies of endometriosis. *Human Reproduction Update, 6*(1), 37–44.

Bolick, D.R., & Hellman, D.J. (1998). Laboratory implementation and efficacy assessment of ThinPrep cervical cancer screening system. *Acta Cytologica, 42*(1), 209–213.

Bosch, F.X., Lorincz, A., Muñoz, N., Meijer, C.J., & Shah, K.V. (2002). The causal relationship between human papilloma virus and cervical cancer. *Journal of Clinical Pathology, 55*(4), 244–265.

Bosch, F.X., Manos, M.M., Munoz, N., Sherman, M., Jansen, A.M., Peto, J. et al. (1995). Prevalence of human papillomavirus in cervical cancer: A worldwide perspective. International Biological Study on Cervical Cancer (IBBSCC) study group. *Journal of the National Cancer Institute, 87*(11), 796–802.

Boyce, E.A., & Kohn, E.C. (2005). Ovarian cancer in the proteomics era: Diagnosis, prognosis, and therapeutics targets. *International Journal of Gynecological Cancer, 15*(Suppl. 3), 266–273.

Brewer, M.A., Ranger-Moore, J., Baruche, A., Alberts, D.S., Greene, M., Thompson, D., et al. (2005). Exploratory study of ovarian intraepithelial neoplasia. *Cancer Epidemiology, Biomarkers and Prevention, 14*(2), 299–305.

Brewster, W.R., Hubbell, F., Largent, J., Ziogas, A., Lin, F., Howe, S., et al. (2005). Feasability of management of high grade cervical lesions in a single visit. *JAMA, 294*(17), 2182–2187.

Brinton, L.A., Schairer, C., Haenszel, W., Stolley, P., Lehman, H.F., Levine, R., et al. (1986). Cigarette smoking and invasive cervical cancer. *JAMA, 255*(23), 3265–3269.

Buys, S.S., Partridge, E., Greene, M.H., Prorok, P.C., Reding, D., Riley, T.L., et al. (2005). Ovarian cancer screening in the Prostate, Lung, Colorectal and Ovarian (PLCO) cancer screening trial: Findings from the initial screen of a randomized trial. *American Journal of Obstetrics and Gynecology, 193*(5), 1630–1639.

Casey, M.J., Synder, C., Bewtra, C., Narod, S.A., Watson, P., & Lynch, H.T. (2005). Intra-abdominal carcinomatosis after prophylactic oophorectomy in women of hereditary breast ovarian cancer syndrome kindreds associated with *BRCA1* and *BRCA2* mutations. *Gynecologic Oncology, 97*(2), 457–467.

Castellsagué, X., Diaz, M., Sanjose, S., Muñoz, N., Herrero, R., Franceschi, S., et al. (2006). Worldwide human papillomavirus etiology of cervical adenocarcinoma and its cofactors: Implications for screening and prevention. *Journal of the National Cancer Institute, 98*(5), 303–315.

Chacho, M.S., Mattie, M.E., & Schwartz, P.E. (2003). Cytohystologic correlation rates between conventional Papanicolaou smears and Thin-Prep cervical cytology: A comparison. *Cancer, 99*(3), 135–140.

Chen, L.M., Yang, K.Y., Little, S.E., Cheung, M.K., & Caughey, A.B. (2007). Gynecologic cancer prevention in Lynch syndrome/hereditary nonpolyposis colorectal cancer families. *Obstetrics and Gynecology, 110*(1), 18–25.

Chen, S., Iversen, E.S., Friebel, T., Finkelstein, D., Weber, B.L., Eisen, A., et al. (2006). Characterization of *BRCA1* and *BRCA2* mutations in a largé United States sample. *Journal of Clinical Oncology, 24*(6), 863–871.

Chua, K.L., & Hjerpe, A. (1996). Persistence of human papillomavirus (HPV) infections preceding cervical cancer. *Cancer, 77*(1), 121–127.

Clifford, G.M., Smith, J.S., Plummer, M., Munoz, M., & Franceschi, S. (2003). Human papillomavirus types in invasive cervical cancer worldwide: A meta-analysis. *British Journal of Cancer, 88*(1), 63–73.

Collaborative Group on Epidemiological Studies of Ovarian Cancer. (2008). Ovarian cancer and oral contraceptives: Collaborative reanalysis of data from 45 epidemiological studies including 23,257 women with ovarian cancer and 87,303 controls. *Lancet, 371*(9609), 303–314.

Cooper, J.M., & Stegmann, B.J. (2005). Clinical evaluation of abnormal uterine bleeding. In G. Coukos & S.C. Rubin (Eds.), *Cancer of the uterus* (pp. 195–228). New York: Marcel Dekker.

Coughlin, S.S., Breslau, E.S., Thompson, T., & Benard, V.B. (2005). Physician recommendation for Papanicolaou testing among U.S. women, 2000. *Cancer Epidemiology, Biomarkers and Prevention, 14*(5), 1143–1148.

Daly, M.B., & Ozols, R.F. (2002).The search for predictive patterns in ovarian cancer: Proteomics meets bioinformatics. *Cancer Cell, 1*(2), 111–112.

Danforth, K.N., Tworoger, S.S., Hecht, J.L., Rosner, B.A., Colditz, G.A., & Hankinson, S.E. (2007). Breast-feeding and risk of ovarian cancer in two prospective cohorts. *Cancer Causes and Control, 18*(5), 517–523.

Denny, L., Kuhn, L., De Souza, M., Pollack, A.E., Dupree, W., & Wright, T.C., Jr. (2005). Screen-and-treat approaches for cervical cancer prevention in low-resource settings. *JAMA, 294*(17), 2173–2181.

Dickler, M.N., & Norton, L. (2001). The MORE trial: Multiple outcomes for raloxifene evaluation—breast cancer as a secondary end point: Implications for prevention. *Annals of the New York Academy of Sciences, 949,* 134–142.

Dubinsky, T.J. (2004). Value of sonography in the diagnosis of abnormal vaginal bleeding. *Journal of Clinical Ultrasound, 32*(7), 348–353.

Duska, L.R., Garrett, A., Rueda, B.R., Haas, J., Chang, Y., & Fuller, A.F. (2001). Endometrial cancer in women 40 years old or younger. *Gynecologic Oncology, 83*(2), 388–393.

Fahey, M.T., Irwig, L., & Macaskill, P. (1995). Meta-analysis of Pap test accuracy. *American Journal of Epidemiology, 141*(7), 680–689.

Fairfield, K.M., Hunter, D.J., Colditz, G.A., Fuchs, C.S., Cramer, D.W., Speitzer, F.E., et al. (2004). A prospective study of dietary lactose and ovarian cancer. *International Journal of Cancer, 110*(2), 271–277.

Fairfield, K.M., Willett, W.C., Rosner, B.A., Manson, J.E., Speizer, F.E., & Hankinson, S.E. (2002). Obesity, weight gain, and ovarian cancer. *Obstetrics and Gynecology, 100*(2), 288–296.

Fields, M.M., & Chevlen, E. (2006). Ovarian cancer screening: A look at the evidence. *Clinical Journal of Oncology Nursing, 10*(1), 77–81.

Finch, A., Beiner, M., Lubinski, J., Lynch, H.T., Moller, P., Rosen, B., et al. (2006). Salpingo-oophorectomy and the risk of ovarian, fallopian tube and peritoneal cancers in women with a *BRCA1* or *BRCA2* mutation. *JAMA, 296*(2), 185–192.

Fisher, B., Costantino, J.P., Redmond, C.K., Fisher, E.R., Wickerham, D.L., & Cronin, W.M. (1994). Endometrial cancer in tamoxifen-treated breast cancer patients: Findings from the National Surgical Adjuvant Breast and Bowel Project (NSABP) B-14. *Journal of the National Cancer Institute, 86*(7), 527–537.

Fishman, D.A., Cohen, L., Blank, S.V., Shulman, L., Singh, D., Bozorgi, K., et al. (2005). The role of ultrasound evaluation in the detection of early-stage epithelial ovarian cancer. *American Journal of Obstetrics and Gynecology, 192*(4), 1214–1221.

Folsom, A.R., Mink, P.J., Sellers, T.A., Hong, C.P., Zheng, W., & Potter, J.D. (1995). Hormonal replacement therapy and morbidity and mortality in a prospective study of postmenopausal women. *American Journal of Public Health, 85*(8, Pt. 1), 1128–1132.

Friedenreich, C.M., & Orenstein, M.R. (2002). Physical activity and cancer prevention: Etiologic evidence and biological mechanisms. *Journal of Nutrition, 132*(11), 3456S–3464S.

FUTURE II Study Group. (2007). Quadrivalent vaccine against human papillomavirus to prevent high-grade cervical lesions. *New England Journal of Medicine, 356*(19), 1915–1927.

Gates, M.A., Tworoger, S.S., Hecht, J.L., De Vivo, I., Rosner, B., & Hankinson, S.E. (2007). A prospective study of dietary flavonoid intake and incidence of epithelial ovarian cancer. *International Journal of Cancer, 121*(10), 2225–2232.

Gilbert, L.K., Alexander, L., Grosshans, J.F., & Jolley, L. (2003). Answering frequently asked questions about HPV. *Sexually Transmitted Diseases, 30*(3), 193–194.

Giuliano, A.R., Papenfuss, M., Abrahamsen, M., Denman, C., de Zapien, J.G., Henze, J.L., et al. (2001). Human papilloma virus infection at the United States-Mexico border: Implications for cervical cancer prevention and control. *Cancer Epidemiology, Biomarkers and Prevention, 10*(11), 1129–1136.

Goff, B.A., Mandel, L.S., Drescher, C.W., Urban, N., Gough, S., Schurman, K.M., et al. (2007). Development of an ovarian cancer symptom index: Possibilities for earlier detection. *Cancer, 109*(2), 221–227.

Goff, B.A., Mandel, L.S., Melancon, C.H., & Muntz, H.G. (2004). Frequency of symptoms of ovarian cancer in women presenting to primary care. *JAMA, 291*(22), 2705–2712.

Grady, D., Ettinger, B., Moscarelli, E., Plouffe, L., Sarkar, S., Ciaccia, A., et al. (2004). Safety and adverse effects associated with raloxifene: Multiple outcomes of raloxifene evaluation. *Obstetrics and Gynecology, 104*(4), 837–844.

Grady, D., Gebretsadik, T., Kerlikowske, K., Ernster, V., & Petitti, D. (1995). Hormone replacement therapy and endometrial cancer risk: A meta-analysis. *Obstetrics and Gynecology, 85*(2), 304–313.

Hecht, J.L., & Mutter, G.L. (2006). Molecular and pathologic aspects of endometrial carcinogenesis. *Journal of Clinical Oncology, 24*(29), 783–791.

Hensley, M.L., Castiel, M., & Robson, M.E. (2000). Screening for ovarian cancer: What we know, what we need to know. *Oncology, 14*(11), 1601–1607.

Herbst, A.L. (2001). Intraepithelial neoplasia of the cervix: Etiology, screening, diagnostic techniques, management. In M.A. Stenchever, W. Droegemueller, A. Herbst, & D. Mishell (Eds.), *Comprehensive gynecology* (4th ed., pp. 857–888). St. Louis, MO: Mosby.

Hildesheim, A., Schiffman M.H., Gravitt, P.E., Glass, A.G., Greer, C.E., Zhang, T., et al. (1994). Persistence of type-specific Papillomavirus infection among cytologically normal women. *Journal of Infectious Disease, 169*(2), 235–240.

Ho, G.Y., Bierman, R., Beardsley, L., Chang, C.J., & Burk, R.D. (1998). Natural history of cervico-vaginal papillomavirus infection in young women. *New England Journal of Medicine, 338*(7), 423–428.

Ho, G.Y., Kadish, A.S., Burk, R.D., Basu, J., Palan, P.R., Mikhail, M., et al. (1998). HPV 16 and cigarette smoking as risk factors for high-grade cervical intra-epithelial neoplasia. *International Journal of Cancer, 78*(3), 281–285.

Holowaty, P., Miller, A.B., Rohan, T., & To, T. (1999). Natural history of dysplasia of the uterine cervix. *Journal of the National Cancer Institute, 91*(3), 252–258.

Jemal, A., Siegel, R., Ward, E., Hao, Y., Xu, J., Murray, T., et al. (2008). Cancer statistics, 2008. *CA: A Cancer Journal for Clinicians, 58*(2), 71–96.

Kauff, N.D., Domchek, S.M., Friebel, T.M., Robson, M.E., Lee, J., Garber, J.E., et al. (2008). Risk-reducing salpingo-oophorectomy for the prevention of *BRCA1*- and *BRCA2*-associated breast and gynecologic cancer: A multicenter, prospective study. *Journal of Clinical Oncology, 26*(8), 1331–1337.

Kehoe, S.M., & Kauff, N.D. (2007). Screening and prevention of hereditary gynecologic cancers. *Seminars in Oncology, 34*(5), 406–410.

Koralek, D.O., Bertone-Johnson, E.R., Leitzmann, M.F., Sturgeon, S.R., Lacey, J.V., Schairer, C., et al. (2006). Relationship between calcium, lactose, vitamin D, and dairy products and ovarian cancer. *Nutrition and Cancer, 56*(1), 22–30.

Koutsky, L. (1997). Epidemiology of genital human papillomavirus infection. *American Journal of Medicine, 102*(5A), 3–8.

Koutsky, L.A., & Kiviat, N.B. (1999). Genital human papilomavirus. In K.K. Holmes, P.F. Sparling, & P.A. Mardh (Eds.), *Sexually transmitted diseases* (pp. 347–359). New York: McGraw-Hill.

Kramer, B.S. (2004). The science of early detection. *Urologic Oncology, 22*(4), 344–347.

Kushi, L.H., Byers, T., Doyle, C., Bandera, E.V., McCullough, M., McTiernan, A., et al. (2006). American Cancer Society guidelines on nutrition and physical activity for cancer prevention: Reducing the risk of cancer with healthy food choices and physical activity. *CA: A Cancer Journal for Clinicians, 56*(5), 254–281.

Lacey, J.V., Brinton, L.A., Leitzmann, M.F., Mouw, T., Hollenbeck, A., Schatzkin, A., et al. (2006). Menopausal hormone therapy and ovarian cancer risk in the National Institutes of Health-AARP Diet and Health Study Cohort. *Journal of the National Cancer Institute, 98*(19), 1397–1405.

Lamb, J.D., Garcia, R.L., Goff, B.A., Paley, P.J., & Swisher, E.M. (2006). Predictors of occult neoplasia in women undergoing risk-reducing salpingo-oophorectomy. *American Journal of Obstetrics and Gynecology, 194*(6), 1702–1709.

Lancaster, J.M., Powell, C.B., Kauff, N.D., Cass, I., Chen, L.M., Lu, K.H., et al. (2007). Society of Gynecologic Oncologists Education Committee statement on risk assessment for inherited gynecologic cancer predispositions. *Gynecologic Oncology, 107*(2), 159–162.

Lindor, N.M., Petersen, G.M., Hadley, D.W., Kinney, A.Y., Miesfeldt, S., Lu, K.H., et al. (2006). Recommendations for the care of individuals with an inherited predisposition to Lynch syndrome: A systematic review. *JAMA, 296*(12), 1506–1517.

Littman, A.J., Voigt, L.F., Beresford, S.A., & Weiss, N.S. (2001). Recreational physical activity and endometrial cancer risk. *American Journal of Epidemiology, 154*(10), 924–933.

Lukanova, A., Toniolo, P., Lundin, E., Micheli, A., Akhmedkhanov, A., Muti, P., et al. (2002). Body mass index in relation to ovarian cancer: A multi-centre nested case-control study. *International Journal of Cancer, 99*(4), 603–608.

Madison, T., Schottenfeld, D., James, S.A., Schwartz, A.G., & Gruber, S.B. (2004). Endometrial cancer: Socioeconomic status and racial/ethnic differences in stage at diagnosis, treatment, and survival. *American Journal of Public Health, 94*(12), 2104–2111.

Mahon, S.M. (2000). Principles of cancer prevention and early detection. *Clinical Journal of Oncology Nursing, 4*(4), 169–176.

Manhart, L.E., & Koutsky, L.A. (2002). Do condoms prevent genital HPV infection, external genital warts, or cervical neoplasia? A meta-analysis. *Sexually Transmitted Diseases, 29*(11), 725–735.

Markowitz, L.E., Dunne, E.F., Saraiya, M., Lawson, H.W., Chesson, H., Unger, E.R., et al. (2007). Quadrivalent human papillomavirus vaccine: Recommendations of the Advisory Committee on Immunization Practices (ACIP). *Morbidity and Mortality Weekly Report: Recommendations and Report, 56*(RR-2), 1–24.

Martin, V.R. (2007). Ovarian cancer: An overview of treatment options. *Clinical Journal of Oncology Nursing, 11*(2), 201–207.

Martin, V.R., & Cherry, C. (2006). Ovarian cancer. In K.H. Dow (Ed.), *Nursing care of women with cancer* (pp. 96–119). St. Louis, MO: Elsevier Mosby.

Maxwell, G.L., Tian, C., Risinger, J., Brown, C.L., Rose, G.S., Thigpen, J.T., et al. (2006). Racial disparity in survival among patients with advanced/recurrent endometrial adenocarcinoma: A Gynecologic Oncology Group study. *Cancer, 107*(9), 2197–2205.

Mays, R., Zimer, G., Winston, Y., Kee, R., Dickes, J., & Su, L. (2000). Human papilomavirus, genital warts, Pap smears and cervical cancer: Knowledge and beliefs of adolescent and adult women. *Health Care for Women International, 21*(5), 361–374.

Medverd, J.R., & Dubinsky, T.J. (2002). Cost analysis model: US versus endometrial biopsy in evaluation of peri- and postmenopausal abnormal vaginal bleeding. *Radiology, 222*(3), 619–627.

Melnikow, J., Nuovo, J., Willan, A.R., Benjamin, K., Chan, M., & Howell, L.P. (1998). Natural history of cervical squamous intraepithelial lesions: A meta-analysis. *Obstetrics and Gynecology, 92*(4, Pt. 2), 727–735.

Miller, K., Blumenthal, P., & Blanchard, K. (2004). Oral contraceptives and cervical cancer: Critique of a recent review. *Contraception, 69*(5), 347–351.

Miller, B.A., Kolonel, L.N., Bernstein, L., Young, J.L., Jr., Swanson, G.M., West, D., et al. (Eds.). (1996). *Racial/ethnic patterns of cancer in the United States 1988–1992* (NCI Publication No. 96-4104). Bethesda, MD: National Cancer Institute. Retrieved February 18, 2009, from http://seer.cancer.gov/publications/ethnicity

Mills, P.K., Riordan, D.G., Cress, R.D., & Young, H.A. (2004). Perineal talc exposure and epithelial ovarian cancer risk in the Central Valley of California. *International Journal of Cancer, 112*(3), 458–464.

Moleshi, R., Chu, W., Karlan, B., Fishman, D., Risch, H., Fields, A., et al. (2000). *BRCA1* and *BRCA2* mutation analysis of 208 Ashkenazi Jewish women with ovarian cancer. *American Journal of Human Genetics, 66*(4), 1259–1272.

Mor, G., Visintin, I., Lai, Y., Zhao, H., Schwartz, P., Rutherford, T., et al. (2005). Serum protein markers for early detection of ovarian cancer. *Proceedings of the National Academy of Sciences of the United States of America, 102*(21), 7677–7682.

Moradi, T., Weiderpass, E., Signorello, L.B., Persson, I., Nyrén, O., & Adami, H.O. (2000). Physical activity and postmenopausal endometrial cancer risk (Sweden). *Cancer Causes and Control, 11*(9), 829–837.

Moreno, V., Bosch, F.X., Muñoz, N., Meijer, C.J., Shah, K.V., Walboomers, J.M., et al. (2002). Effect of oral contraceptives on risk of cervical cancer in women with human papillomavirus infection: The IARC multicentric case-control study. *Lancet, 359*(9312), 1085–1092.

Moscicki, A.B., Schiffman, M., Kjaer, S., & Villa, L.L. (2006). Chapter 5: Updating the natural history of HPV and anogenital cancer. *Vaccine, 24*(Suppl. 3), S42–S51.

Muñoz, N. (2003). Valor del test del virus del papiloma humano en el diagnóstico y cribado de la neoplasia cervical [Value of human papillomavirus testing in the diagnosis and screening of cervical neoplasia]. *Medicina Clinica, 121*(12), 455–456.

Narod, S.A., Dube, M.P., Klijn, J., Lubinski, J., Lynch, H.T., Ghadrian, P., et al. (2002). Oral contraceptives and the risk of breast cancer in *BRCA1* and *BRCA2* mutation carriers. *Journal of the National Cancer Institute, 94*(23), 1773–1779.

National Cancer Institute. (2008a). *Endometrial cancer (PDQ®): Prevention and early detection* (Health professional version). Retrieved March 8, 2008, from http://www.cancer.gov/cancertopics/pdq/screening/endometrial/healthprofessional

National Cancer Institute. (2008b). *Ovarian cancer (PDQ®): Prevention and early detection* (Health professional version). Retrieved March 8, 2008, from http://www.cancer.gov/cancertopics/pdq/treatment/ovarianepithelial/healthprofessional

National Comprehensive Cancer Network. (2009a). *Colorectal Cancer Screening* [v.1.2009]. Retrieved July 2, 2009, from http://www.nccn.org/professionals/physician_gls/PDF/colorectal_screening.pdf

National Comprehensive Cancer Network. (2009b). *NCCN Clinical Practice Guidelines in Oncology™: Ovarian cancer* [v.1.2009]. Retrieved July 2, 2009, from http://www.nccn.org/professionals/physician_gls/PDF/ovarian.pdf

Netter, F.H. (2006). *Atlas of human anatomy* (4th ed., p. 373). Philadelphia: Elsevier Saunders.

Omerod, K. (2002). Gynecologic cancers. In K. Jennings Dozier & S. Mahon (Eds.), *Cancer prevention, detection and control: A nursing perspective* (pp. 539–575). Pittsburgh, PA: Oncology Nursing Society.

O'Rourke, J., & Mahon, S.M. (2003). A comprehensive look at early detection of ovarian cancer. *Clinical Journal of Oncology Nursing, 7*(1), 41–47.

Ovarian cancer: Screening, treatment, and follow-up. (1994). *National Institute of Health Consensus Statement, 12*(3), 1–30.

Ozols, R.F., Daly, M., Klein-Szanto, A., Hamilton, T.C., Bast, R.C., Jr., & Brewer M.A. (2003). Specific keynote: Chemoprevention of ovarian cancer: The journey begins. *Gynecologic Oncology, 88*(1, Pt. 2), S59–S66.

Ozols, R.F., Rubin, S.C., Thomas, G.M., & Robboy, S.J. (2005). Epithelial ovarian cancer. In W.J. Hoskins, C.A. Perez, & R.C. Young (Eds.), *Principles and practice of gynecologic oncology* (4th ed., pp. 895–988). Philadelphia: Lippincott Williams & Wilkins.

Parazzini, F., La Vecchia, C., Bocciolone, L., & Franceschi, S. (1991). The epidemiology of endometrial cancer. *Gynecologic Oncology, 41*(1), 1–16.

Parslov, M., Lidegaard, O., Klintorp, S., Pedersen, B., Jonsson, L., Eriksen, P.S., et al. (2000). Risk factors among young women with endometrial cancer: A Danish case-control study. *American Journal of Obstetrics and Gynecology, 182*(1, Pt. 1), 23–29.

Penn, I. (2000). Cancers in renal transplant recipients. *Advances in Renal Replacement Therapy, 7*(2), 147–156.

Pike, M.C., & Ross, R.K. (2000). Progestins and menopause: Epidemiological studies of risks of endometrial and breast cancer. *Steroids, 65*(10–11), 659–654.

Piver, M.S. (2002). Hereditary ovarian cancer. Lessons from the first twenty years of the Gilda Radner Familial Ovarian Cancer. *Gynecologic Oncology, 85*(1), 9–17.

Prentice, R.L., Thomson, C.A., Caan, B., Hubbell, F.A., Anderson, G.L., Beresford, S.A., et al. (2007). Low-fat dietary pattern and cancer incidence in the Women's Health Initiative Dietary Modification Randomized Controlled Trial. *Journal of the National Cancer Institute, 99*(20), 1534–1543.

Purdie, D.M. (2003). Epidemiology of endometrial cancer. *Reviews in Gynaecological Practice, 3*(4), 217–220.

Rebbeck, T.R., Lynch, H.T., Neuhasuen, S.L., Narod, S.A., Van'tVeer, I., Garber, J.E., et al. (2002). Prophylactic oophorectomy in carriers of *BRCA1* or *BRCA2* mutations. *New England Journal of Medicine, 346*(21), 1616–1622.

Ries, L., Eisner, M., & Kosary, C. (2004). *Cancer statistics review.* Bethesda, MD: National Cancer Institute.

Robson, M.E. (2002). Clinical considerations in the management of individuals at risk for hereditary breast and ovarian cancer. *Cancer Control, 9*(6), 457–465.

Ronnett, B., Seidman, J.D., Zaino, R.J., Ellenson, L.H., & Kurman, R.J. (2005). Pathology of endometrial hyperplasia and carcinoma. In G. Coukos & S.C. Rubin (Eds.), *Cancer of the uterus* (pp. 93–147). New York: Marcel Dekker.

Saslow, D., Runowitz, C.D., Solomon, D., Moscicki, A.B., Smith, R.A., Eyre, H.J., et al. (2002). American Cancer Society guideline for the early detection of cervical neoplasia and cancer. *CA: A Cancer Journal for Clinicians, 52*(6), 342–362.

Satagopan, J.M., Boyd, J., Kauff, N.D., Robson, M., Scheuer, L., Narod, S., et al. (2002). Ovarian cancer risk in Ashkenazi Jewish carriers of *BRCA1* and *BRCA2* mutations. *Clinical Cancer Research, 8*(12), 3776–3781.

Schafer, A., Friedman, W., Meilke, M., Schwartländer, B., & Koch, M.A. (1991). The increased frequency of cervical dysplasia-neoplasia in women infected with the human immunodeficiency virus as related to the degree of immunosuppression. *American Journal of Obstetrics and Gynecology, 164*(2), 593–599.

Schiffman, M.H., Bauer, H.M., Hoover, R.N., Glass, A.G., Cadell, D.M., Rush, B.B., et al. (1993). Epidemiologic evidence showing that human papillomavirus infection causes most cervical intraepithelial neoplasia. *Journal of National Cancer Institute, 85*(12), 958–964.

Schildkraut, J.M., Calingaert, B., Marchbanks, P.A., Moorman, P.G., & Rodriguez, G.C. (2002). Impact of progestin and estrogen potency in oral contraceptives on ovarian cancer risk. *Journal of the National Cancer Institute, 94*(1), 32–38.

Schmeler, K., Soliman, P.T., Sun, C.C., Slomovitz, B.M., Gershenson, D.M., & Lu, K.H. (2005). Endometrial cancer in young, normal-weight women. *Gynecologic Oncology, 99*(2), 388–392.

Schouten, L.J., Rivera, C., Hunter, D.J., Spiegelman, D., Adami, H.O., Arslan A., et al. (2008). Height, body mass index, and ovarian cancer: A pooled analysis of 12 cohort studies. *Cancer Epidemiology, Biomarkers, and Prevention, 17*(4), 902–912.

Siddiqui, M.A., & Perry, C.M. (2006). Human papillomavirus quadrivalent (types 6, 11, 16, 18) recombinant vaccine (Gardasil). *Drugs, 66*(9), 1263–1271.

Smith, J.F., Brownlow, M., Brown, M., Kowaski, R., Esser, M.T., Ruiz, W., et al. (2007). Antibodies from women immunized with Gardasil cross-neutralize HPV 45 pseudovirions. *Human Vaccines, 3*(4), 109–116.

Smith, R.A., Cokkinides, V., & Eyre, H.J. (2003). American Cancer Society guidelines for the early detection of cancer, 2003. *CA: A Cancer Journal for Clinicians, 53*(1), 27–43.

Smith, R.A., von Eschenbach, A.C., Wender, R., Levin, B., Byers, T., Rothenberger, D., et al. (2001). American Cancer Society guidelines for the early detection of cancer: Update of early detection guidelines for prostate, colorectal, and endometrial cancers. *CA: A Cancer Journal for Clinicians, 51*(1), 38–75.

Solomon, D., Breen, N., & McNeel, B.A. (2007). Cervical cancer screening rates in the United States and the potential impact of implementation screening guidelines. *CA: A Cancer Journal for Clinicians, 57*(1), 105–111.

Sonoda, Y., & Barakat, R.R. (2006). Screening and the prevention of gynecologic cancer: Endometrial cancer. *Best Practice and Research. Clinical Obstetrics and Gynaecology, 20*(2), 363–377.

Stoler, M.H. (2002) New Bethesda terminology and evidence-based management guidelines for cervical cytology. *JAMA, 287*(16), 2140–2141.

Strate, L.L., & Syngal, S. (2005). Hereditary colorectal cancer syndromes. *Cancer Causes and Control, 16*(3), 201–213.

Terry, K.L., Titus-Ernstoff, L., McKolanis, J.R., Welch, W.R., Finn, O.J., & Cramer, D.W. (2007).Incessant ovulation, mucin 1 immunity, and risk for ovarian cancer. *Cancer Epidemiology, Biomarkers and Prevention, 16*(1), 30–35.

Thompson, D., & Eaton, D. (2001). Variations in cancer risks, by mutation position in *BRCA2* mutation carriers. *American Journal of Human Genetics, 68*(2), 410–419.

Thurmond, A., Mendelson, E., Böhm-Vélez, M., Bree, R., Finberg, H., Fishman, E.K., et al. (2000). Role of imaging in abnormal vaginal bleeding. American College of Radiology. ACR Appropriateness Criteria. *Radiology, 215*(Suppl. 8), 3–7.

Tiffen, J.M., & Mahon, S.M. (2006). Educating women regarding the early detection of endometrial cancer: What is the evidence? *Clinical Journal of Oncology Nursing, 10*(1), 102–104.

Trimble, C.L., Genkinger, J.M., Burke, A.E., Hoffman, S.C., Helzlsouer, K.J., Diener-West, M., et al. (2005). Active and passive cigarette smoking and the risk of cervical neoplasia. *American Journal of Obstetrics and Gynecology, 105*(1), 174–181.

Tworoger, S.S., Fairfield, K.M., Colditz, G.A., Rosner, B.A., & Hankinson, S.E. (2007). Association of oral contraceptive use, other contraceptive methods, and infertility with ovarian cancer risk. *American Journal of Epidemiology, 166*(8), 894–901.

Tworoger, S.S., Gertig, D.M., Gates, M.A., Hecht, J.L., & Hankinson, S.E. (2008). Caffeine, alcohol, smoking, and the risk of incident epithelial ovarian cancer. *Cancer, 112*(5), 1169–1177.

U.S. Centers for Disease Control and Prevention. (2007). *Human papilloma virus: HPV information for clinicians.* Atlanta, GA: Author. Retrieved February 12, 2009, from http://www.cdc.gov/std/hpv/common-clinicians/ClinicianBro-fp.pdf

U.S. Preventive Services Task Force. (2003). Screening for cervical cancer: Recommendations and rationale. *American Family Physician, 67*(8), 1759–1766.

van Leeuwen, F.E., Benraadt, J., Coebergh, J.W., Kiemeney, L.A., Gimbrère, C.H., Otter, R., et al. (1994). Risk of endometrial cancer after tamoxifen treatment of breast cancer. *Lancet, 343*(8895), 448–452.

van Nagell, J.R., Jr., DePriest, P.D., Ueland, F.R., DeSimone, C.P., Cooper, A.L., McDonald, J.M., et al. (2007).Ovarian cancer screening with annual transvaginal sonography: Findings of 25,000 women screened. *Cancer, 109*(9), 1887–1896.

Vasen, H.F., Möslein, G., Alonso, A., Bernstein, I., Bertario, L., Blanco, I., et al. (2007). Guidelines for the clinical management of Lynch syndrome (hereditary non-polyposis cancer). *Journal of Medical Genetics, 44*(6), 353–362.

Vasen, H.F., Stormorken, A., Menko, F.H., Nagengast, F.M., Kleibeuker, J.H., Griffioen, G., et al. (2001). MSH2 mutation carriers are at higher risk of cancer than MLH1 mutation carriers: A study of hereditary nonpolyposis colorectal cancer families. *Journal of Clinical Oncology, 19*(20), 4074–4080.

Villa, L.L., Costa, R.L., Petta, C.L., Andrade, R.P., Ault, K.A., Giuliano, A.R., et al. (2006). Prophylactic quadrivalent human papillomavirus (types 6, 11, 16, 18) L1 virus-like particle vaccine in young women: A randomized double-blind placebo-controlled multicentre phase II efficacy trial. *Lancet Oncology, 6*(5), 271–278.

Vine, M.F., Ness, R.B., Calingaert, B., Schildkraut, J.M., & Berchuck, A. (2001). Types and duration of symptoms prior to diagnosis of invasive or borderline ovarian tumor. *Gynecologic Oncology, 83*(3), 466–471.

Walboomers, J.M., Jacobs, M.V., Manos, M.M., Bosch, F.X., Kummer, J.A., Shah, K.V., et al. (1999). Human papillomavirus is a necessary cause of invasive cervical cancer worldwide. *Journal of Pathology, 189*(1), 12–19.

Walsh, J.C. (2006). The impact of knowledge, perceived barriers and perceptions of risk on attendance for a routine cervical smear. *European Journal of Contraception and Reproductive Health Care, 11*(4), 291–296.

Whittemore, A.S., Balise, R.R., Pharoah, P.D., Dicioccio, R.A., Oakley-Girvan, I., Ramus, S.J., et al. (2004). Oral contraceptive use and ovarian cancer risk among carriers of *BRCA1* or *BRCA2* mutations. *British Journal of Cancer, 91*(11), 1911–1915.

Winer, R.L., Hughes, J.P., Feng, Q., O'Reilly, S., Kiviat, N.B., Holmes, K.K., et al. (2006). Condom use and the risk of genital human papillomavirus infection in young women. *New England Journal of Medicine, 354*(25), 2645–2654.

Winer, R.L., Kiviat, N.B., Hughes, J.P., Adam, D.E., Lee, S.K., Kuypers, J.M., et al. (2005). Development and duration of human papillomavirus lesions, after initial infection. *Journal of Infectious Diseases, 191*(5), 731–738.

Winer, R.L., Lee, S.K., Hughes, J.P., Adam, D.E., Kiviat, N.B., & Koutsky, L.A. (2003). Genital human papillomavirus infection: Incidence and risk factors in a cohort of female university students. *American Journal of Epidemiology, 157*(3), 218–226.

Wong, C., Hempling, R.E., Piver, M.S., Natarajan, N., & Mettlin, C.J. (1999). Perineal talc exposure and subsequent epithelial ovarian cancer: A case-control study. *Obstetrics and Gynecology, 93*(3), 372–376.

Woodman, C., Collins, S., Winter, H., Bailey, A., Ellis, J., Prioer, P., et al. (2001). Natural history of cervical human papillomavirus infection in young women: A longitudinal cohort study. *Lancet, 3*(57), 1831–1847.

World Health Organization Collaborative Study of Neoplasia and Steroid Contraceptives. (1993). Invasive cervical cancer and combined oral contraceptives: Results from a multinational study. *International Journal of Cancer, 55*(2), 228–236.

Zhou, X.C., Dowdy, S.C., Podratz, K.C., & Jiang, S.W. (2007). Epigenetic considerations for endometrial cancer prevention, diagnosis and treatment. *Gynecologic Oncology, 107*(1), 143–153.

Zunzunegui, M.V., Kink, M.C., Coria, C.F., & Charlet, J. (1986). Male influence on cervical cancer risks. *American Journal of Epidemiology, 123*(2), 302–307.

CHAPTER 4

Preinvasive Disease of the Cervix, Vulva, and Vagina

Eileen Fusco, MSN, APRN-BC, AOCNP®

Introduction

Cervical cancer continues to be a major concern worldwide, killing 270,000 women yearly (World Health Organization, 2007). It is the second most common cause of cancer-related deaths in women worldwide. The impact is felt predominantly in the developing world, particularly in Africa, Asia, and Central and South America, where 80% of the cancers are diagnosed (Ferlay, Bray, Pisani, & Parkin, 2001). These areas lack population-based routine screening programs where early detection of precursor cervical lesions could lead to successful treatment (Parkin, Bray, Ferlay, & Pisani, 2005).

Preinvasive Disease

In 1886, Sir John Williams identified a noninvasive squamous intraepithelial lesion that was termed *carcinoma in-situ*. In 1966, Richart proposed the term *cervical intraepithelial neoplasia* (CIN) to encompass all forms of precursor cervical lesions. Initially, the focus was on treating all lesions termed CIN, thinking that these lesions were occurring in a continuum. However, over the last decade, the pathogenesis of cervical precursor lesions has evolved, and it is recognized that the CIN designation is composed of two distinct entities.

The first entity is the product of an infection with human papillomavirus (HPV) and is reflective of that infection as it displays a marked cytopathic effect that consists of nuclear atypia, nuclear enlargement, and koilocytosis. *Koilocytosis* has been described in the literature for many years as the cellular changes associated with HPV infections and correlates with condyloma (a wart on the skin or a mucous membrane, usually of the genitals or anus) or a low-grade change (Meisels, Roy, Fortier, & Morin, 1979). These HPV-related infections represent only about 1% of all genital HPV infections and are not considered precursor oncogenic lesions (Dunne et al., 2007; Weinstock, Berman, & Cates, 2004). The second entity is considered a precancerous change (and should be treated as such) and is associated with a type of oncogenic HPV infection.

The natural history of CIN was evaluated in a meta-analysis by Ostor in 1993. His review encompassed almost 14,000 patients. The initial diagnosis of CIN was made by biopsy, cytology, or a combination of both. In this extensive review, Ostor noted that 60% of patients with CIN I will revert to normal. In patients who had CIN III, about 30% will revert to normal.

In 1998, a second meta-analysis by Melnikow et al. revealed that progression to cancer was 0.25% with atypical squamous cells of undetermined significance (ASCUS), 0.15% with a low-grade epithelial lesion (LSIL), and 1.44% with a high-grade epithelial lesion (HSIL). Regression to normal occurred in 68% of the patients with ASCUS, 47% of those with LSIL, and 35% of those with HSIL. Multiple studies suggest that a woman with ASCUS has a very low risk of developing an invasive lesion. The risk of having a preinvasive lesion confirmed by biopsy is estimated at 5%–17%, but this increases to 24%–94% in women with ASC-H (atypical cells, cannot rule out high grade), confirming that this category should be treated as preinvasive (Crum et al., 1999; Sherman, Solomon, Schiffman, & ASCUS-LSIL Triage Study Group, 2001; Solomon, Breen, & McNeel, 2007).

Evaluation of the Cervix

See Chapter 3 for pathophysiology of cervical cancer, Pap smear technique, HPV, and HPV vaccine for prevention.

The Bethesda System

The terminology used to describe preinvasive lesions of the lower genital tract has evolved over the last 50 years. The first term used to describe precursor lesions was *dysplasia* (Reagan & Harmonic, 1956). Richart (1967) redefined dysplasia into three classifications of CIN I, II, and III, and these terms are still used. However, as the biology of preinvasive lesions evolved, the terminology changed again and three classifications were merged into two, as squamous intraepithelial lesions (SIL) I and II. The current terminology used to describe cervical and vaginal cytology results is the Bethesda System (TBS), and it, too, has undergone several revisions since its introduction in 1988. TBS was the first attempt to standardize the reporting language of cervical cytology to clinicians. The most recent revision, TBS 2001, conveyed cervical cytology results to practitioners in a new way, integrating the knowledge of the natural history of HPV infection and diagnostic terminology. Initially, the focus of TBS was designed to identify all squamous epithelial lesions, including low-grade lesions. With the more recent information about LSIL representing a self-limited HPV infection, a shift occurred and began to focus on the screening and detection of HSIL, and this is reflected in TBS 2001 (Solomon, Davey, et al., 2002).

The most important component of TBS evaluates specimen adequacy as either satisfactory or unsatisfactory. This is an effort at quality assurance and speaks to the size of the sample itself. Also addressed in specimen adequacy is the presence or absence of the transformation zone (TZ) because the majority of CINs occur there. The terminology "satisfactory but limited by" has been eliminated. Factors that might limit the nature of the specimen and make it unsatisfactory are the presence of blood or an infection or a lack of sampling of the TZ components. It has been shown that the presence of endocervical cells in the sample is a quality indicator of the sampling, increasing the detection of cervical abnormalities (Minzter, Curtis, Resnick, & Morrell, 1999). In another study by Mitchell in 2001, the presence of endocervical cells in two consecutive Pap specimens had a higher rate of detection of a CIN II lesion than if no endocervical cells were detected on the sampling.

The second part of TBS provides an interpretation of the results related to SIL or malignancy and if atrophy, reactivity, or infection is present. A negative interpretation of results is self-explanatory.

The third component of TBS is a new modification. It groups together cells that look abnormal to the cytologist. Two new cell classifications were added: ASCUS and ASC-H. ASCUS is the terminology used to describe atypical squamous cells of undetermined significance, and ASC-H describes atypical squamous cells—cannot rule out high-grade lesion. This second designation (ASC-H) is most likely associated with a cervical neoplasm and not a transient infection with HPV (Sherman et al., 2001). The next category of epithelial cell abnormalities encompasses noninvasive lesions, which are placed in two tiers, LSIL and HSIL (Solomon, Schiffman, et al., 2002).

The previous category of AGUS was replaced by atypical glandular cells (AGC) and includes an attempt to identify the cell of origin such as the endocervix or the endometrium. This category is meant to reflect the numbers of potentially high-grade lesions that can be associated with this category (Soofer & Sidawy, 2000). Endocervical adenocarcinoma in situ (AIS) and AGC favor neoplasia and are separate categories (Solomon, Davey, et al., 2002). Figure 4-1 is a comprehensive list of TBS.

TBS served as the basis for new guidelines for management of abnormal cervical cytology results. From 2002 to 2003, several new screening guidelines were published by the American Cancer Society (Saslow et al., 2002), the American College of Obstetricians and Gynecologists (ACOG) (2003), and U.S. Preventive Services Task Force (2008).

In summary:

1. All three organizations agree that screening should begin coincident with the onset of sexual activity, when the risk of transient HPV infection is the highest and the risk of cervical cancer is low.
2. Two out of three groups recommend stopping screening at age 65 or 70 if there has been negative screening for three consecutive years.
3. Screening interval recommendations vary, but women older than 30 years with a negative cytology result and a positive HPV high-risk type should have both tests repeated in 6–12 months.
4. All three guidelines recommend against routine cervical screening for women after a hysterectomy unless the surgery was performed for a gynecologic cancer.

A study by Solomon et al. (2007) was published in an attempt to determine the impact of these new screening guidelines. Based on population projections, 75 million Pap tests will be performed in 2010. If the guidelines are implemented, this number will be reduced by half.

Diagnostic Tests

If the Pap smear is reported as having any atypical squamous or glandular cells or squamous intraepithelial le-

Figure 4-1. The 2001 Bethesda System

Specimen Adequacy
- Satisfactory (presence of transformation zone/endocervical component)
- Unsatisfactory (reasons stated)

Interpretation/Result
- Negative for intraepithelial lesion or malignancy
- Or positive for
  - Atrophy
  - Reactivity
  - Infection

Epithelial Cell Abnormalities
- Atypical squamous cell of undetermined significance (ASCUS)
- Atypical squamous cell (ASC-H)
- Low-grade epithelial lesion (LSIL)
- High-grade epithelial lesion/carcinoma in situ (HSIL/CIS)
- Squamous cell carcinoma (SCC)

Note. Based on information from Solomon, Davey, et al., 2002.

sions, further diagnostic testing is required depending on the classification of the abnormal cells.

HPV-DNA testing can be performed to identify the presence or absence of HPV and if present, the types of virus (see Chapter 3, Table 3-1, for types and association with specific genital lesions). In April 2005, ACOG published a practice bulletin that endorsed using the HPV-DNA testing in conjunction with cytology for cervical screening. This reflexive testing has been made easier with the introduction of the ThinPrep® Pap Test. This test is approved by the U.S. Food and Drug Administration (FDA) as a platform for HPV-DNA testing directly from the ThinPrep collection vial. The cells are still collected in the same way with no additional discomfort. The cells are rinsed into a vial filled with a preservative solution. This procedure ensures that the cells are released more readily into the liquid, capturing virtually all the cells.

The second test recommended by ACOG for any woman with abnormal squamous cells is a colposcopy. This can be done as part of the pelvic examination in an outpatient office setting. A colposcopy is the examination of the cervix with a colposcope after the application of a 3%–5% acetic acid solution to the cervix. A colposcope is a binocular microscope with variable magnifications and a green light filter that allows for visualization of areas on the cervix that may be indicative of CIN.

The colposcopic exam of the cervix assists in the evaluation of the TZ. It allows the detection of abnormal vascular patterns, punctuate lesions, surface contour and demarcation of lesions, or white epithelium. The application of a dilute acetic acid solution enhances the visualization of dysplastic lesions. The goal of a successful colposcopic exam is to view the TZ in its entirety, as this is where the majority of CIN lesions will occur. This is more difficult in older women, as the normal changes of aging cause the squamocolumnar junction (SCJ) to lie upward in the endocervical canal. The exam is noted to be satisfactory or unsatisfactory based on the complete visualization of the TZ or any lesion noted. Any lesion noted is biopsied guided by colposcopic visualization. HPV previously had been associated with cauliflower-like lesions or condyloma. It is recognized that HPV infection can be associated with a flat white lesion on the cervix that can best be seen with a colposcope. The numbers of colposcopically directed biopsies taken during the exam are determined by what is visualized by the examiner. Incomplete evaluation of the SCJ makes the colposcopy unsatisfactory, and further attempts to evaluate the abnormality will be needed (Wright, Lickrish, & Shier, 1995) (see Table 4-1 for abnormal colposcopic findings).

Endocervical curettage (ECC) or scraping is a tissue specimen obtained from the endocervical canal using a curette (biopsy) or brush (cytology). This may be performed to evaluate the area in the endocervical canal that is not visible to the examiner. These samples are submitted separately to pathology. Additional cervical sampling is performed occasionally (see Figure 4-2 for reasons).

Table 4-1. Abnormal Colposcopic Findings

Type	Characteristics
Aceto-white epithelium	Focal, transient whiteness, flat, or projections
Atrophy	Epithelium thinned by lack of estrogen
Inflammation	May be caused by infection
Leukoplakia	Focal, white epithelium, elevated
Mosaicism	Focal, vessels form block-like pattern
Punctation	Focal, increase in vessel caliber and spacing
Transformation zone not seen	May be because of age or prior surgery

Note. Based on information from Wright et al., 1995.

If the Pap result shows AGC or AIS, these glandular cells may be migrating down through the cervical canal from the uterus and indicate the presence of endometrial hyperplasia or carcinoma. A tissue sample from inside the uterus during an office endometrial biopsy may be done or may be obtained during a dilation and curettage in the operating room.

Vulvar Intraepithelial Neoplasia

Vulvar cancers account for about 4% of the gynecologic cancers diagnosed annually, and women in the seventh to eighth decade of life are at the most risk (Jemal et al., 2008). Women in all age groups may develop HPV-associated condyloma or warts in the vulvar area but are most susceptible between the ages of 20–24 years. Condyloma generally is associated with low-risk types of HPV. The majority of lesions are seen on the labia minora, the anus, and at the introitus. Lesions are most often multifocal and may or may not be pigmented. They may be asymptomatic but can be associated with symptoms such as pruritus or pain and may present with a lump or bleeding (Jones, Rowan, & Stewart, 2005).

Just as squamous cell cancer of the cervix is preceded by preinvasive lesions, squamous cell vulvar cancer is preceded by precursor lesions. The terminology used to describe preinvasive lesions of both the vulva and the vagina parallel those used for the cervix (Wright & Richart, 1997). Thus, vulvar intraepithelial neoplasia (VIN) is a premalignant condition of the vulva. VIN shares the same microscopic characteristics as CIN. Diagnostic tests may include a vulvar colposcopy and biopsy of any suspicious lesions. The International Society for the Study of

Figure 4-2. Reasons for Additional Cervical Sampling

1. Unable to perform colposcopy
2. Unsatisfactory colposcopy
3. Endocervical curettage result positive for cervical intraepithelial neoplasia
4. Discrepancy between the Pap and the biopsy result

Note. Based on information from Wright et al., 1995.

Vulvovaginal Diseases has published a grading system, using similar nomenclature as TBS (Ridley et al., 1989).

Jones et al. (2005) demonstrated in a case-series study of more than 400 women that VIN was strongly associated with HPV infection and cigarette smoking. Thirty percent of the women had been treated previously for preinvasive or invasive cervical cancer.

Vaginal Intraepithelial Neoplasia

Vaginal lesions often accompany CIN, but unlike the cervix, the vagina has no TZ. Incorporation of HPV may occur with injury to tissue during sexual activity. Women with CIN should have a thorough vaginal examination, including vaginal colposcopy. These lesions are often asymptomatic. Studies indicate that these lesions have the same features as CIN and the same potential for invasion (Lenehan, Meffe, & Lickrish, 1986; Sillman et al., 1997). The majority of the lesions are found in the upper third of the vagina. It can occur coincidentally with abnormal cervical cytology.

Risk Factors for Premalignant Vaginal and Vulvar Lesions

The risk factors for these lesions are similar to those for cervical lesions (see Chapter 3). An additional risk factor for vaginal lesions is prior treatment for a cervical cancer. More than 50% of the women with vaginal neoplasia studied by Daling et al. (2002) in a population-based case-control study of 156 women had a prior hysterectomy.

Currently, no treatment exists to eliminate HPV. An infection with HPV is often transient, as stated previously. It resolves in the majority of cases without intervention in about a year. Hildesheim et al. (1994) found in their study that about one-third of the young women who had persistent infections were infected with oncogenic HPV types.

Management of Preinvasive Disease

The underlying concepts in the management of clinically significant, preinvasive cervical disease are that excision or ablation of a high-grade lesion before it becomes invasive will decrease the possibility of the lesion progressing to cancer (Cox, 2002). Clinical significance is determined using HPV testing, colposcopy, and tissue sampling. The concept of a continuum of HPV infection progressing from CIN I to CIN III has been refuted because studies have demonstrated that low-grade lesions will regress over time if a woman's immune system is normal (Nasiell, Nasiell, & Vaclavinkova, 1983; Ostor, 1993; Shafi et al., 1997).

The challenge that practitioners face is how to identify a lesion that will regress over time as opposed to one that will lead to a cancer without doing invasive, expensive tests on large numbers of patients. Several studies have been done to address this challenge.

In 2003, the ASCUS/LSIL Triage Study (ALTS) Group published a randomized controlled trial (RCT) that enrolled more than 3,000 women (ALTS Group, 2003a). The goal was to compare initial management strategies with in women with ASCUS. Women were enrolled onto one of three arms:

1. Immediate colposcopy
2. HPV triage/cytology (referral to colposcopy if enrollment triage cytology was positive or missing)
3. Conservative management (no intervention and continue to screen, unless cytology was HSIL).

In this RCT, it was found that a single enrollment HPV test identified more than 90% of the patients with CIN III. The diagnosis of CIN III was equivalent in all three arms, but in the HPV arm, it was diagnosed sooner. In this study, women who were on the HPV triage arm avoided colposcopy without a decrease in the detection of CIN III lesions (Schiffman & Solomon, 2003).

Women with ASCUS who were HPV negative in this trial were followed for two years. Using combined cytology and HPV testing, the negative predictive value was almost 100%. In this group of women, the risk for progression to cancer is extremely low, and they may return to annual screening with cytology and/or HPV testing (Safaeian, Solomon, Wacholder, Schiffman, & Castle, 2007).

A number of women with LSIL may regress to normal. In an attempt to identify the group destined to regress, the ALTS group also published the results of a randomized trial in 2003 that focused on the management of the LSIL lesions (ALTS Group, 2003b; Schiffman & Solomon, 2003). The trial enrolled women who had LSIL results on Pap smears. They were placed on one of three arms:

1. Immediate colposcopy
2. HPV-based triage and repeat cytology
3. Conservative management.

Interestingly, the HPV triage arm closed early because more than 80% of the women referred were HPV positive, and large numbers were referred to colposcopy. Immediate colposcopy yielded only 56% sensitivity in detecting CIN III. In the conservative management arm, repeat cytology was performed and had the lowest percentage of CIN II or greater, possibly reflecting regression of lesions over time. This study was unable to make a recommendation regarding the management of women with LSIL identified on Pap smears with HPV infection. Repeating Pap smears alone was not a viable triage method as too few were negative.

In an effort to clarify the question, Guido, Schiffman, Solomon, and Burke (2003) did a prospective review of patients with LSIL or patients with ASCUS and HPV infection. The review did not identify a definitive management strategy.

Based on the results of the ALTS trial and newly published TBS terminology, the American Society for Colposcopy and Cervical Pathology (ASCCP) published consensus guidelines for the triage and management of women with abnormal cervical cytology results. Recommendations for follow-up of women with abnormal cervical cytology are listed in Table 4-2. HPV DNA testing was considered reasonable to add to cervical cytology in women older than 30 years of age (Wright et al., 2007). Detailed algorithms can be found on the ASCCP Web site. Their recommendations for women with a Pap test result that was ASC-H are that these women have a repeat cytology performed, perferably with reflexive DNA testing for HPV done to assess for high-risk types of HPV. Women with HSIL and AGC should be referred for immediate colposcopic evaluation and possible excision or surgical treatment.

Table 4-2. Management of Women With Abnormal Cervical Cytology

Type	Procedure
AGC	Colposcopy Endocervical sampling Possible excisional procedure
AIS	Colposcopy Endocervical sampling Endometrial sampling Possible excisional procedure
ASC-H	Colposcopy Repeat cytology Review cytology
ASCUS	Repeat cytology Reflexive HPV-DNA testing Colposcopy
HSIL	Review of cytology results Colposcopy Colposcopically directed biopsy Endocervical sampling Diagnostic excisional procedure
LSIL	Repeat cytology Colposcopy Endocervical sampling

AGC—atypical glandular cells; AIS—adenocarcinoma in situ; ASC-H—atypical squamous cells cannot rule out high grade; ASCUS—atypical squamous cells of undetermined significance; HSIL—high-grade epithelial lesion; LSIL—low-grade epithelial lesion

Note. Based on information from American College of Obstetricians and Gynecologists, 2005.

Excision Treatment

Two types of cervical excision may be done for HSIL as part of diagnosis and treatment. The advantage of excision rather than ablative treatment is that the tissue is preserved for histologic examination that may be useful to determine further treatment decisions (Spinelli, 2000).

The first type is a loop electro excision procedure (LEEP). This may be done as an office procedure. The LEEP uses a thin wire loop electrode that is attached to a power source. The loop emits a painless electrical current that quickly cuts away the affected cervical tissue in the immediate area of the loop wire. This causes the abnormal cells to rapidly heat and burst and separates the tissue as the loop wire moves through the cervix. This allows removal of tissue to further assess an abnormal Pap, or it may be treatment for an abnormal Pap. This technique allows the practitioner to send the excised tissue to the laboratory for further evaluation, which ensures that the lesion was removed completely, as well as allowing for a more accurate assessment of the abnormal area.

The second type of excision is a cervical cone biopsy. A *cone biopsy* or *conization* is a surgical procedure in which an inverted cone-shaped tissue sample from the cervix is removed for examination. This procedure usually is an outpatient surgical procedure to diagnose cervical cancer or to remove cancerous or precancerous tissue. This procedure excises more tissue than the LEEP because is removes tissue from the SCJ of the cervix and abnormal areas on the exocervix and the endocervical canal. This allows a better perspective of the extent of invasion and can be all the treatment needed, or it may provide pathologic information that may identify the need for more surgery to ensure total removal of the cancer.

If invasive carcinoma is found histologically in either of these excision specimens, more extensive surgery and possible chemo-radiation therapy is recommended (see Chapter 5).

Cervical glandular lesions have received increasing attention over the years. In 1952, Helper, Dockerty, and Randall described cellular changes adjacent to invasive cancer. This work was expanded on by Freidell and McKay (1953) when they described glandular lesions that were atypical but noninvasive. Soofer and Sidawy (2000) looked at more than 87,000 patient records at their institution covering a five-year period with less than 1% of the patients reviewed having AGC. High-grade lesions were found in 25% of that group and may occur after a long time period. Workup may not be complete without a diagnostic cone procedure.

Ablative Treatment

Two types of ablative therapy currently are used. These therapies usually are reserved for treatment of low-grade SIL and condylomas of the cervix, vulva, or vagina or for the treatment of persistent preinvasive disease after excisional treatments in these sites.

Cryotherapy uses liquid nitrogen to freeze the tissue. A probe is placed on the lesion and when activated freezes the tissue that leads to tissue necrosis. This is an inexpensive treatment that can be done in an office setting (Cox, 2002; Temple, 2000).

Laser therapy uses a carbon dioxide laser beam mounted on a colposcope to visualize and treat the entire TZ of the cervix. The laser beam is absorbed by water that causes vaporization of the SIL and the entire target tissue. This therapy also is used to treat low-grade SIL or persistent condyloma of the vulva or vagina. The procedure usually is performed in an outpatient surgical setting (DiSaia & Creasman, 2002; Spinelli, 2000).

Premalignant Vaginal and Vulvar Lesions

A literature search revealed no systematic reviews or RCTs on the treatment of premalignant vaginal or vulvar lesions.

In vulvar disorders, several cohort studies have been published reviewing laser treatment versus local excision. Management strategies may be based on the patient symptoms. Treatments may include excision, laser, applications of medications such as imiquimod or 5-fluorouracil (5-FU), or a combination of modalities. Jones et al. (2005) observed that 52% of the women with multifocal disease required subsequent treatments. Herod, Schafi, Rollason, Jordan, and Luesley (1996) stated that recurrence in the local excision group was significantly lower than that of the laser group and the difference was statistically significant. A retrospective review by Hillemanns, Wang, Staehle, Michels, and Dannecker (2006), confirmed this, and the risk of recurrence was significantly greater in those patients with multifocal and high-grade disease.

Treatment of vaginal disorders generally is conservative to preserve a functioning vagina. Examinations may be complicated by atrophy or postoperative changes. In a postmenopausal patient with a low-grade vaginal lesion (VAIN I), topical vaginal estrogen can be used. If the lesion persists, the disease can be treated with topical 5% 5-FU.

Special Considerations

An unsatisfactory colposcopy in any patient should always prompt further investigation. At the minimum, it should include a review of the cytology result to confirm the abnormality and following the published guidelines.

The dual infection of HIV and HPV is associated with unique management issues. Numerous studies have supported that the combination will produce an increased risk of cervical cancer, a higher prevalence of HPV, and a higher incidence of CIN (Cuzick, Terry, Ho, Hollingworth, & Anderson, 1992; Delmas et al., 2000). HIV infection is associated with significantly higher HPV loads in those patients with severe CIN and higher still in those women with advanced HIV disease, causing the course of the disease to be more aggressive (Weissenborn et al., 2003). Women who are HIV positive with abnormal cervical cytology should be referred for colposcopy regardless of the status of their infection or the level of their viremia.

The management of AGC requires an aggressive evaluation. Because of the inaccessibility of glandular cells in the endocervical canal and their lack of visibility on colposcopy, these patients should be referred to a gynecologic oncologist for management.

Medical and surgical management of vulvar and vaginal neoplasia is poorly defined. Because of the inability to collect large numbers of patients to compare and evaluate interventions, a collaborative approach toward research in these areas is essential (Buck & Guth, 2003; Todd & Luesley, 2005).

One of the challenges clinicians face to this day is the barriers to cervical cancer screening. They vary across the world, from country to country, and even within countries themselves with diverse populations and socioeconomic statuses. Barriers to screening are lack of knowledge, poverty, lack of access to the healthcare system and new technologies, and personal healthcare behaviors (Miller et al., 1996).

Walsh (2006) attempted to examine the impact of knowledge, perceived barriers, and risk on attendance at a screening clinic using a prospective design. Participants were sent questionnaires and letters inviting them to a free visit with cervical smear test. The questionnaires covered information concerning previous experiences with screening, knowledge, perception of risk and barriers, as well as socioeconomic information. Of the 3,000 participants, 41% returned their questionnaires. Less than half the women who responded identified the fact that the Pap smear could prevent cancer. Many thought it was used to detect infection. Only 17% of the women contacted accepted the invitation and had an examination performed. Previous unpleasant experiences and poor perception of risk also were barriers to attendance.

A study published in 2005 by Brewster et al. attempted to overcome some of the previously listed barriers. In an RCT of 3,521 women, an attempt was made to educate and simplify the screening process by using a single-visit approach. Women were provided with results of Pap tests on the day of the procedure with explanations of the importance of follow-up. In the group of women who were randomized to the single-visit approach, if the Pap was significant for an abnormal cytology, with either HSIL or AGUS, an excision was performed at the time of the visit. Despite the intensive efforts to educate and treat these women in a timely fashion, only 36% overall returned for the follow-up screening the following year.

Denny et al. (2005) also published a screen and treat approach to cervical cancer prevention in South Africa. The RCT had advantages for the low resource setting, as it was not reliant on cytology-based screening and colposcopy services. Using nurses as examiners for HPV screening and direct visualization, the entire assessment was completed in one visit. This study did result in high rates of follow-up.

These three studies highlight the continued difficulty practitioners face worldwide. The unique availability of the cervix to visual inspection and cytologic and histologic sampling has led to improved overall cure rates of cervical cancer nationally and worldwide.

Summary

Cervical cancer serves as a model of a cancer that has an identifiable precursor lesion, CIN, a slow progression to cancer, a minimally invasive screening test that is inexpensive and readily available, and an identified causal factor that is modifiable. The identification of the causative factor, the burden of HPV disease, and the understanding of the natural history of the disease has presented an opportunity for practitioners for teaching. Cervical cancer is not a sexually transmitted disease. The cancer is not transmitted; only the virus is, and therein lies the challenge for healthcare providers. Nurses need to clearly communicate to female patients that their sexual practices as well as the practices of their sexual partners place them at risk for HPV. As the onset of sexual activity frequently occurs during adolescence, our challenge is to educate both mothers and daughters. It involves an exchange of intimate information from patients to ascertain risk factors. It involves an intimate examination that very often is difficult for women. It involves diagnostic techniques that are invasive and frightening.

Oncology nurses are in a unique situation, as they can be effective in all the educational areas needed for women. Newly acquired scientific information about HPV and a new vaccine provide a unique opportunity for them to educate women confidently and accurately about how to keep themselves healthy. It is also an opportunity to eradicate cervical cancer across the globe.

References

American College of Obstetricians and Gynecologists. (2003). Cervical cytology screening. ACOG Practice Bulletin, Number 45, August 2003. *International Journal of Gynecology and Obstetrics, 83*(2), 237–247.

American College of Obstetricians and Gynecologists. (2005). *ACOG Practice Bulletin No. 61: Human papillomavirus clinical management guidelines for obstetrician-gynecologists.* Washington, DC: Author.

ASCUS-LSIL Triage Study (ALTS) Group. (2003a). Results of a randomized trial on the management of cytology interpretations of atypical squamous cells of undetermined significance. *American Journal of Obstetrics and Gynecology, 188*(6), 1383–1392.

ASCUS-LSIL Triage Study (ALTS) Group. (2003b). A randomized trial on the management of low-grade squamous intraepithelial lesion cytology interpretations. *American Journal of Obstetrics and Gynecology, 188*(6), 1393–1400.

Brewster, W.R., Hubbell, F.A., Largent, J., Ziogas, A., Lin, F., Howe, S., et al. (2005). Feasibility of management of high-grade cervical lesions in a single visit. *JAMA, 294*(17), 2182–2187.

Buck, H.W., & Guth, K.J. (2003). Treatment of vaginal intraepithelial neoplasia (primarily low grade) with imiquimod 5% cream. *Journal of Lower Genital Tract Disease, 7*(4), 290–293.

Cox, T.J. (2002). Management of women with cervical cancer precursor lesions. *Obstetrics and Gynecology Clinics of North America, 29*(4), 787–816.

Crum, C.P., Genest, D.R., Krane, J.F., Hogan, C., Sun, D., Bellerose, B., et al. (1999). Sub-classifying atypical squamous cells in Thin-Prep cervical cytology correlates with detection of high-risk human papillomavirus DNA. *American Journal of Clinical Pathology, 112*(3), 384–390.

Cuzick, J., Terry, G., Ho, L., Hollingworth, T., & Anderson, M. (1992). Human papillomavirus type 16 in cervical smears as predictor of high-grade cervical intraepithelial neoplasia. *Lancet, 339*(8799), 959–960.

Daling, J.R., Madeleine, M.M., Schwartz, S.M., Shera, K.A., Carter, J.J., McKnight, B., et al. (2002). A population-based study of squamous cell vaginal cancer: HPV and cofactors. *Gynecologic Oncology, 84*(2), 263–270.

Delmas, M.C., Larsen, C., van Benthem, B., Hamers, F.F., Bergeron, C., Poveda, J.D., et al. (2000). Cervical squamous intraepithelial lesions in HIV-infected women: Prevalence, incidence and regression. *AIDS, 14*(12), 1775–1784.

Denny, L., Kuhn, L., De Souza, M., Pollack, A.E., Dupree, W., & Wright, T.C., Jr. (2005). Screen and treat approaches for cervical cancer prevention in low-resource settings. *JAMA, 294*(17), 2173–2181.

DiSaia, P.J., & Creasman, W.T. (Eds.). (2002). *Clinical gynecologic oncology* (6th ed., pp. 1–50). St. Louis, MO: Mosby.

Dunne, E.F., Unger, E.R., Sternberg, M.R., McQuillan, G., Swan, D.C., Patel, S.S., et al. (2007). Prevalence of HPV infection among females in the U.S.: A national health and nutrition examination survey (NHANES), 2003-2004. *JAMA, 297*(8), 813–819.

Ferlay, J., Bray, F., Pisani, P., & Parkin, D.M. (2001). *Globocan 2000: Cancer incidence, mortality and prevalence worldwide* [version 1.0, IARC Cancerbase no. 5]. Lyons, France: IARC Press.

Friedell, G.H., & McKay, D.G. (1953). Adenocarcinoma in situ of the endocervix. *Cancer, 6*(5), 887–897.

Guido, R., Schiffman, M., Solomon, D., & Burke, L. (2003). ASCUS-LSIL Triage study group: Postcolposcopy management strategies for patients referred with low-grade squamous intraepithelial lesions or human papillomavirus DNA-positive atypical squamous cells of undetermined significance: A two-year prospective study. *American Journal of Obstetrics and Gynecology, 188*(6), 1401–1405.

Helper, T.K., Dockerty, M.B., & Randall, L.M. (1952). Primary adenocarcinoma of the cervix. *American Journal of Obstetrics and Gynecology, 63*(4), 800–880.

Herod, J., Shafi, M.I., Rollason, T., Jordan, J.A., & Luesley, D.M. (1996). Vulvar intraepithelial neoplasia: Long term follow-up of treated and untreated women. *British Journal of Obstetrics and Gynaecology, 103*(5), 446–452.

Hildesheim, A., Schiffman M.H., Gravitt, P.E., Glass, A.G., Greer, C.E., Zhang, T., et al. (1994). Persistence of type-specific Papillomavirus infection among cytologically normal women. *Journal of Infectious Disease, 169*(2), 235–240.

Hillemanns, P., Wang, X., Staehle, S., Michels, W., & Dannecker, C. (2006). Evaluation of different treatment modalities for vulvar intraepithelial neoplasia (VIN): CO_2 laser vaporization, photodynamic therapy, excision and vulvectomy. *Gynecologic Oncology, 100*(2), 271–275.

Jemal, A., Siegel, R., Ward, E., Hao, Y., Xu, J., Murray, T., et al. (2008). Cancer statistics, 2008. *CA: A Cancer Journal for Clinicians, 58*(2), 71–96.

Jones, R.W., Rowan, D., & Stewart, A. (2005). Vulvar intraepithelial neoplasia: Aspects of the natural history and outcome in 405 women. *Obstetrics and Gynecology, 106*(6), 1319–1326.

Lenehan, P.M., Meffe, F., & Lickrish, G.M. (1986).Vaginal intraepithelial neoplasia: Biologic aspects and management. *Obstetrics and Gynecology, 68*(3), 333–337.

Meisels, A., Roy, M., Fortier, M., & Morin, C. (1979). Condylomatous lesions of the cervix: Morphologic and colposcopic diagnosis. *American Journal of Diagnostic Gynecology and Obstetrics, 1,* 109–116.

Melnikow, J., Nuovo, J., Willan, A.R., Chan, B.K., & Howell, L.P. (1998). Natural history of cervical squamous intraepithelial lesions: A meta-analysis. *Obstetrics and Gynecology, 92*(4, Pt. 2), 727–735.

Miller, B.A., Kolonel, L.N., Bernstein, L., Young, J.L., Jr., Swanson, G.M., West, D., et al. (Eds.). (1996). *Racial/ethnic patterns of cancer in the United States 1988–1992* [NIH Publication No. 96-4104]. Bethesda, MD: National Cancer Institute. Retrieved March 6, 2009, from http://seer.cancer.gov/publications/ethnicity

Mintzer, M., Curtis, P., Resnick, J.C., & Morrell, D. (1999). The effect of the quality of Papanicolaou smears on the detection of cytologic abnormalities. *Cancer, 87*(3), 113–117.

Mitchell, H.S. (2001). Longitudinal analysis of histologic high-grade disease after negative cervical cytology according to endocervical status. *Cancer, 93*(4), 237–240.

Nasiell, K., Nasiell, M., & Vaclavinkova, V. (1983). Behavior of moderate cervical dysplasia during long-term follow-up. *Obstetrics and Gynecology, 61*(5), 609–614.

Ostor, A.G. (1993). Natural history of cervical intraepithelial neoplasia: A critical review. *International Journal of Gynecological Pathology, 12*(2), 186–192.

Parkin, D.M., Bray, F., Ferlay, J., & Pisani, P. (2005). Global cancer statistics, 2002. *CA: A Cancer Journal for Clinicians, 55*(2), 74–108.

Reagan, J.W., & Harmonic, M.J. (1956). The cellular pathology in carcinoma in situ: A cytohistopathological correlation. *Cancer, 9*(2), 385–402.

Richart, R.M. (1966). Influence of diagnostic and therapeutic procedures on the distribution of cervical intraepithelial neoplasia. *Cancer, 19*(11), 1635–1638.

Richart, R.M. (1967). Natural history of cervical intraepithelial neoplasia. *Clinical Obstetrics and Gynecology, 10*(4), 748–784.

Richart, R.M. (1973). Cervical intraepithelial neoplasia: A review. *Pathology Annual, 8,* 301–328.

Ridley, C.M., Frankman, O., Jones I.S.C., Pincus, S.H., Wilkinson, E.J., Fox, H., et al. (1989). New nomenclature for vulvar disease. International Society for the Study of Vulvar Disease. *Human Pathology, 20*(5), 495–496.

Safaeian, M., Solomon, D., Wacholder, S., Schiffman, M., & Castle, P. (2007). Risk of precancer and follow-up management strategies for women with human papillomavirus-negative atypical squamous cells of undetermined significance. *Obstetrics and Gynecology, 109*(6), 1325–1331.

Saslow, D., Runowicz, C.D., Solomon, D., Moscicki, A.B., Smith, R.A., Eyre, H.J., et al. (2002). American Cancer Society guideline for the early detection of cervical neoplasia and cancer. *CA: A Cancer Journal for Clinicians, 52*(6), 342–362.

Schiffman, M., & Solomon, D. (2003). Findings to date from the ASCUS-LSIL Triage Study (ALTS). *Archives of Pathology and Laboratory Medicine, 127*(8), 946–949.

Shafi, M.I., Luesley, D.M., Jordan, J.A., Dunn, J.A., Rollason, T.P., Yates, M. (1997). Randomised trial of immediate versus deferred treatment strategies for the management of minor cervical cytological abnormalities. *British Journal of Obstetrics and Gynaecology, 104*(5), 590–594.

Sherman, M.E., Solomon, D., Schiffman, M., & ASCUS-LSIL Triage Study Group. (2001). Qualification of ASCUS: A comparison of equivocal LSIL and equivocal HSIL cervical cytology in the ASCUS-LSIL Triage Study. *American Journal of Clinical Pathology, 116*(3), 386–394.

Sillman, F.H., Fruchter, R.G., Chen, Y.S., Camilien, L., Sedlis, A., & McTique, E. (1997). Vaginal intraepithelial neoplasia: Risk factors for persistence, recurrence, and invasion and its management. *American Journal Obstetrics and Gynecology, 176*(1, Pt. 1), 93–99.

Solomon, D., Breen, N., & McNeel, B.A. (2007). Cervical cancer screening rates in the United States and the potential impact of implementation screening guidelines. *CA: A Cancer Journal for Clinicians, 57*(2), 105–111.

Solomon, D., Davey, D., Kurman, R., Moriarty, A., O'Connor, D., Prey, M., et al. (2002). The 2002 Bethesda System—Terminology for reporting results of cervical cytology. *JAMA, 287*(16), 2114–2119.

Solomon, D., Schiffman, M., & Tarone, R. (2002). ASCUS-LSIL Triage Study (ALTS) conclusions reaffirmed: Response to a November 2001 commentary. *Obstetrics and Gynecology, 99*(4), 671–674.

Soofer, S.B., & Sidawy, M.K. (2000). Atypical glandular cells of undetermined significance: Clinically significant lesions and means of patient follow-up. *Cancer, 90*(4), 207–214.

Spinelli, A. (2000). Preinvasive diseases of the cervix, vulva and vagina. In G. Moore, L. Almadrones, B. Colvin-Huff, L. Gossfeld, & J. Eriksson (Eds.), *Women and cancer: A gynecologic oncology nursing perspective* (2nd ed., pp. 50–81). Sudbury, MA: Jones and Bartlett.

Temple, S. (2000). Cervical cancer. In C.H. Yarbro, M.H. Frogge, & M. Goodman (Eds.), *Cancer nursing: Principles and practice* (6th ed., pp. 1137–1154). Sudbury, MA: Jones and Bartlett.

Todd, R.W., & Luesley, D.M. (2005). Medical management of vulvar intraepithelial neoplasia. *Journal of Lower Genital Tract Disease, 9*(4), 206–212.

U.S. Preventive Services Task Force. (2008). *The guide to clinical preventive services, 2008* (2nd ed.). Rockville, MD: Agency for Healthcare Research and Quality. Retrieved June 5, 2009, from http://www.ahrq.gov/clinic/pocketgd08/pocketgd08.pdf

Walsh, J. (2006). The impact of knowledge, perceived barriers and perceptions of risk on attendance for a routine cervical smear. *European Journal of Contraception and Reproductive Health Care, 11*(4), 291–296.

Weinstock, H., Berman, S., & Cates, W., Jr. (2004). Sexually transmitted diseases among American youth: Incidence and prevalence estimates, 2000. *Perspectives in Sexual Reproductive Health, 36*(1), 6–10.

Weissenborn, S.J., Funke, A.M., Hellmich, M., Mallmann, P., Fuchs, P.G., et al. (2003). Oncogenic human papillomavirus DNA loads in human immunodeficiency virus positive women with high-grade cervical lesions are strongly elevated. *Journal of Clinical Microbiology, 41*(6), 2763–2767.

World Health Organization. (2007). *Cervical cancer, human papillomavirus (HPV), and HPV vaccines: Key points for policy-makers and health professionals.* Geneva, Switzerland: Author. Retrieved

March 2, 2009, from http://www.who.int/reproductive-health/publications/cervical_cancer_keypoints/cerv_cancer_hpv_keypts.pdf

Wright, T.C., & Richart, R.M. (1997). Pathogenesis and diagnosis of preinvasive lesions of the lower genital tract. In W. Hoskins, C. Perez, & R. Young (Eds.), *Principles and practice of gynecologic oncology* (2nd ed., pp. 675–715). Philadelphia: Lippincott Raven.

Wright, T.C., Jr., Massad, L.S., Dunton, C.J., Spitzer, M., Wilkinson, E.J., & Solomon, D. (2007). 2006 Consensus guideline for the management of women with abnormal cervical cancer screening tests. *American Journal of Obstetrics and Gynecology, 197*(4), 346–355.

Wright, V.C., Lickrish, G.M., & Shier, R.M. (Eds.). (1995). *Basic and advanced colposcopy—Part 1: A practical handbook for diagnosis* (2nd ed.). Houston, TX: Biomedical Communications.

CHAPTER 5

Invasive Cervical Cancer

Sharon Schwartz, MSN, CRNP

Introduction

According to the American Cancer Society (ACS, 2008), an estimated 11,050 new cases of invasive cervical cancer will be diagnosed in 2008 in the United States, with 3,870 deaths. For women aged 20–39 years, cervical cancer remains the second leading cause of cancer deaths following breast cancer. From 2003–2005, the average age at diagnosis was 48 years (Ries et al., 2007). Based on Surveillance, Epidemiology and End Results (SEER) data, 1 in 145 American women will be diagnosed with cervical cancer in their lifetime (Ries et al.).

Unlike other gynecologic cancers, a screening test is available for cervical cancer. The Pap smear screening test for cervical cancer was introduced in 1941 (Idestrom, Milsom, Andersson-Ellstrom, & Athlin, 2006). The Pap smear allows for detection and treatment of preinvasive and early lesions. Early detection of cervical cancer is named as a health indicator for *Healthy People 2010*, which is an ongoing project to define health priorities for the United States by the U.S. Department of Health and Human Services (2002). This is important because, when detected early, cervical cancer has a high cure rate and less morbidity. In areas such as the United States, where screening is inexpensive and widespread, the incidence and mortality of cervical cancer has declined. Cervical cancer was once the leading cause of death for women in the United States; since the Pap smear was introduced, the incidence of cervical cancer has decreased 74% (see Figure 5-1) (ACS, 2008; Ries et al., 2007; U.S. Centers for Disease Control and Prevention [CDC], 2009).

Even in the United States where screening is prevalent, populations of women do not receive the recommended screening and proper treatment of preinvasive lesions. The prognosis for cervical cancer is greatly dependent on the extent of disease at diagnosis. The current death rate is higher than it should be in the United States, reflecting that 33% of American women are not screened and treated appropriately (see Figure 5-2).

Globally, cervical cancer remains the second leading cause of cancer deaths in women after breast cancer. Internationally, 370,000 new cases were diagnosed annually with a 50% mortality rate. In some parts of the world, it is the leading cause of death in women. Approximately 60% of women who develop cervical cancer in the developing world either have not had any screening or had none in the past five years (Herrero et al., 2000; Molano et al., 2002; Yang, Bray, Parkin, Sellors, & Zhang, 2004).

The etiology and risk factors for cervical cancer, as well as screening guidelines, are discussed in Chapter 3.

Types of Cervical Cancer and Histology

The most frequently occuring types of cervical cancer are squamous cell cancer and adenocarcinoma of the cervix. Squamous cell cancers often arise from the portio of the cervix, whereas adenocarcinomas originate in the endocervical glands of the cervix. The area on the cervix where these two different cell types meet is the squamocolumnar junction (SCJ). This area of the cervix is dynamic. Over the course of a woman's life, the glandular cells are replaced by squamous cells in response to hormonal changes. This process is called metaplasia. The SCJ is vulnerable to infection; this is often the point of entry for human papillomavirus (HPV) and the site where dysplasia develops. Squamous cell carcinoma is the most frequent type of cervical cancer diagnosed, accounting for 74% of diagnoses (Kleinerman, Kosary, & Hildesheim, 2006). See Table 5-1 for a listing of all the histologic types of cervical cancer.

Signs, Symptoms, and Diagnosis of Cervical Cancer

The most common symptom of invasive cervical cancer is irregular bleeding. One study found that 56% of women with cervical cancer presented with irregular bleeding (Pretorius,

Figure 5-1. Cervical Cancer Incidence Rates

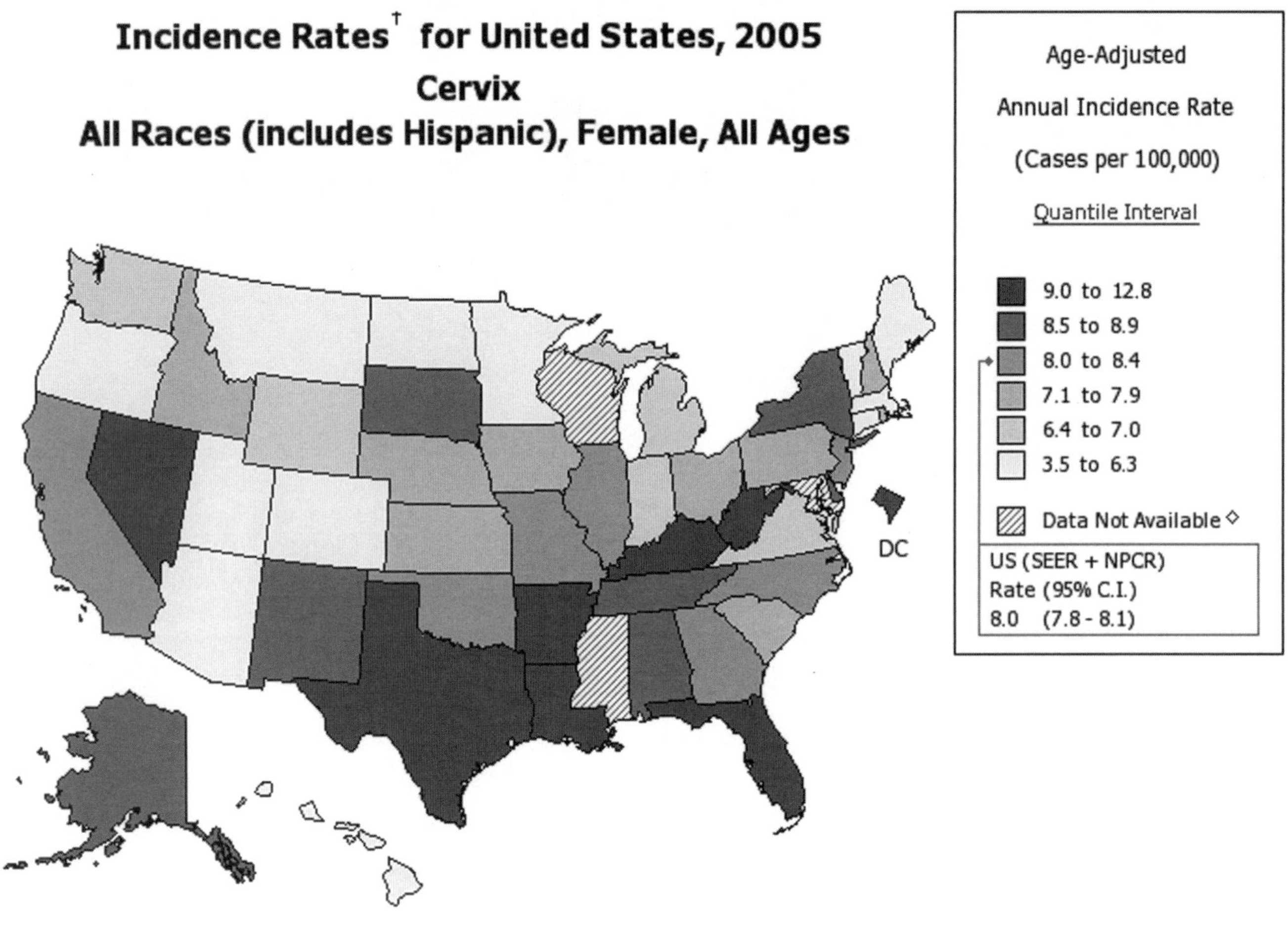

Created by statecancerprofile.cancer.gov on 05/18/2009 6:33 pm.

State Cancer Registries may provide more current or more local data.

Data presented on the State Cancer Profiles Web Site may differ from statistics reported by the State Cancer Registries (for more information).

† Incidence rates (cases per 100,000 population per year) are age-adjusted to the 2000 US standard population (19 age groups: <1, 1-4, 5-9. ..., 80-84, 85+). Rates are for invasive cancer only (except for bladder which is invasive and in situ) or unless otherwise specified.

Rates calculated using SEER*Stat. Population counts for denominators are based on Census populations as modified by NCI. The US populations included with the data release have been adjusted for the population shifts due to hurricanes Katrina and Rita for 62 counties and parishes in Alabama, Mississippi, Louisiana, and Texas (See US Population Data – 1969-2005 for more information.)

◊Data not available for this combination of geography, cancer site, age and race/ethnicity.

Because of the impact on Louisiana's population for the July – December 2005 time period due to Hurricanes Katrina/Rita, SEER excluded Louisiana cases diagnosed for that six month time period. So the count has been suppressed due to data consistency issues.

Note. From "State Cancer Profiles," by National Cancer Institute and U.S. Centers for Disease Control and Prevention, 2009. Retrieved May 5, 2009, from http://www.statecancerprofiles.cancer.gov/map/map.withimage.php?00&001&057&00&2&1&1&1&6&0#map

Figure 5-2. Cervical Cancer Death Rates

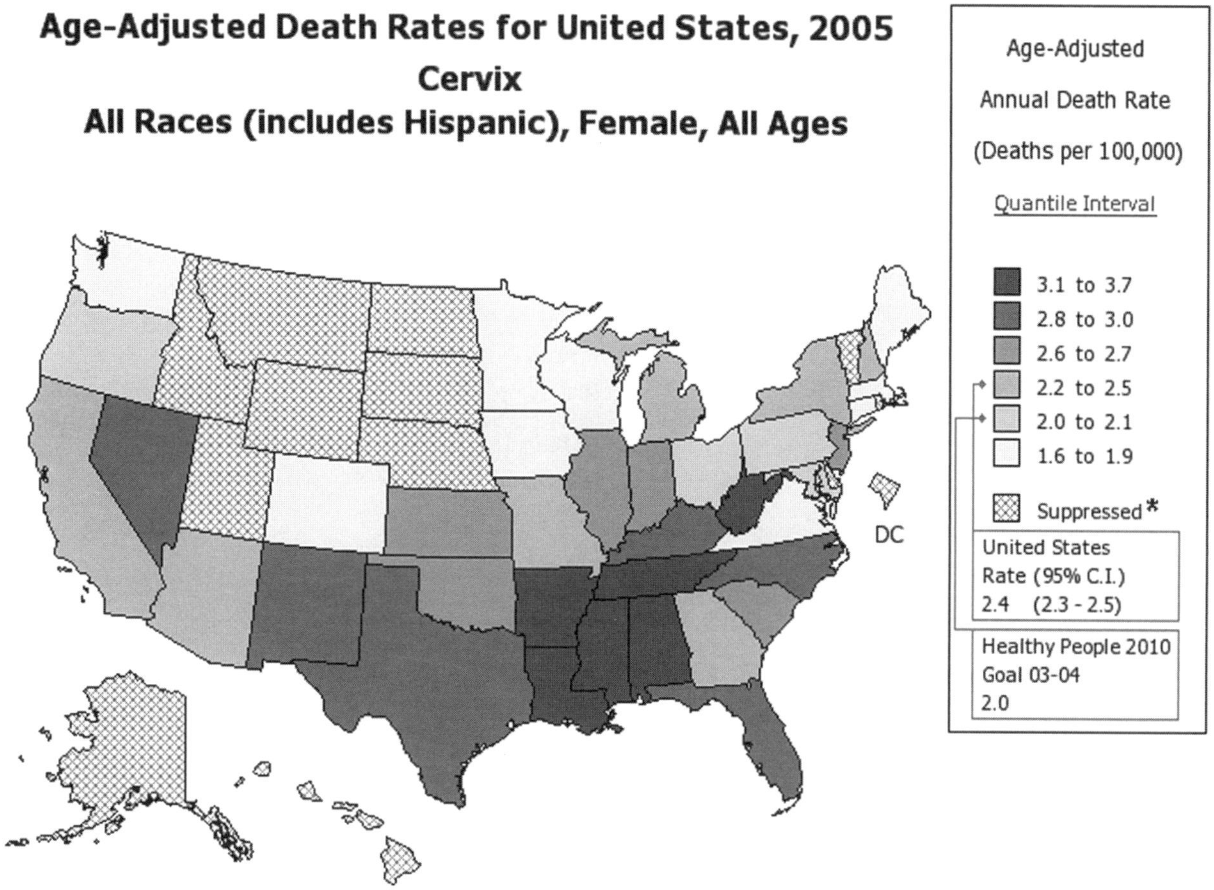

Created by statecancerprofile.cancer.gov on 05/18/2009 6:40 pm.

State Cancer Registries may provide more current or more local data.

Data presented on the State Cancer Profiles Web Site may differ from statistics reported by the State Cancer Registries (for more information).

Source: Death data provided by the National Vital Statistics System public use data file. Death rates calculated by the National Cancer Institute using SEER*Stat. Death rates (deaths per 100,000 population per year) are age-adjusted to the 2000 US standard population (19 age groups: <1, 1-4, 5-9. ..., 80-84, 85+). The Healthy People 2010 goals are based on rates adjusted using different methods but the differences should be minimal. Population counts for denominators are based on Census populations as modified by NCI. The US populations included with the data release have been adjusted for the population shifts due to hurricanes Katrina and Rita for 62 counties and parishes in Alabama, Mississippi, Louisiana, and Texas (See US Population Data – 1969-2005 for more information.)

*Data have been suppressed to ensure confidentiality and stability of rate estimates. Counts are suppressed if fewer than 16 cases were reported in a specific area-sex-race category.

**Data have been suppressed for states with a population below 50,000 per sex for American Indian/Alaska Native or Asian/Pacific Islanders because of concerns regarding the relatively small size of these populations in some states.

Healthy People 2010 Goal 03-04: Reduce the death rate from cancer of the uterine cervix to 2.0.

Healthy People 2010 Objectives provided by the Centers for Disease Control and Prevention.

Because of the impact on Louisiana's population for the July – December 2005 time period due to Hurricanes Katrina/Rita, SEER excluded Louisiana cases diagnosed for that six month time period. So the count has been suppressed due to data consistency issues.

Note. From "State Cancer Profiles," by National Cancer Institute and U.S. Centers for Disease Control and Prevention, 2009. Retrieved May 5, 2009, from http://www.statecancerprofiles.cancer.gov/map/map.withimage.php?00&001&057&00&2&2&1&1&6&0#map

Table 5-1. Histologic Cell Types of Cervical Cancer

Cell Type	Characteristics
Squamous cell carcinoma keratinizing and nonkeratinizing	70%–75% of all cervical cancers Originates in squamous cells on portio of cervix
Verrucous carcinoma	Associated with HPV type 6 Rare subtype of well-differentiated squamous cancer
Adenocarcinoma	20%–25% of cervical cancers Derived from glandular endocervix
Adenoma malignum	Well-differentiated adenocarcinoma; May be difficult to recognize as carcinoma 1% of adenocarcinomas
Adenoid cystic carcinoma	More aggressive type of adenocarcinoma Occurs predominantly in African American women of high parity in their 60s and 70s
Clear cell adenocarcinoma	Aggressive cell type
Endometrioid adenocarcinoma	Contains a mixture of squamous and glandular cells 3%–5% of cervical cancers
Adenosquamous carcinoma	Poorly differentiated adenosquamous carcinoma Extremely aggressive
Neuroendocrine carcinoma	1/3 of small cell carcinomas of the cervix High frequency of LVSI, lymph node metastasis, and recurrence Poor prognosis Chemotherapy must be a part of the treatment plan because of the aggressive nature of this type of cervical cancer
Small cell carcinoma	–
Undifferentiated carcinoma	–

HPV—human papillomavirus; LVSI—lymph-vascular space invasion

Note. Based on information from Pecorelli & Odicino, 2003; Randall et al., 2005; Reynolds, 2002.

Semrad, Watring, & Fotheringham, 1991). This can include bleeding between periods (metrorrhagia) and postcoital bleeding. The amount of bleeding may range from spotting to frank bleeding. Many women also complain of a persistent vaginal discharge, which is often described as whitish, blood tinged, and malodorous. Late signs and symptoms include unilateral pelvic pain radiating to the leg (resulting from disease to the pelvic sidewall), leakage of urine or stool into the vagina (vesicovaginal or rectovaginal fistula), fatigue, and weight loss (Hacker, 2005).

Women often present with no symptoms at all. The first sign of an abnormality may be an abnormal Pap smear. The cervix may appear normal on gross examination. This is especially true of lesions in the endocervix that may not be visible. To investigate an abnormal pap smear, the examination may include colposcopy. Using a colposcope, the cervix is examined under magnification using different lenses and filters to identify areas of abnormality. The entire SCJ should be visualized for a colposcopy to be considered satisfactory. Abnormal areas may appear white after the application of acetic acid, or the green filter of the colposcope may reveal abnormal blood vessels on the cervix. The most abnormal-looking lesion should be biopsied. In addition, endocervical curettage (ECC) should be performed as an additional diagnostic tool. ECC allows for collecting cells from the endocervical canal where abnormalities may not be evident on examination (Reynolds, 2002). A colposcopy may be performed during pregnancy but not an ECC (Partridge et al., 2008).

Once the disease progresses, lesions may be visible on the cervix on gross examination. Early lesions may appear as normal ectropion (the normal extrusion of glands on the portio of the cervix), or they may appear as an exophytic lesion. These lesions are often quite friable and may cause excessive bleeding during the examination. Any gross lesion should be biopsied (Apgar, Rubin, & Brotzman, 2002; Randall, Michael, Ver Morken, & Stehman, 2005).

A excisional biopsy, either a loop electrosurgical excision procedure (LEEP) or a cold knife conization (CKC) of the cervix. The type of procedure depends on the location and type of lesion being treated. If the lesion is on the ectocervix and a squamous lesion is suspected, a LEEP may be sufficient. However, during a LEEP, tissue is removed for pathology and the edges are cauterized—leaving an effect on the tissue. A CKC produces clear tissue margins sometimes needed for diagnosing invasion and margin status. If the lesion is suspected to be in the endocervix or is glandular in nature, a CKC is a better choice. The CKC is the recommended procedure in cases such as

- When a cervical biopsy reveals carcinoma in situ but invasion cannot be ruled out
- When a cervical biopsy shows microinvasive cancer
- When colposcopy results do not correlate with Pap smear results (when the Pap result is more severe than colposcopic biopsies reveal).

Excisional biopsy of the cervix will determine the presence and extent of invasion for treatment planning. During the pelvic examination, a barrel-shaped enlargement of the cervix may be palpable on examination. If disease involves the parametria, nodularity of the uterosacral and cardinal ligaments often is noted. Disease involving these ligaments may cause the cervix to lose mobility and become fixed (Randall et al., 2005).

Cervical Cancer Staging

Cervical cancer is the only remaining gynecologic cancer that is not staged based on surgical pathology, with the exception of gestational trophoblastic disease (see Appendix). Staging of cervical cancer is accomplished clinically based on physical examination. The stage is most often assigned at the time of primary diagnosis. Accurate staging is imperative in treatment planning. Surgery is not the primary means of staging because it is not indicated for advanced disease and because radiation is used as primary treatment even in some early-stage cervical cancers (Pecorelli & Odicino, 2003).

Understanding the typical course of the disease will help to make sense of the staging system. Cervical cancer follows a typical pattern of spread to other organs. It is spread via direct extension to adjacent organs, through the lymphatic system and the bloodstream. Once cells break through the basement membrane of the epithelium, they invade the stroma. Direct extension of cancer cells may proceed to lateral structures such as the cardinal and uterosacral ligaments, ascend to the endometrium, descend to invade the vagina, invade the bladder anteriorly, or invade the pouch of Douglas and rectum posteriorly (Trimble, Harlan, & Clegg, 2005). Lymphatic spread of cervical cancer typically follows from the pelvic sidewall nodes to the common iliac nodes and then to the para-aortic nodes and sometimes up to the scalene and supraclavicular nodes. The most common distant metastatic sites for cervical cancer are the liver, lungs, and bone (Potish, Twiggs, Okagaki, Prem, & Adcock, 1985).

Currently, two staging systems are in use. The first is the International Federation of Gynecology and Obstetrics (FIGO) method, which is the most universally accepted staging method. This method of staging by examination allows for consistency between patients managed by surgery and those managed by radiation and chemotherapy (LaPolla, Schlaerth, Gaddis, & Morrow, 1986). The other staging system adopted by the American Joint Committee on Cancer (AJCC) and the International Union Against Cancer is based on the tumor, node, metastasis (TNM) system (Greene et al., 2002). Patients who undergo surgery for cervical cancer will keep their initial FIGO clinical staging classification but may also have TNM information from the surgical pathology (Stehman et al., 2007).

Although FIGO clinical staging is employed for consistency, it is not always accurate. A Gynecologic Oncology Group (GOG) study group evaluated women treated with primary surgery and compared their initial FIGO stage to their TNM stage at the time of surgery. This revealed errors in FIGO clinical staging ranging from 24% to 67%. However, little evidence has demonstrated improved overall survival from surgical staging (Lagasse, Creasman, Shingleton, Ford, & Blessing, 1980). Studies comparing clinical staging to surgical staging have shown a tendency to overestimate the extent of disease during surgery. Lai et al. (2003) reported in a prospective study with a small number of patients that invasive staging was detrimental to the patient. Another retrospective study by Marnitz et al. (2005) showed that the prognosis for women with advanced disease who had lymph node staging and debulking was identical to those without surgery. These same studies have not been found to change patient survival, and the future of surgical staging in cervical cancer remains investigational (Creasman, 1995; Pecorelli & Odocino, 2003).

According to FIGO (Quinn et al., 2006), the method for staging may include

- Inspection
- Palpation
- Colposcopy
- ECC
- Hysteroscopy
- Examination under anesthesia with cystoscopy and sigmoidoscopy
- IVP of the ureters
- Chest x-ray (CXR).

Diagnostic modalities such as computed tomography (CT), positron emission tomography (PET), and magnetic resonance imaging (MRI) can be useful for treatment planning but are not to be used in staging (Pecorelli & Odocino, 2003). Physical examination is the first piece of evidence for staging (Creasman, 1995; Greene et al., 2002; Shepherd, 1996). However, each imaging modality has limitations in staging cervical cancer. CT is not as effective in identifying parametrial involvement whereas MRI is better in localizing the tumor as well as parametrial extension. However, MRI is less effective in evaluating lymph nodes and distant metastasis (Grigsby, 2007). Pecorelli and Odicino (2003, p. 391) noted that "only if the rules for clinical staging are strictly observed will it be possible to compare results among clinicians and institutions and by differing modes of therapy."

Because CT, MRI, and PET are not universally accessible, they are not yet part of clinical staging. However, Russell et al. (1996) showed that the traditional FIGO staging procedures such as proctoscopy or sigmoidoscopy are becoming less common. Hricak et al. (2005) studied CT and MRI for use in initial staging of cervical cancer. They found that CT and MRI imaging improves the accuracy of clinical staging. As these tests become more available, they may become an official part of staging.

Treatment

The overall prognosis of invasive cervical cancer correlates directly to the FIGO stage. However, other indicators affect overall survival. A woman's prognosis depends on size of the tumor, lymph node status, performance status, and cell type. Positive lymph nodes, bulky tumors, parametrial extension, depth of tumor invasion, lymph-vascular space invasion (LVSI), and aggressive cell types (poorly differentiated, small cell, and neuroendocrine tumors) are poor prognostic indicators (Randall et al., 2005).

Treatment options are based on the woman's initial staging. The initial treatment depends on the extent of disease at diagnosis and individual variables. The woman's age and comorbidities must be taken into account when deciding on the method of treatment. Definitive surgery typically is reserved for early-stage disease. However, radiation therapy also may be used as primary treatment in early stages. Both surgery and primary radiation with concomitant chemotherapy have been proven equally effective in treating early cervical cancer. More advanced cases usually are treated with combination radiotherapy and chemotherapy. Chemotherapy is used as a radiosensitizer when radiation therapy is employed and also for metastatic and recurrent disease (Schneider & Kohler, 2007). The many subtleties involving the extent of the cancer and the women's overall status must be taken into consideration when making treatment plans. For this reason, any woman diagnosed with cervical cancer should see at least one gynecologic oncologist to ensure proper treatment (Malzoni, Tinelli, Cosentino, Perone, & Vicario, 2007).

Advantages and disadvantages of each modality must be evaluated based on patient-specific criteria. Surgery offers preservation of the ovaries and avoidance of RT-related side effects such as vaginal stenosis and gastrointestinal (GI) side effects. Surgery may not be an option in women with comorbid disease or bulky tumors. When surgery is part of the plan of care, the type of hysterectomy that is performed depends on the extent of the lesion. A simple (extrafascial) hysterectomy may be used in very early disease, usually stage IA1. Except for these early lesions, the standard of care for surgical management of cervical cancer is a radical hysterectomy. This is generally performed when cervical cancer is limited to early-stage disease (stage IA2 to IB1). A radical hysterectomy differs from a simple hysterectomy because the connective tissue surrounding the uterus and cervix and upper vagina are removed and surgery includes a full pelvic lymphadenectomy. This is necessary because of the typical pattern of metastasis in cervical cancer. Left untreated, cancer cells from the cervix will migrate out to the pelvic sidewalls.

Piver, Rutledge, and Smith (1974) described five classes of radical hysterectomy based on how much tissue is dissected and excised during surgery. These classes are described as follows.

- Class I—This class describes a total hysterectomy with removal of all cervix, a small amount of tissue around the cervix, and a small vaginal margin (also known as an *extrafascial* hysterectomy or *simple* hysterectomy).
- Class II—This type of hysterectomy removes the uterus, cervix, upper one-third of the vagina, and paracervical tissues. The uterine artery is ligated where it crosses over the ureter; the uterosacral and cardinal ligaments are divided midway toward their attachment to sacrum and the pelvic sidewall (also known as a *modified radical* hysterectomy).
- Class III—This surgery includes resection of the parametrial tissues to the pelvic sidewall. The uterine artery is ligated at its origin from the superior vesical or internal iliac artery; uterosacral and cardinal ligaments are resected at their attachments to the sacrum and pelvic sidewall; and the upper one-half of the vagina is resected. This surgery also should include a pelvic and para-aortic lymph node dissection.
- Class IV—This is a more extensive version of class III. The ureter is dissected completely from the vesicouterine ligament, the superior vesical artery is sacrificed, and three-fourths of the vagina is resected. This is not as common as the other procedures because patients with disease requiring this level of dissection should be treated with radiation.
- Class V—This surgery includes resection of a portion of the bladder or distal ureter with ureteral reimplantation into the bladder.

Class III is the standard type of radical hysterectomy for stages IB and IIA. For patients with stage I cancer with less than 5 mm of invasion, a class II operation can be utilized (Hacker, 2005; Pikaart et al., 2007; Randall, 2005). Radical hysterectomy is a technically challenging surgery and should only be performed by an experienced gynecologic oncologist (Malzoni et al., 2007).

Aside from general surgery risks, such as hemorrhage, infection, thromboembolic events, wound breakdown, ileus, and bowel obstructions, radical hysterectomy has specific morbidities. Surgical complications specific to radical hysterectomy may include (Hacker, 2005)

- Urinary dysfunction
- Fistula formation
- Urinary tract infections
- Ureteral obstruction
- Lymphocysts
- Lymphedema.

Bladder dysfunction following radical hysterectomy is the most common complication, and it may be prolonged. Many patients will go home from the hospital with an indwelling catheter. About 75% will have return to normal bladder function within one to two weeks following surgery and most will be back to normal by three weeks. Sexual dysfunction also is common after radical hysterectomy because part of the length of the vagina is removed. This is especially pronounced when followed with adjuvant RT (Hacker, 2005; Grigsby & Perez, 1991; LaPolla et al., 1986).

RT is advantageous for women who cannot tolerate surgery and for those with bulky disease or larger tumors. RT causes acute inflammation of the normal tissue while treating tumor. During treatment, cystitis and diarrhea are common side effects of radiation on the bladder and bowel. Acute inflammation can become chronic, which may lead to morbidities such as colitis, proctitis, and enteritis. These side effects eventually can lead to vesicovaginal or rectovaginal fistulas or possibly bowel obstructions in some women (Rose, 2003). Significant lymphedema may occur from surgical lymphadenectomy or blockage of lymph channels from disease or effects of radiation, or a combination of these (Fiorica et al., 1990). Early intervention with physical therapy can decrease the severity of lymphedema and help manage the effects (see Chapter 14 for long-term symptom management of lymphedema).

Sexual function is a major component of quality-of-life indicators for women with cervical cancer. Studies have shown that 30%–63% of survivors of cervical cancer experience problems with sexual function (Donovan et al., 2007). Radical hysterectomy shortens the length of the vagina, and studies have shown that even without adjuvant radiation, this effect on the length of the vagina affects sexual function. One study showed that after radical hysterectomy 11% of previously sexually active women did not resume sexual relations. For those who did, 35% had persistent dyspareunia. However, studies have demonstrated women who have surgery alone (no adjuvant radiation) have less sexual dysfunction (Vistad et al., 2006). RT leads to vaginal stenosis often requiring the use of a dilator to maintain patency. Brand, Bull, and Cakis, 2006, showed that vaginal stenosis occurs in up to 38% of women treated with RT, with patients older than 50 years most at risk. This is a major cause of long-term sexual dysfunction in patients with cervical cancer (Bruner et al., 1993). They found that frequency of intercourse decreased while dyspareunia increased and led to decreased sexual satisfaction.

Treatment modalities must be chosen carefully, as both surgery and RT are associated with significant, sometimes long-term, consequences. Because 50%–60% of surgical patients will require adjuvant chemotherapy, treatment decisions should be made to decrease the patient's exposure to multiple therapeutic modalities and their associated consequences (Randall et al., 2005). Both modalities of treatment, surgery and RT, have proven to be equally effective in treating early cervical cancer (Landoni et al., 1997). The decision for surgery is based on the individual's treatment goals. Younger, healthy women usually opt for definitive surgery to preserve fertility options and optimum sexual function, whereas primary radiation is used in patients who present a surgical risk (Pecorelli, 2000).

Microinvasive Disease and Early Invasive Cervical Carcinoma (IA1–IB1)

Microinvasive disease only can be identified microscopically; any gross lesion should be classified as IB. Microinvasive lesions less than 3 mm are classified as FIGO IA1 (Pecorelli & Odocino, 2003, Quinn et al., 2006). Patients with microinvasive disease require a cone biopsy for definitive diagnosis and staging. In stage IA1 cervical cancer, conization of the cervix may be all that is required to treat the patient. This means the depth of invasion must be less than 3 mm and less than 7 mm in diameter with negative ECC and no vascular or lymphatic invasion (Pecorelli & Odocino; Quinn et al.). As long as the margins are negative, more extensive treatment is unnecessary at this point, but the patient must be followed closely with Pap smears at 4 months, 10 months, and then annually (if all follow-up Pap smears are negative) (Kleinerman et al., 2006). Conservative therapy such as this usually is performed in women wishing to preserve fertility. For those women with positive margins or positive ECC, the physician may attempt to perform a larger cone biopsy to achieve negative margins and to avoid more extensive surgery. If a larger cone biopsy does not attain negative margins or LVSI is noted, the woman should be treated as a stage IA2. A simple hysterectomy (no extra dissection of parametrial tissue) is the standard treatment for women with IA1 disease who have completed childbearing because these women have a very low risk of metastasis to lymph nodes (0.5%–1.2%). After surgery, the risk of recurrence is about 1% with an overall five-year survival rate of 99% (Gray, 2008).

Oophorectomy in women with microinvasive disease is optional and may be avoided in those who wish to retain ovarian function. A seven-year retrospective review by Owens et al. (1989) showed no ovarian metastases in women with microinvasive disease who underwent oophorectomy at the time of surgery. None of the patients who kept their ovaries developed metastatic disease or needed surgery for ovarian pathology. Owens' group also demonstrated that women who had their ovaries surgically moved out of the potential field of radiation (transposed) retained ovarian function. This provides women the possibility of using advanced reproductive technology to conceive with their own eggs. (However, a gestational carrier would be needed after a hysterectomy.)

For those women with early disease (FIGO IA) who are not surgical candidates, intracavitary radiation is effective and does not require supplementation with external beam treatment (Grigsby & Perez, 1991; Randall, 2005).

If the cone biopsy does not attain negative margins or LVSI is noted, the woman should be managed as stage IA2. Stage IA2 disease is still microinvasive with a tumor size 3–5 mm in depth and less than 7 mm in diameter. Women with IA2 disease have a higher chance of nodal metastasis (5%–7%). Risk for recurrence is 3%–5% and overall survival at 5 years is 96% (Gray, 2008). A radical hysterectomy is indicated in women with IA2 to IIA FIGO stages. The type of radical hysterectomy employed is a Piver type III, which involves removing the central lesion with wide excision of the parametrial and paravaginal tissue along with the upper vagina, ligating the uterine artery at its origin; and dissecting the ureters free from the cardinal ligaments (Pikaart et al., 2007). Women who are not good candidates for the class III radical hysterectomy can receive either low-dose brachytherapy (LDR) or high-dose brachytherapy (HDR) in addition to pelvic RT along with platinum-based chemotherapy (Nag et al., 2000, 2002).

Radical Trachelectomy

Statistical trends from SEER (up to 2005) data show that women are delaying childbearing and that of the 2008 estimates of new cervical cancer diagnoses in the United States, 11,070 women younger than age 45 will account for 22% of the new cases (Reis et al., 2007). These trends intersect as women who are delaying completing their families are diagnosed with invasive cervical cancer. To meet the needs of these women, fertility-sparing treatments for invasive cervical cancer have been developed. For those women who wish to preserve fertility but are beyond IA1 disease, radical trachelectomy may be an option. In this surgery, the uterus and ovaries are spared, the cervix and parametrial tissue are removed, and a cervical cerclage is placed. Lymph nodes are evaluated laparoscopically at the beginning of the procedure. As long as the nodes are negative, the surgery proceeds to remove the cervix and parametrial tissue and then a cervical cerclage is placed. This technique was developed by Dargent in 1994 and continues to be refined by a select number of gynecologic oncologists (Dargent, Brun, Roy, & Remi, 1994). The surgery can be performed with either an abdominal or vaginal approach depending on the preference and experience of the surgeon. Nearly half of all women with cervical cancer younger than 40 years old are candidates for radical trachelectomy (Leitao & Chi, 2005).

Radical trachelectomy is reserved for those patients younger than 40 years old who have disease ranging from IA1 with LVSI to IB1 stage cervical carcinoma (see Figure 5-3 for criteria). In a review of eight series on radical trachelectomy by Sonoda, Chi, Carter, Barakat, and Abu Rustum (2008), of the 548 women who had the procedure, the overall recurrence rate was 4%; 75% of those women who attempted pregnancy conceived on their own, and 60% delivered at term. The spontaneous abortion rate (SAB) was similar to that of the general population. The second trimester SAB rate was higher when the surgery was first developed, but the use of cervical cerclage has decreased the amount of losses. These women need to deliver via Caesarean section because of the permanent cerclage placement (Mathevet, Laslo de Kaszon, & Dargent, 2003). Women need to be selected carefully for this procedure as well as carefully counseled that this is not the standard approach for IA2-IB disease and that recurrence and pregnancy complications are risks. It is essential that a multidisciplinary management plan is utilized, including a reproductive endocrinologist and an obstetrician who specializes in high-risk pregnancies, along with a gynecologic oncologist experienced in radical trachelectomy (Saunders, Ferrier, & Ryan, 1996).

Figure 5-3. Selection Criteria for Radical Trachelectomy Candidates

- Confirmed cervical cancer
- Stage IA1 with LVSI or IA2–IB1
- Squamous or adenocarcinoma histology
- Age younger than 40
- No history of infertility
- Lesion smaller than 2 cm
- No evidence of metastasis
- Cervical length longer than 2 cm
- Desire for future fertility
- Post conization 4–6 weeks

LVSI—lymph-vascular space invasion

Note. Based on information from Abu-Rustum & Sonoda, 2007; Gray, 2008; Sonoda et al., 2008.

The Role of Minimally Invasive Surgery

As in other fields, gynecologic oncology has made many strides in the past five years to perform less-invasive surgery without compromising overall survival. With respect to cervical cancer, advances have been made toward minimally invasive surgery, although it is not yet the standard. Some centers are performing laparoscopic-assisted radical vaginal hysterectomy. Candidates must be chosen carefully. The ideal candidate should have a tumor that is less than 4 cm in diameter (may include stages IA1 to small IIA), histologically proven negative lymph nodes, and negative LVSI. The lymph nodes are first sampled through a laparoscopic approach and then, if the nodes are proven negative, they proceed with the laparoscopic-assisted radical vaginal hysterectomy (Gil-Moreno et al., 2005; Jackson et al., 2004; Malzoni et al., 2007; Ramirez, Slomovitz, Soliman, Coleman, & Levenback, 2006; Spirtos, Eisenkop, Schlaerth, & Ballon, 2002; Spirtos, Schlaerth, Kimball, Leiphart, & Ballon, 1996).

Hertel et al. (2003) reported an overall survival rate of 98% with laparoscopic radical hysterectomy. Spirtos et al. (2002) reported that laparoscopic radical hysterectomy with lymph node dissection can be performed with the same results as open surgery provided the surgeon has experience in laparoscopic procedures. Their group had a recurrence rate of 10% and a five-year survival rate of 89.7% (Spirtos et al.). Sardi, Vidaurreta, Bermudez, and di Paola (1999) reported an overall survival rate of 100% for stage IA, 88% for stage IB2, and 85% for stage IB2 after laparoscopic radical hysterectomy.

The benefits of minimally invasive surgery include shorter hospital stays, smaller incisions (meaning easier wound healing), along with a quicker return to activities. Centers performing laparoscopic-assisted radical hysterectomies report lower incidences of blood loss during surgery as well as decreased rates of bowel and bladder dysfunction following surgery (Jackson et al., 2004). Spirtos et al. (2002) found not only that survival was equivalent to open radical hysterectomy but also that there was less long-term bladder dysfunction. Other centers performing laparoscopic radical hysterectomies also have reported lower incidences of bladder and bowel dysfunction following surgery (Ramirez et al., 2006). Although this seems like a positive, it also raises questions regarding how much tissue is removed during this surgery compared to a traditional radical hysterectomy. Is the same amount of tissue evaluated, and if not, does this pose a higher risk for recurrence? Longer follow-up of women who undergo laparoscopic radical hysterectomies is needed to answer these questions before laparoscopic surgery becomes standard of care (Gil-Moreno et al., 2005; Jackson et al., 2004; Malzoni et al., 2007; Pikaart et al., 2007; Ramirez et al., 2006; Spirtos et al., 2002).

Currently, laparoscopic-assisted radical hysterectomies also are performed using the da Vinci® (Intuitive Surgical, Inc.) robot. This is essentially the same as laparoscopy but offers better instrumentation and visualization. A few multicenter studies suggest robotic radical hysterectomies have similiar benefits as laparoscopic procedures, such as decreased blood loss, shorter hospital stays, and less complications (Obermair et al., 2008). These studies also demonstrated that during a robotic radical hysterectomy, the same number of lymph nodes were sampled as during traditional open surgery (Lowe, Chamberlain, Kamelle, Johnson, & Tillmanns, 2009).

Adjuvant Radiation Therapy After Surgery

Information from surgical staging can classify patients as low, intermediate, or high risk of recurrence. Adjuvant RT is indicated in patients with high or intermediate risk following surgery. High-risk patients are those with positive lymph nodes, positive or close resection margins, and parametrial involvement. Intermediate risk features include large tumor size, deep cervical stromal invasion, and positive LVSI (Estape et al., 1998; Vigliotti et al., 1992). Low-risk patients have none of those features and do not require adjuvant RT.

The GOG 92 clinical trial studied women with IB cancer of the cervix after radical hysterectomy to identify those with intermediate and high risk for recurrence and to determine if adjuvant RT would increase survival in those patients (Morris et al., 1999; Sedlis et al., 1999). Of those who received adjuvant RT, 15% experienced a recurrence, compared to 28% without adjuvant RT, and this was a statistically significant reduction in recurrence. The progression-free survival at two years was 79% in women without RT after surgery and 88% in women who received adjuvant RT after surgery (Sedlis et al.).

Women receiving RT for cervical cancer often receive concomitant chemotherapy with a platinum-based agent. Chemotherapy acts as a sensitizing agent for RT. This is important because one of the challenges with RT and cervical cancer is the hypoxic nature of cervical tumors. Radiation works by ionizing, or activating, oxygen. This creates free radicals that bind to cellular DNA and break it, resulting in cell death. Higher levels of hemoglobin and oxygen perfusion are associated with better radiation outcomes (Rose, Bundy, et al., 1999). Six GOG studies confirmed the survival benefit of a platinum-based chemotherapeutic agent in addition to RT over RT alone (Keys, 1999; Morris et al., 1999; Pearcey et al., 2002; Peters, 2000; Rose, Bundy, et al.; Whitney et al., 1999). For those patients with high-risk features, the four-year progression-free interval improves from 63% to 80% with the addition of platinum (Atlan et al., 2002).

Local Disease (Stages IB–IIA)

Stage IB cervical cancer ranges from microinvasive tumors to visible lesions. Microinvasive tumors are not visible to the examiner without magnification. Microinvasive tumors with a depth of stromal invasion greater than 5 mm or a diameter greater than 7 mm (microinvasive but beyond IA2) are considered IB. IB tumors also encompass visible lesions of less than 4 cm (IB1) and those greater than 4 cm (IB2). Women with IB disease have a 15% risk of spread to the lymph nodes (Gray, 2008). The generally accepted treatment for stages up to IB and IB1 is class III radical hysterectomy with lymph node dissection. If the patient is not a surgical candidate, pelvic RT with concurrent chemoradiation and brachytherapy would be the primary treatment.

Primary treatment for IB2 disease (a visible tumor larger than 4 cm) is controversial. Studies show that IB2 bulky tumors have a greater incidence of recurrence and decreased overall survival, regardless of primary treatment choice (Creasman, 1995; Finan et al., 1996; Kristensen, Abeler, Risberg, Trop, & Bryne, 1999; Trattner et al., 2001). According to National Comprehensive Cancer Network (NCCN) guidelines, either radical hysterectomy or primary chemoradiation is appropriate (Greer et al., 2008). Advantages for initial surgical treatment in bulky cervical cancer include

- Tumor removal eliminates the need for brachytherapy as part of adjuvant RT
- Any bulky lymph nodes can be removed during surgery
- Surgical pathology may reveal other risk factors that warrant additional further treatment. However, adjuvant RT is often required.

Because of the size of IB2 tumors (larger than 4 cm), the potential for adjuvant chemoradiation is high. A study by Landoni et al. (1997) showed that 87% of women treated with primary surgery needed adjuvant RT and experienced significant morbidities as a result of both modalities. The disadvantages for women who undergo both radical surgery and adjuvant chemoradiation include an increased risk of major and minor GI and genitourinary complications, lymphocysts, and lymphedema (Fiorca et al., 1990). Vaginal stenosis, and subsequent sexual dysfunction, is common in women who receive RT. As many as 38% of women experienced vaginal stenosis following RT with the highest incidence in women older than age 50 (Brand, Bull, & Cakir, 2006).

It is important to individualize care for women with bulky stage IB disease to maximize their survival potential and minimize morbidity. The current standard of care for these patients is external beam radiation plus intracavitary brachytherapy with concurrent platinum chemotherapy (Morice et al., 2007). Some advocate for neoadjuvant chemoradiotherapy followed by radical hysterectomy. Ferrandina et al. (2007) found that local control was very high (73%) after chemoradiotherapy followed by surgery especially in stages IB2 and II patients. However, exposure to three different types of treatment means managing the morbidities associated with each (Estape et al., 1998; Finan et al., 1996; LaPolla et al., 1986).

Locally Advanced Disease (FIGO IIB–IVA)

Locally advanced cervical cancer is classified as beyond the cervix but not out of the pelvis (FIGO IIB–IVA). Treatment at this stage is limited to chemoradiation. Surgery is not indicated because achieving negative margins is difficult due to the lateral spread of disease to the parametria. Effective radiation includes a combination of external whole-pelvic RT and brachytherapy treatment. The whole-pelvic dose is 45–50.4 Gy followed by brachytherapy for a total of more than 80 Gy (Rose, 2003; Stehman et al., 2007). It is important for women receiving RT to have their treatments on time because delay has a direct relationship to pelvic control and overall survival (Lanciano, Pajak, Martz, & Hanks, 1993). All women receiving RT should be considered for concurrent treatment with cisplatin chemotherapy.

For women with parametrial involvement not yet extending to the pelvic sidewall (IIB), RT in combination with chemotherapy is the treatment of choice. Studies suggest that adding cisplatin to RT in patients with stage IB2–IVA cervical cancer increases overall survival from 30% to 50% (Keys et al., 1999; Morris et al., 1999; Rose, 2003; Thomas, 1999; Whitney et al., 1999). Current NCCN guidelines recommend radiation therapy and concurrent cisplatin-based chemotherapy treatment (alone or in combination with 5-fluorouracil) for IIB–IVA disease (Greer et al., 2008).

Completion Surgery After Chemoradiation

Some data suggest that neoadjuvant chemoradiotherapy followed by hysterectomy and excision of grossly positive lymph nodes for stages IB2–II disease improves local control and reduces recurrence rates (Morice et al., 2007). Women who received primary chemoradiation and underwent surgery were found to have residual disease in as many as 60% of pathology specimens. These studies suggest that surgery following chemoradiation for bulky IB tumors decreases recurrence rates, although it has no effect on overall survival (Keys et al., 2003; Paley et al., 2000). Ferrandina et al. (2007) found that local control reached 73% when chemoradiation was followed by surgery, especially in women with IB2 and II staged cancer. However, the woman is exposed to three treatment modalities, each with their own morbidities with no current benefit in overall survival. More studies are needed to show the advantages of this treatment plan.

Stage III–IVB and Recurrent Disease

For women with stage III disease (involving unilateral or bilateral pelvic sidewalls), the prognosis is better for smaller size original tumors (less than 4 cm) and unilateral pelvic sidewall involvement. The recommended treatment of choice is concurrent chemoradiation (Creasman, 1995; Greer et al., 2008).

A woman is classified with stage IVA cervical cancer when disease has spread to adjacent organs (bladder or rectum). The treatment for stage IVA disease is concurrent chemoradiation. This involves intracavitary radiation and external beam radiation combined with cisplatin or fluorouracil (Rose, 2003).

Stage IVB involves disease spread to distant organs, and treatment is considered palliative. Systemic chemotherapy is the treatment modality for IVB or recurrent cervical cancer (Tao et al., 2008).

Approximately 35% of patients with cervical cancer will experience persistent or recurrent disease. The prognosis for these patients is poor with a one-year survival rate of 15%–20% (Cadron et al., 2007). Local recurrence limited to the vagina, uterus, or pelvic cavity most often is discovered within two to three years after initial treatment. The main risk factor associated with a central recurrence is the size of the original tumor. Bulkier tumors were more likely to recur locally. However, recurrences may occur after 10–15 years, and some think these are actually new primary cancers (Eifel, Jhingran, Brown, Levenback, & Thames, 2006). Signs of recurrent disease include (Hacker, 2005)

- Abnormal Pap smear
- A palpable tumor in the pelvis or the abdomen
- Ulceration of the vagina or irradiated cervix
- Pain
- Unilateral lower extremity edema
- Vaginal bleeding or discharge
- Supraclavicular adenopathy
- Ascites
- Unexplained weight loss
- Progressive ureteral obstruction
- Cough.

The most common distant sites for metastases are the lungs, para-aortic lymph nodes, and bones (Panek et al., 2007). The main risk factor for distant recurrences is parametrial disease at the time of original staging (Werner-Wasik et al., 1995). Recurrent cervical cancer has a very poor prognosis. Average survival is nine months following a recurrence, even with treatment (Pectasides, Kamposioras, Papaxoinis, & Pectasides, 2008). If the woman with recurrent cervical cancer has not received prior RT, chemoradiation may offer a chance for cure. RT can be targeted to unradiated areas for palliation. Those women with a central recurrence after RT may be candidates for pelvic exenteration (Eifel et al., 2006). See Chapter 12 for a more complete discussion of this complicated treatment modality.

As previously stated, chemotherapy is the appropriate treatment modality for IVB and recurrent cervical cancer. Cisplatin has shown the most activity in cervical cancer, with a response rate of 13%–19%, progression-free survival of 2.8–3.2 months, and overall survival of 6.5–8.8 months

(Moore, 2008). Other single-agent regimens have been studied without any increase in survival or decrease in toxicity (Tao et al., 2008). The GOG studied different agents in combination with cisplatin, but much work needs to be done to identify better regimens. The addition of topotecan showed benefit (an increase in survival time by 2.9 months) but also showed bone marrow suppression and less activity in those who previously have received cisplatin in combination with RT (Monk et al., 2009). Currently, a multicenter GOG study is assessing the activity of several regimens (cisplatin plus different agents) to find a regimen with more activity for advanced and recurrent cervical cancer (Tao et al.). In the meantime, patients may be included in clinical trials in addition to receiving current cisplatin regimens (Pecorelli & Odicino, 2003; Randall et al., 2005; Rose, 2003).

Follow-Up Care

Women treated for cervical cancer must have regular follow-up. NCCN guidelines recommend that women should be evaluated every three months for one year, every four months the following year, every six months for the next three years and then annually. These visits should include interval history, physical examination, and Pap smears. No current recommendations include regular chest x-rays, but imaging should be ordered for any suspected recurrence (Greer et al., 2008).

Special Situations

Cervical Cancer and Pregnancy

Invasive cervical cancer occurs in 0.05% of pregnancies (ACS, 2008). The primary symptom, as in nonpregnant patients, is bleeding. This is often attributed to pregnancy complications. All pregnant women should be screened with a Pap smear at initiation of care, and abnormalities should be evaluated employing colposcopy (Swensen et al., 2004). A cone biopsy should be performed if invasion is suspected, but the woman must be aware of the potential for miscarriage. If invasive cancer is diagnosed during pregnancy, management is dependent on the stage of the disease as well as the gestational age of the fetus. Careful multidisciplinary care plans must be developed with the obstetricians, neonatologists, and oncologists. The patient and her family must always be fully informed about her choices and their consequences for both herself and her baby. MRI can be safely used in pregnancy to help with treatment plans. Cervical cancer diagnosed up to 20 weeks of pregnancy ideally should be treated immediately. The patient should be offered definitive surgical treatment including radical hysterectomy with the pregnancy left in situ or chemoradiation. Clearly, both options would mean termination of the pregnancy. If the patient is unwilling to terminate the pregnancy, studies have shown that delaying treatment to complete the pregnancy does not have an effect on survival in early-stage cervical cancer (Sood et al., 2000). However, the effect of delaying treatment on the prognosis is unclear for more advanced cancer. Patients who are diagnosed after 28 weeks can delay treatment until delivery. Alternatively, neoadjuvant chemotherapy may be considered to prevent progression of disease. To avoid birth defects, chemotherapy should not be given until after 12 weeks of pregnancy (Greer et al., 2008). Short-term follow up of women treated with chemotherapy during pregnancy has not demonstrated any congenital defects; however, long-term studies are not available (Swensen et al.). Delivery once fetal lung maturity is accomplished is recommended. Patients with invasive cervical cancer should have Caesarean section births to avoid hemorrhage of the dilating cancerous cervix. A Caesarean radical hysterectomy and lymphadenectomy is the treatment of choice for patients with stage IA2–IIA disease once fetal lung maturity is achieved (ACS, 2008; Creasman, 1995; Hacker, 2005; Pecorelli, 2000; Randall et al., 2005; Swensen et al.).

Incidental Disease

For women who have surgery for an assumed benign gynecologic reason and are given a diagnosis of invasive cervical cancer, further treatment is based on the extent of disease. Workup should include a history and physical, complete blood count with platelets, liver and kidney function tests, CXR, MRI, and CT or PET/CT. Patients with microinvasive (IA1) disease who had a simple hysterectomy require no further treatment. Women whose pathology showed microinvasion plus LVSI should receive treatment based on margin status. If the surgical margins were negative, completion surgery (e.g., radical parametrectomy, upper vaginectomy, and lymphadenectomy) or chemoradiation is recommended. If the woman had a supracervical hysterectomy, either a trachelectomy with lymphadenectomy, provided she is otherwise healthy, or RT that includes vaginal brachytherapy should be performed. Positive vaginal margins should be treated with brachytherapy (Greer et al., 2008). Treatment is more complicated in cervical stump cancer regardless of treatment modality. For women with more advanced disease who are no longer surgical candidates, chemoradiation is warranted (Randall et al., 2005).

Palliative Care

Palliative care for progressive disease is challenging. Symptoms are consistent with the location of the disease and often cause embarrassment and pain. Symptoms may include

- Ulceration of the cervix or vagina that may cause discharge and foul odor

- Tissue necrosis or invasion into vessels that may cause hemorrhage
- Fistulas from the bladder or rectum that may develop into the vagina causing urine or stool incontinence
- Pain can be a result of invasion into the lumbar sacral plexus, soft tissues of the pelvis, or bony metastasis
- Ureteral involvement that may cause hydronephrosis and eventual kidney failure.

Providing adequate pain control, autonomy, and comfort with dignity for the patient is the ultimate goal of palliative care (Cain, Heintz, & Swarte, 1995; Rose, Blessing, Gershenson, & McGehee, 1999).

Future Directions

Many questions remain unanswered in the treatment of cervical cancer regardless of stage. Radiation for treatment of cervical cancer is limited by the fact that cervical tumors are often hypoxic, whereas radiation works best with oxygen perfused tumors. The GOG phase III trial evaluating a new chemotherapeutic agent (tirapazamine) has shown greater effect in hypoxic tissue (Morice et al., 2007). Minimally invasive and fertility-sparing surgical techniques are innovative and provide hope for less morbidity and a better quality of life but need further study and refining of techniques. If studies continue to show equivalence to radical hysterectomy, these fertility-sparing and more cosmetically appealing techniques may become the new standard of care.

The value of PET/CT in the diagnosis of primary cervical cancer and recurrence needs to be defined. It is becoming more common for initial staging as well as to aid in identifying recurrence because PET/CT is more sensitive than traditional CT or MRI in detecting lymphatic spread. Because lymphatic spread is one of the main mechanisms for metastasis of cervical cancer, this is significant. Brooks et al. (2009) suggest that using PET for surveillance can identify recurrence when the patient is asymptomatic and the tumor is localized. Medicare includes cervical cancer as one of the diagnoses for which they will pay for PET; therefore, it is becoming more common. As imaging improves and becomes more widely available, official staging criteria may incorporate more radiologic methods to aid in the correct diagnosis and optimal management of patients (Gold, 2008).

Of particular interest are studies of recurrent cervical cancer where management is a challenge. The current standard of treatment for recurrent disease is single-agent cisplatin. However, studies are currently evaluating combined regimens, for example, cisplatin plus topotecan. A current phase III trial within the GOG evaluates different combinations to discover the most effective one for recurrent disease (Moore, 2008).

Biologic agents are a new possibility in management of cervical, especially recurrent, cancer. Bevacizumab, a recombinant, humanized, anti-VEGF, monoclonal antibody, has been shown to inhibit the growth of solid tumors by cutting off their blood supply. Studies adding bevacizumab to chemotherapeutic regimens for recurrent and persistent cervical cancer are under way (GOG 227C) (Monk et al., 2009). Another biologic agent that has been identified as a possible addition to treatment for recurrent disease is erlotinib. Erlotinib is a tyrosine kinase (epidermal growth factor) inhibitor. GOG 227D is evaluating its use for the treatment of recurrent disease (Cadron et al., 2007).

Summary

Cervical cancer is a disease that presents opportunities and challenges for nurses during its trajectory from prevention to end-stage care. There have been many significant developments in cervical cancer treatment but still many unmet needs. Cervical cancer is one of the only cancers for which a screening test and a preventive vaccine are available. Nurses are involved in educating patients and the public about the importance of regular screening that can help to prevent this disease or find it in its early, most treatable form. Primary prevention, in the form of the HPV vaccine, is now available but is not universally accepted. Nurses can be involved in public education and reforming public policy with regard to the vaccination of appropriate candidates, particularly the underserved who may not have access to care or the ability to pay for the vaccine and may be at higher risk of developing the disease. Nurses have a role in secondary prevention, with education regarding early diagnosis, the importance of regular gynecologic follow-up of cervical cancer, and prevention of sequelae. Tertiary prevention seeks to limit the degree of disability. Here, nurses interact with women at all stages of cervical cancer to help improve their quality of life in areas of pain management, sexual function, fertility preservation, lymphedema management, and hygiene and self-care.

Many quality-of-life studies of patients after cervical cancer noted that these women perceived that they were not given enough information about short- and long-term side effects (Clemmens et al., 2008; Vistad et al., 2006). Providing women with information and anticipatory guidance through all phases of diagnosis and treatment is a key role for nurses who are involved in caring for patients with cervical cancer. Nurses also contribute to the care of women who participate in research studies that seek to identify emerging treatments for cervical cancer. Finally, nurses are involved in the discussions of palliative care and hospice with women and their families at the end stage of disease. Nurses seek to ensure each woman's maximum quality of life and dignity in death.

References

Abu-Rustum, N.R., & Sonoda, Y. (2007). Fertility-sparing radical abdominal trachelectomy for cervical carcinoma. *Gynecologic Oncology, 104*(2, Suppl. 1), 56–59.

American Cancer Society. (2008). *What are the key statistics about cervical cancer?* Retrieved May 5, 2009, from http://www.cancer.org/docroot/CRI/content/CRI_2_4_1X_What_are_the_key_statistics_for_cervical_cancer_8.asp

Apgar, B.S., Rubin, M.M., & Brotzman, G.L. (2002). Principles and technique of the colposcopic examination. In B.S. Apgar, G.L. Brotzman, & M. Spitzer (Eds.), *Colposcopy principles and practice* (pp. 115–132). Philadelphia: Saunders.

Atlan, D., Touboul, E., Deniaud-Alexandre, E.D., Lefranc, J.P., Antoine, J.M., Jannett, D., et al. (2002). Operable stages IB and II cervical carcinomas: A retrospective study comparing preoperative uterovaginal brachytherapy and postoperative brachytherapy. *International Journal of Radiation Oncology, Biology, Physics, 54*(3), 780–793.

Brand, A.H., Bull, C.A., & Cakir, B. (2006). Vaginal stenosis in patients treated with radiotherapy for carcinoma of the cervix. *International Journal of Gynecological Cancer, 16*(1), 288–293.

Brooks, R.A., Rader, J.S., Dehdashti, F., Mutch, D.G., Powell, M.A., Thaker, P.H., et al. (2009). Surveillance FDG-PET detection of asymptomatic recurrences in patients with cervical cancer. *Gynecologic Oncology, 112*(1), 104–109.

Bruner, D.W., Lanciano, R., Keegan, M., Corn, B., Martin, E., & Hanks, G.E. (1993). Vaginal stenosis and sexual function following intracavitary radiation for the treatment of cervical and endometrial carcinoma. *International Journal of Radiation Oncology, Biology, Physics, 27*(4), 825–830.

Cain, J.M., Heintz, P.M., & Swarte, N.B. (1995). End of life care. In W.J. Hoskins, C.A. Perez, R.C. Young, R.R. Barakat, M. Markman, & M.E. Randall (Eds.), *Principles and practice of gynecologic oncology* (4th ed., pp. 1343–1359). Philadelphia: Lippincott Williams & Wilkins.

Cadron, I., Van Gorp, T., Amant, F., Leunen, K., Neven, P., & Vergote, I. (2007). Chemotherapy for recurrent cervical cancer. *Gynecologic Oncology, 107*(1, Suppl. 1), S113–S118.

Clemmens, D.A., Knafl, K., Lev, E.L., & McCorkle, R. (2008). Cervical cancer: Patterns of long-term survival. *Oncology Nursing Forum, 35*(6), 897–903.

Creasman, W.T. (1995). New gynecologic cancer staging. *Gynecologic Oncology, 58*(2), 157–158.

Dargent, D., Brun, J., Roy, M., & Remi, I. (1994). Pregnancies following radical trachelectomy for invasive cervical cancer. *Gynecologic Oncology, 54*(1), 105.

Donovan, K.A., Taliaferro, L.A., Alvarez, E.M., Jacobsen, P.B., Roetzheim, R.G., & Wenham, R.M. (2007). Sexual health in women treated for cervical cancer: Characteristics and correlates. *Gynecologic Oncology, 104*(2), 428–434.

Eifel, P.J., Jhingran, A., Brown, J., Levenback, C., & Thames, H. (2006). Time course and outcome of central recurrence after radiation therapy for carcinoma of the cervix. *International Journal of Gynecologic Cancer, 16*(3), 1106–1111.

Estape, R.E., Angioli, R., Madrigal, M., Janicek, M., Gomez, C., Penalaver, M., et al. (1998). Close vaginal margins as a prognostic factor after radical hysterectomy. *Gynecologic Oncology, 68*(3), 229–232.

Ferrandina, G., Legge, F., Fagotti, A., Fanfani, F., Distefano, M., Morganti, A., et al. (2007). Preoperative concomitant chemoradiotherapy in locally advanced cervical cancer: Safety, outcome, and prognostic measures. *Gynecologic Oncology, 107*(1, Suppl. 1), S127–S132.

Finan, M.A., DeCesare, S., Fiorica, J.V., Chambers, R., Hoffman, M.S., Kline, R.C., et al. (1996). Radical hysterectomy for stage IB1 vs. IB2 carcinoma of the cervix: Does the new staging system predict morbidity and survival? *Gynecologic Oncology, 62*(2), 139–147.

Fiorica, J.V., Roberts, W.S., Greenberg, H., Hoffman, M.S., LaPolla, J.P., & Cavanagh, D. (1990). Morbidity and survival patterns in patients after radical hysterectomy and postoperative adjuvant pelvic radiotherapy. *Gynecologic Oncology, 36*(3), 343–347.

Gil-Moreno, A., Puig, O., Perez-Benavente, M.A., Diaz, B., Verges, R., De la Torre, J., et al. (2005). Total laparoscopic radical hysterectomy (type II–III) with pelvic lymphadenectomy in early invasive cervical cancer. *Journal of Minimally Invasive Gynecology, 12*(2), 113–120.

Gold, M.A. (2008). PET in cervical cancer—implications for "staging," treatment planning, assessment of prognosis, and prediction of response. *Journal of the National Comprehensive Cancer Network, 6*(1), 37–45.

Gray, H.J. (2008). Primary management of early stage cervical cancer (IA1–IB) and appropriate selection of adjuvant therapy. *Journal of the National Comprehensive Cancer Network, 6*(1), 47–52.

Greene, F.L., Page, D.L., Fleming, I.D., Fritz, A.G., Balch, C.M., Haller, D.G., et al. (Eds.). (2002). *AJCC cancer staging manual* (6th ed.). New York: Springer.

Greer, B.E., Koh, W.J., Abu-Rustum, N., Bookman, M.A., Bristow, R.E., Campos S., et al. (2008). Cervical cancer, clinical practice guidelines in oncology. *Journal of the National Comprehensive Cancer Network, 6*(1), 14–36.

Grigsby, P.W., & Perez, C.A. (1991). Radiotherapy alone for medically inoperable carcinoma of the cervix: Stage IA and carcinoma in situ. *International Journal of Radiation Oncology, Biology, Physics, 21*(2), 375–378.

Hacker, N.F. (2005). Cervical cancer. In J.S. Berek & N.F. Hacker (Eds.), *Practical gynecologic oncology* (4th ed., pp. 337–395). Philadelphia: Lippincott Williams & Wilkins.

Herrero, R., Hildesheim, A., Bratti, C., Sherman, M.E., Hutchinson, M., Morales, J., et al. (2000). Population-based study of human papillomavirus infection and cervical neoplasia in rural Costa Rica. *Journal of the National Cancer Institute, 92*(6), 464–474.

Hertel, H., Kohler, C., Michels, W., Possover, M., Tozzi, R., & Schneider, A. (2003). Laparoscopic-assisted radical vaginal hysterectomy (LARVH): Prospective evaluation of 200 patients with cervical cancer. *Gynecologic Oncology, 90*(3), 505–511.

Hricak, H., Gatsonis, C., Chi, D.S., Amendola, M.A., Brandt, K., Schwartz, L.H., et al. (2005). Role of imaging in pretreatment evaluation of early invasive cervical cancer: Results of the intergroup study American College of Radiology Imaging Network 6651–Gynecologic Oncology Group 183. *Journal of Clinical Oncology, 23*(36), 9329–9337.

Idestrom, M., Milsom, I., Andersson-Ellstrom, A., & Athlin, E. (2006). Cervical cancer screening—"For better or worse . . .": Women's experience of screening. *Cancer Nursing, 29*(6), 453–460.

Jackson, K.S., Das, N., Naik, R., Lopes, A.D., Godfrey, K.A., Hatem, M.H., et al. (2004). Laparoscopically assisted radical vaginal hysterectomy vs. radical abdominal hysterectomy for cervical cancer: A match controlled study. *Gynecologic Oncology, 95*(3), 655–661.

Keys, H.M., Bundy, B.N., Stehman, F.B., Muderspach, L.I., Chafe, W.E., Suggs, C.L., III, et al. (1999). Cisplatin, radiation, and adjuvant hysterectomy compared with radiation and adjuvant hysterectomy for bulky stage IB cervical carcinoma. *New England Journal of Medicine, 340*(15), 1154–1161.

Keys, H.M., Bundy, B.N., Stehman, F.B., Okagaki, T., Gallup, D.G., Burnett, A.F., et al. (2003). Radiation therapy with and without extrafascial hysterectomy for bulky stage IB cervical carcinoma: A randomized trial of the Gynecologic Oncology Group. *Gynecologic Oncology, 89*(3), 343–353.

Kleinerman, R.A., Kosary, C., & Hildesheim, A. (2006). New malignancies following cancer of the cervix uteri, vagina and vulva. In R.E. Curtis, D.M. Freedman, E. Ron, L.A.G. Ries, D.G. Hacker, B.K. Edwards, et al. (Eds.), *New malignancies among cancer survivors: SEER Cancer Registries, 1973–2000* [NIH Publication No. 05-5302] (pp. 207–229). Bethesda, MD: National Cancer Institute. Retrieved March 30, 2009, from http://seer.cancer.gov/publications/mpmono/Ch08_Uteri.pdf

Kristensen, G.B., Abeler, V.M., Risberg, B., Trop, C., & Bryne, M. (1999). Tumor size, depth of invasion, and grading of the invasive tumor front are the main prognostic factors in early squamous cell cervical carcinoma. *Gynecologic Oncology, 74*(2), 245–251.

Lagasse, L.D., Creasman, W.T., Shingleton, H.M., Ford, J.H., & Blessing, J.A. (1980). Results and complications of operative staging in cervical cancer: Experience of the Gynecologic Oncology Group. *Gynecologic Oncology, 9*(1), 90–98.

Lai, C.H., Huang, K.G., Hong, J.H., Lee, C.L., Chou, H.H., Chang, T.C., et al. (2003). Randomized trial of surgical staging (extraperitoneal or laparoscopic) versus clinical staging in locally advanced cervical cancer. *Gynecologic Oncology, 89*(1), 160–167.

Lanciano, R.M., Pajak, T.F., Martz, K., & Hanks, G.E. (1993). The influence of treatment time on outcome for squamous cell cancer of the uterine cervix treated with radiation: A patterns-of-care study. *International Journal of Radiation Oncology, Biology, Physics, 25*(3), 391–397.

Landoni, F., Maneo, A., Colombo, A., Placa, F., Milani, R., Perego, P., et al. (1997). Randomised study of radical surgery versus radiotherapy for stage Ib–IIa cervical cancer. *Lancet, 350*(9077), 535–540.

LaPolla, J.P., Schlaerth, J.B., Gaddis, O., & Morrow, C.P. (1986). The influence of surgical staging on the evaluation and treatment of patients with cervical carcinoma. *Gynecologic Oncology, 24*(2), 194–206.

Leitao, M.M., & Chi, D.S. (2005). Fertility-sparing options for patients with gynecologic malignancies. *Oncologist, 10*(8), 613–622.

Lowe, M.P., Chamberlain, D.H., Kamelle, S.A., Johnson, P.R., & Tillmanns, T.D. (2009). A multi-institutional experience with robotic-assisted radical hysterectomy for early stage cervical cancer. *Gynecologic Oncology, 113*(2), 191–194.

Malzoni, M., Tinelli, R., Cosentino, F., Perone, C., & Vicario, V. (2007). Feasibility, morbidity, and safety of total laparoscopic radical hysterectomy with lymphadenectomy: Our experience. *Journal of Minimally Invasive Gynecology, 14*(5), 584–590.

Marnitz, S., Kohler, C., Roth, C., Fuller, J., Hinkelbein, W., & Schneider, A. (2005). Is there a benefit of pretreatment laparoscopic transperitoneal surgical staging in patients with advanced cervical cancer? *Gynecologic Oncology, 99*(3), 536–544.

Mathevet P., Laslo de Kaszon, E., & Dargent, D. (2003). Préservation de fertilité dans le premier cancer cervical [Fertility preservation in early cervical cancer]. *Gynécologie, Obstétrique et Fertilité, 31*(9), 706–712.

Molano, M., Posso, H., Weiderpass, E., van den Brule, A.J., Ronderos, M., Franceschi, S., et al. (2002). Prevalence and determinants of HPV infection among Colombian women with normal cytology. *British Journal of Cancer, 87*(3), 324–333.

Monk, B.J., Sill, M.W., Burger, R.A., Gray, H.J., Buekers, T.E., & Roman, L.D. (2009). Phase II trial of bevacizumab in the treatment of persistent or recurrent squamous cell carcinoma of the cervix: A gynecologic oncology group study. *Journal of Clinical Oncology, 27*(7), 1069–1074.

Moore, D.H. (2008). Chemotherapy for advanced, recurrent and metastatic cervical cancer. *Journal of the National Comprehensive Cancer Network, 6*(1), 53–57.

Morice, P., Uzan, C., Zafrani, Y., Delpech, Y., Gouy, S., & Haie-Meder, C. (2007). The role of surgery after chemoradiation therapy and brachytherapy for stage IB2–II cervical cancer. *Gynecologic Oncology, 107*(1, Suppl. 1), S122–S124.

Morris, M., Eifel, P.J., Lu, J., Grigsby, P. W., Levenback, C., Stevens, R.E., et al. (1999). Pelvic radiation with concurrent chemotherapy compared with pelvic and para-aortic radiation for high-risk cervical cancer. *New England Journal of Medicine, 340*(15), 1137–1143.

Nag, S., Chao, C., Erickson, B., Fowler, J., Gupta, N., Martinez, A., et al. (2002). The American Brachytherapy Society recommendations for low-dose-rate brachytherapy for carcinoma of the cervix. *International Journal of Radiation Oncology, Biology, Physics, 52*(1), 33–48.

Nag, S., Erickson, B., Thomadsen, B., Orton, C., Demanes, J.D., & Petereit, D. (2000). The American Brachytherapy Society recommendations for high-dose-rate brachytherapy for carcinoma of the cervix. *International Journal of Radiation Oncology, Biology, Physics, 48*(1), 201–211.

Obermair, A., Gebski, V., Frumovitz, M., Soliman, P.T., Schmeler, K.M., Levenback, C., & Ramirez, P.T. (2008). A phase III randomized clinical trial comparing laparoscopic or robotic radical hysterectomy with abdominal radical hysterectomy in patients with early stage cervical cancer. *Journal of Minimally Invasive Gynecology, 15*(5), 584–588.

Owens, S., Roberts, W.S., Fiorica, J.V., Hoffman, M.S., LaPolla, J.P., & Cavanagh, D. (1989). Ovarian management at the time of radical hysterectomy for cancer of the cervix. *Gynecologic Oncology, 35*(3), 349–351.

Paley, P.J., Goff, B.A., Minudri, R., Greer, B.E., Tamimi, H.K., & Koh, W.J. (2000). The prognostic significance of radiation dose and residual tumor in the treatment of barrel-shaped endophytic cervical carcinoma. *Gynecologic Oncology, 76*(3), 373–379.

Panek, G., Gawrychowski, K., Sobiczewski, P., Derlatka, P., Danska-Bidzinska, A., Gmyrek, L., et al. (2007). Results of chemotherapy for pulmonary metastases of carcinoma of the cervix in patients after primary surgical and radiotherapeutic management. *International Journal of Gynecologic Cancer, 17*(5), 1056–1061.

Partridge, E.E., Abu-Rustum, N., Campos, S., Fahey, P.J., Greer, B.E., Lele, S.M., et al. (2008). Cervical cancer screening. *Journal of the National Comprehensive Cancer Network, 6*(1), 58–82.

Pearcey, R., Brundage, M., Drouin, P., Jeffrey, J., Johnston, D., Lukka, H., et al. (2002). Phase III trial comparing radical radiotherapy with and without cisplatin chemotherapy in patients with advanced squamous cell cancer of the cervix. *Journal of Clinical Oncology, 20*(4), 966–972.

Pecorelli, S. (2000). Cancer of the cervix uteri. *International Journal of Gynecology and Obstetrics, 70*, 37–58.

Pecorelli, S., & Odicino, F. (2003). Cervical cancer staging. *Cancer Journal, 9*(5), 390–394.

Pectasides, D., Kamposioras, K., Papaxoinis, G., & Pectasides, E. (2008). Chemotherapy for recurrent cervical cancer. *Cancer Treatment Reviews, 34*(7), 603–613.

Peters, W.A., III, Liu, P.Y., Barrett, R.J., II, Stock, R.J., Monk, B.J., Berek, J.S., et al. (2000). Concurrent chemotherapy and pelvic radiation therapy compared with pelvic radiation therapy alone as adjuvant therapy after radical surgery in high-risk early-stage cancer of the cervix. *Journal of Clinical Oncology, 18*(8), 1606–1613.

Pikaart, D.P., Holloway, R.W., Ahmad, S., Finkler, N.J., Bigsby, G.E., Ortiz, B.H., et al. (2007). Clinical-pathologic and morbidity analyses of Types 2 and 3 abdominal radical hysterectomy for cervical cancer. *Gynecologic Oncology, 107*(2), 205–210.

Piver, M.S., Rutledge, F., & Smith, J.P. (1974). Five classes of extended hysterectomy for women with cervical cancer. *Obstetrics and Gynecology, 44*(2), 265–272.

Potish, R.A., Twiggs, L.B., Okagaki, T., Prem, K.A., & Adcock, L.L. (1985). Therapeutic implications of the natural history of advanced cervical cancer as defined by pretreatment surgical staging. *Cancer, 56*(4), 956–960.

Pretorius, R., Semrad, N., Watring, W., & Fotheringham, N. (1991). Presentation of cervical cancer. *Gynecologic Oncology, 42*(1), 48–53.

Quinn, M.A., Benedet, J.L., Odicino, F., Maisonneuve, P., Beller, U., Creasman, W.T., et al. (2006). Carcinoma of the cervix uteri. FIGO 6th Annual Report on the Results of Treatment in Gynecological Cancer. *International Journal of Gynaecology and Obstetrics, 95*(Suppl. 1), S43–S103.

Ramirez, P.T., Slomovitz, B.M., Soliman, P.T., Coleman, R.L., & Levenback, C. (2006). Total laparoscopic radical hysterectomy and lymphadenectomy: The M. D. Anderson Cancer Center experience. *Gynecologic Oncology, 102*(2), 252–255.

Randall, M.E., Michael, H., Ver Morken, J., & Stehman, F. (2005). Uterine cervix. In W.J. Hoskins, C.A. Perez, R.C. Young, R.R. Barakat, M. Markman, & M.E. Randall (Eds.), *Principles and practice of gynecologic oncology* (4th ed., pp. 743–822). Philadelphia: Lippincott Williams & Wilkins.

Reynolds, R.K. (2002). Squamous cervical cancer: Invasion and microinvasion. In B.G. Apgar, G.L. Brotzman, & M. Spitzer (Eds.), *Colposcopy: Principles and practice* (pp. 279–300). Philadelphia: Saunders.

Ries, L.A.G., Melbert, D., Krapcho, M., Mariotto, A., Miller, B.A., Feuer, E.J., et al. (Eds.). (2007, November). SEER stat fact sheets: Cervix uteri. *SEER cancer statistics review, 1975–2005*. Bethesda, MD: National Cancer Institute. Retrieved March 30, 2009, from http://seer.cancer.gov/statfacts/html/cervix.html

Rose, P.G. (2003). Stage IIB–IVA cancer of the cervix. *Cancer Journal, 9*(5), 404–414.

Rose, P.G., Blessing, J.A., Gershenson, D.M., & McGehee, R. (1999). Paclitaxel and cisplatin as first-line therapy in recurrent or advanced squamous cell carcinoma of the cervix: A Gynecologic Oncology Group study. *Journal of Clinical Oncology, 17*(9), 2676–2680.

Rose, P.G., Bundy, B.N., Watkins, E.B., Thigpen, J.T., Deppe, G., Maiman, M.A., et al. (1999). Concurrent cisplatin-based radiotherapy and chemotherapy for locally advanced cervical cancer. *New England Journal of Medicine, 340*(15), 1144–1153.

Russell, A.H., Shingleton, H.M., Jones, W.B., Fremgen, A., Winchester, W.P., Clive, R., et al. (1996). Diagnostic assessments in patients with invasive cancer of the cervix: A National Patterns of Care Study of the American College of Surgeons. *Gynecologic Oncology, 63*(2), 159–165.

Sardi, J., Vidaurreta, J., Bermudez, A., & di Paola, G. (1999). Laparoscopically assisted Schauta operation: Learning experience at the Gynecologic Oncology Unit, Buenos Aires University Hospital. *Gynecologic Oncology, 75*(3), 361–365.

Saunders, D.M., Ferrier, A.J., & Ryan, J. (1996). Fertility preservation in female oncology patients. *International Journal of Gynecologic Cancer, 6*(3), 161–167.

Schneider, A., & Kohler, C. (2007). Disease-based therapy of patients with cervical cancer. *Gynecologic Oncology, 107*(1, Suppl. 1), S16–S17.

Sedlis, A., Bundy, B.N., Rotman, M.Z., Lentz, S.S., Muderspach, L.I., & Zaino, R.J. (1999). A randomized trial of pelvic radiation therapy versus no further therapy in selected patients with stage IB carcinoma of the cervix after radical hysterectomy and pelvic lymphadenectomy: A Gynecologic Oncology Group Study. *Gynecologic Oncology, 73*(2), 177–183.

Shepherd, J.H. (1996). Cervical and vulva cancer: Changes in FIGO definitions of staging. *British Journal of Obstetrics and Gynaecology, 103*(5), 405–406.

Sonoda, Y., Chi, D. S., Carter, J., Barakat, R.R., & Abu-Rustum, N.R. (2008). Initial experience with Dargent's operation: The radical vaginal trachelectomy. *Gynecologic Oncology, 108*(1), 214–219.

Sood, A.K., Sorosky, J.I., Mayr, N., Anderson, B., Buller, R.E., & Niebyl, J. (2000). Cervical cancer diagnosed shortly after pregnancy: Prognostic variables and delivery routes. *Obstetrics and Gynecology, 95*(6, Pt. 1), 832–838.

Spirtos, N.M., Eisenkop, S.M., Schlaerth, J.B., & Ballon, S.C. (2002). Laparoscopic radical hysterectomy (type III) with aortic and pelvic lymphadenectomy in patients with stage I cervical cancer: Surgical morbidity and intermediate follow-up. *American Journal of Obstetrics and Gynecology, 187*(2), 340–348.

Spirtos, N.M., Schlaerth, J.B., Kimball, R.E., Leiphart, V.M., & Ballon, S.C. (1996). Laparoscopic radical hysterectomy (type III) with aortic and pelvic lymphadenectomy. *American Journal of Obstetrics and Gynecology, 174*(6), 1763–1767.

Stehman, F.B., Ali, S., Keys, H.M., Muderspach, L.I., Chafe, W.E., Gallup, D.G., et al. (2007). Radiation therapy with or without weekly cisplatin for bulky stage 1B cervical carcinoma: Follow-up of a Gynecologic Oncology Group trial. *American Journal of Obstetrics and Gynecology, 197*(5), 503.e1–506.e6.

Swensen, R.E., Goff, B.A., Koh, W.J., Petersdorf, S.H., Douglas, J.G., Swisher, E.M., et al. (2004). Cancer in the pregnant patient. In W.J. Hoskins, C.A. Perez, R.C. Young, R.R. Barakat, M. Markman, & M.E. Randall (Eds.), *Principles and practice of gynecologic oncology* (4th ed., pp. 1279–1312). Philadelphia: Lippincott Williams & Wilkins.

Tao, X., Hu, W., Ramirez, P.T., & Kavanagh, J.J. (2008). Chemotherapy for recurrent and metastatic cervical cancer. *Gynecologic Oncology, 110*(3, Suppl. 2), S67–S71.

Thomas, G.M. (1999). Improved treatment for cervical cancer—concurrent chemotherapy and radiotherapy. *New England Journal of Medicine, 340*(15), 1198–2000.

Trattner, M., Graf, A.H., Lax, S., Forstner, R., Dandachi, N., Haas, J., et al. (2001). Prognostic factors in surgically treated stage Ib–IIb cervical carcinomas with special emphasis on the importance of tumor volume. *Gynecologic Oncology, 82*(1), 11–16.

Trimble, E.L., Harlan, L.C., & Clegg, L.X. (2005). Untreated cervical cancer in the United States. *Gynecologic Oncology, 96*(2), 271–277.

U.S. Centers for Disease Control and Prevention. (2009). *United States cancer statistics: 1999–2005 cancer incidence and mortality data.* Atlanta, GA: Author. Retrieved May 5, 2009, from http://apps.nccd.cdc.gov/uscs

U.S. Department of Health and Human Services. (2002). *Healthy people 2010* (2nd ed.). McLean, VA: International Medical Publishing, Inc.

Vigliotti, A.P., Wen, B.C., Hussey, D.H., Doornbos, J.F., Staples, J.J., Jani, S.K., et al. (1992). Extended field irradiation for carcinoma of the uterine cervix with positive periaortic nodes. *International Journal of Radiation Oncology, Biology, Physics, 23*(3), 501–509.

Vistad, I., Fossa, S.D., & Dahl, A.A. (2006). A critical review of patient-rated quality-of-life studies of long-term survivors of cervical cancer. *Gynecologic Oncology, 102*(3), 563–572.

Werner-Wasik, M., Schmid, C.H., Bornstein, L., Ball, H.G., Smith, D.M., & Madoc-Jones, H. (1995). Prognostic factors for local and distant recurrence in stage I and II cervical carcinoma. *International Journal of Radiation Oncology, Biology, Physics, 32*(5), 1309–1317.

Whitney, C.W., Sause, W., Bundy, B.N., Malfetano, J.H., Hannigan, E.V., Fowler, W.C., et al. (1999). Randomized comparison of fluorouracil plus cisplatin versus hydroxyurea as an adjunct to radiation therapy in stage IIB–IVA carcinoma of the cervix with negative para-aortic lymph nodes: A Gynecologic Oncology Group and Southwest Oncology Group study. *Journal of Clinical Oncology, 17*(5), 1339–1348.

Yang, B.H., Bray, F.I., Parkin, D.M., Sellors, J.W., & Zhang, Z.F. (2004). Cervical cancer as a priority for prevention in different world regions: An evaluation using years of life lost. *International Journal of Cancer, 109*(3), 418–424.

CHAPTER 6

Endometrial Cancer

Sheryl Redlin Frazier, RN, MSN, OCN®

Introduction

Endometrial cancer is a neoplasm that occurs within the lining of the uterus known as the endometrium. A variety of other names commonly are used for this disease such as uterine neoplasm or cancer of the uterus, and lay people may understand it best as a cancer of the womb. It is the most common gynecologic malignancy in the United States and accounts for approximately 199,000 cases per year worldwide (Jemal et al., 2008; Parkin, Bray, Ferlay, & Pisani, 2005). Endometrial cancer is typically a consequence of obesity, and as the obesity epidemic spreads worldwide, there is great concern that the global incidence of endometrial cancer will increase as well (Gaudin & Harding, 2003). The problem of obesity and its relationship with endometrial cancer incidence is seen in epidemiologic studies, which have shown that more than 40% of endometrial cancer cases are attributed to being overweight (Kaaks, Lukanova, & Kurzer, 2002). Generalists' and oncology nurses' role is to promote women's awareness of good health practices in order to prevent and detect this cancer.

Bokhman (1983) described two specific types of endometrial cancer that still are used today. Type I, accounting for 90% of endometrial cancers, is associated with prolonged exposure to estrogen, is typically diagnosed in an early stage, and has an excellent prognosis (Amant et al., 2007). Conversely, type II, accounting for 10% of endometrial cancers, has a poorer prognosis related histologically to a higher grade or poorer differentiation, is more often diagnosed at a late stage, has a propensity for metastases, or is a nonendometrioid subtype such as serous or carcinosarcoma (Amant et al., 2007).

Etiology and Epidemiology

Approximately 70% of endometrial cancers occur among women 45–74 years old, with the median age range being 55–64 (American Cancer Society [ACS], 2008a). The lifetime risk among women in the United States is 1 in 41 (ACS, 2008a). ACS estimated that approximately 40,100 new cases would be diagnosed in 2008. In the United States, the incidence has increased significantly from 1975 to 2004, the most remarkable increase occurring from 1975 to 1992 (National Cancer Institute [NCI], 2007). Mostly nonwhite women account for these increases (NCI), and evidence suggests that black women are more likely to be diagnosed at a later stage and have poorer outcomes (Madison, Schottenfeld, James, Schwartz, & Gruber, 2004).

Globally, the incidence of endometrial cancer is 10 times higher in the developed countries of Europe and North America. It is much less common in less developed areas of the world; however, the mortality rate in these areas is higher (Amant et al., 2005). As the incidence of obesity, consumption of Western diets with high fat content, physical inactivity, and life expectancy increase, an increase is anticipated in the worldwide incidence of this cancer (Amant et al., 2005).

As women age, the incidence increases, peaking around 70 years, then the rate declines somewhat. With increasing age, the risk for being diagnosed with more advanced disease also increases. The Surveillance, Epidemiology and End Results (SEER) data for 1988–2001 for early-stage disease (defined as confined to the endometrium or invading less than 50% of the myometrium), which comprised approximately 70% of the total 42,589 cases reviewed, revealed that 64% were women 20–49 years of age, and women 70 years and older accounted for significantly less early-stage disease (Kosary, n.d.). Conversely, older women are more likely to be diagnosed with stage IV disease (9%) when compared with younger women (5%) (Kosary). The SEER data suggest women 20–69 years of age accounted for 19.3% each of stages II, III, and IV, whereas women who were 70 and older accounted for 25% of those stages (Kosary). (See the Appendix for more information regarding staging.) Age, an independent predictor, is associated with higher tumor grade, deeper invasion, more advanced disease, and poorer treatment outcomes and survival (Jolly et al., 2006). As one might anticipate, the morbidity and mortality increases with age and stage, making early diagnosis a priority in order to achieve good outcomes.

ACS (2008c) estimated that approximately 7,470 women would die from endometrial cancer in 2008. When all stages of endometrial cancer are combined, the relative five-year survival rate is approximately 88% (ACS, 2008c). However, the mortality rate has increased since 1988, which may be in part attributed to high-risk histologic subtypes and an increase in the number of cancers that are diagnosed at advanced stages (Ueda et al., 2008). In general, the more advanced the stage, the poorer the grade, and the more advanced the age (coupled with other morbidities such as hypertension, obesity, and diabetes), the greater the decline in survival rates. Obesity and morbid obesity account for more treatment-related complications, shorter overall survival, and, when compared with other women with endometrial cancer, a higher percentage of death from other comorbid conditions (von Gruenigen et al., 2006). Overall survival is directly associated with the disease stage and grade at diagnosis; for example, women who are diagnosed with stage IA or IB and well-differentiated (grade 1) histology, the survival is 99%–100%, but if the histology is grade 3 or poorly differentiated, the five-year survival decreases to 77% (Kosary, n.d.). Likewise, for stage IV the survival rate can be as low as 16.9% for grade 3 to 59.9% for grade 1 (Kosary). Nurses and other healthcare providers have a powerful role in ensuring that the woman with a concern about or risk factors for endometrial cancer be assessed early and treated by a gynecologic oncologist.

Risk Factors

Obesity

Obesity is the greatest risk factor for development of endometrial cancer. More than 60% of adult women in the United States are overweight, with a body mass index (BMI) of 25 or higher, and 33.2% of them are obese, meaning a BMI of 30 or higher (Ogden et al., 2006). A BMI of 30 or higher is a significant risk factor, 3–5 times the general population's risk, and predictive of developing endometrial hyperplasia and cancer (Kaaks et al., 2002). Even more alarming is the fact that the highest fatality rate of all cancers is seen in obese women with endometrial cancer (von Gruenigen et al., 2006). Women who are obese account for more than half of all women diagnosed with endometrial cancer (Bakkum-Gamez, Gonzales-Bosquet, Laack, Mariani, & Dowdy, 2008).

A relationship exists between obesity and a proportionate increase in the amount of circulating estrogen content in the human body that stimulates the endometrial lining to grow and not be shed during normal menstrual cycling, leading to mutations, hyperplasias, and cancer (Soliman et al., 2005). Unopposed estrogen has a similar effect as obesity on the stimulation of the endometrium. Estrogen acts as a promoter of endometrial cellular growth, and progesterone acts as a protector (Mutter, Zaino, Baak, Bentley, & Robboy, 2007). Before 1975, the year of the first reported results of endometrial cancer incidence related to estrogen replacement therapy (ERT), it was general practice for physicians to prescribe unopposed ERT for treatment of menopausal symptoms (Lacey et al., 2005; Sonoda & Barakat, 2006). Although ERT effectively relieved symptoms, the unexpected result was a sharp increase in the incidence of endometrial cancer among these women who had no other known risk factors. In fact, the risk ranged from a 10–20-fold relative risk (Sonoda & Barakat). As a consequence, today, when hormone replacement therapy (HRT) is prescribed for women who have their uterus in place, estrogen is given in combination therapy with a progestational agent and for short duration only.

Tamoxifen is a selective estrogen-receptor response modulator (SERM) used to decrease the risk of recurrent breast cancer or as a preventive measure in women at high risk for developing breast cancer. However, it has been shown to increase the risk for development of endometrial cancer by 2.53 times (Sonoda & Barakat, 2006). Sonoda and Barakat mentioned that a finding of the 2005 National Surgical Adjuvant Breast and Bowel Project study suggested that uterine sarcomas also may be associated with tamoxifen use. Other SERMs that have been investigated have shown mixed effects on the endometrium; however, raloxifene has repeatedly demonstrated a neutral and, in some cases, antiproliferative effect on endometrial tissue (Shelly, Draper, Krishnan, Wong, & Jaffe, 2008). In the STAR (Study of Tamoxifen and Raloxifene) trial, results showed evidence that the raloxifene arm had less incidence of endometrial cancer and hyperplasia than the tamoxifen arm, but not by a statistically significant amount (Shelly et al.). Arzoxifene, used in breast cancer treatment, has shown some efficacy in a Gynecologic Oncology Group (GOG) phase II trial for treating advanced or recurrent endometrial cancer (Shelly et al.). Many SERMs are in clinical development or already have been tested and demonstrated unsatisfactory adverse effects; nevertheless, when women participate in clinical investigations of this class of medications, nurses need to have a wary eye on the potentially adverse gynecologic effects.

Genetic Predisposition

The majority of endometrial cancers (90%–95%) are not related to heredity but occur sporadically, most frequently the result of an environmental exposure (Bakkum-Gamez et al., 2008). However, a subset of women is at a higher risk for developing endometrial cancer because of inherited genetic mutations. Although this subset accounts for only 3%–5% of all endometrial cancers, the lifetime risk in these women is estimated to be 40%–60% (Sonoda & Barakat, 2006). In families who have hereditary cancer syndromes, such as Lynch syndrome or hereditary nonpolyposis colorectal cancer syndrome, the risk for endometrial cancer is significant (Tiffen & Mahon, 2006). Finding a mutation in the *MLH1* and *MSH2* genes, commonly associated with Lynch syndrome, implies the greatest risk (Tiffen & Mahon). Therefore, any woman diagnosed with endometrial cancer should have a family pedigree reviewed particularly for colon, endometrial, and breast cancer. If a woman's history suggests a genetic link, she should be referred for genetic counseling that may include genetic testing and frequent screenings.

Ethnicity

Ethnic differences exist in the incidence and survival rates among women with endometrial cancer. Although the incidence among black women is less, 19.6 per 100,000 women compared to 24.3 per 100,000 in whites, the mortality rate in black women is nearly twice that of white women, at 7.1 per 100,000 compared to 3.9 per 100,000 (NCI, 2007). In a population study conducted by Madison et al. (2004) in Detroit, Michigan, no differences were found in the age at diagnosis among black and white women, but black women were much more likely to be diagnosed at a later stage, with a higher grade and more aggressive histology, and were 2.33 times more likely to die from their disease than their white counterparts. Black women also have a two to three times higher mortality rate than other ethnicities, including Hispanic, American Indian/Alaska Native, and Asian/Pacific Islanders, although the incidence rates were not significantly different (NCI). A recent review of SEER data by Wright et al. (2009) continues to substantiate the evidence that the survival of black women with endometrial cancer is less than that of other women.

Comorbidity

Several comorbid conditions contribute to the risks for development of endometrial cancer. It has been determined that women with diabetes have a relative risk of 2.7 (Soliman et al., 2005). Hypertension, although a common comorbidity, appeared in the Saltzman et al. (2008) study to demonstrate a two-fold increased risk for developing endometrial cancer when paired with diabetes. The combination of factors that are associated with obesity such as insulin resistance, metabolic syndrome, physical inactivity with high "energy" intake, and blood pressure of 140/90 or greater creates a fertile environment for endometrial cancer (Amant et al., 2005). Nulliparity results an overall relative risk of 2.0 (Soliman et al., 2005).

Polycystic ovarian syndrome, a condition involving a set of clinical symptoms that includes polycystic ovaries and a multifactorial metabolic syndrome, seems to contribute to the risk of development of endometrial cancer, particularly in younger women, although the relationship is not yet fully defined (Kaaks et al., 2002; Soliman et al., 2005). Age is an established risk factor for endometrial cancer and is predictive of poorer survival outcomes (Ueda et al., 2008).

Risk Reduction and Protective Effects

Just as exposure to estrogenic effects increases the risk, progestin exposure seems to decrease risk. Pregnancy, for example, provides an environment rich with placental production of progestins and is believed to add a protective benefit against endometrial cancer (Amant et al., 2005). A direct correlation of risk reduction is associated with a woman's total number of pregnancies; for instance, a woman who has never had a child has a two-fold risk of endometrial cancer compared to a woman who has one child (Sonoda & Barakat, 2006). It is possible to deduce that progesterone exerts a protective effect as seen in parity and when used as a mediator for ERT; however, the use of progestins in HRT for menopausal symptoms has raised serious concerns regarding the safety of using estrogen plus progesterone (Sonoda & Barakat). The findings of two large studies of women, the Women's Health Initiative (WHI) (Rossouw et al., 2002) and the Million Women Study (MWS) (Beral, Bull, & Reeves, 2005), suggest that HRT increases the risk of breast and endometrial cancers. Considering the data from the WHI and MWS studies, the overall incidence of breast cancer among women, and the endometrial cancer risk in women with intact uteri, alternative nonhormonal interventions should be recommended to treat menopausal vasomotor symptoms.

The benefit of the use of oral contraceptives in risk reduction has been attributed to the effect that the progestin content is associated with suppression of endometrial tissue growth. Women who have taken 12–23 months of oral contraception have a 40% risk reduction of endometrial cancer, and if the consumption is over a 10-year period, a 60% reduction (Sonoda & Barakat, 2006). A similar study in Sweden (Weiderpass et al., 1999) showed risk reductions of 30%–80% when oral contraception is taken over 3 years or more and 10 years or more, respectively.

Another contraceptive method, the intrauterine device (IUD), was thought to be a potential inducer of endometrial cancer because of its irritative and inflammatory effects on the endometrium. Recent studies have shown no increased risk of cancer but rather suggest a potential benefit for reduction of risk in users of IUDs (Curtis, Marchbanks, & Peterson, 2007; Tao et al., 2006). Even more intriguing and as-yet unproven is the effect of the progestin-secreting IUD in women on HRT or tamoxifen therapy or as an alternative to surgery for women who have endometrial hyperplasia or cancer and are poor surgical candidates (Curtis et al., 2007). Additional studies of IUDs with or without hormone-releasing capabilities and the benefits for risk reduction of endometrial cancers is warranted.

Endometrial cancer is unusual in that smoking tobacco can have a preventive effect. Studies consistently have shown that smoking is associated with a lowered risk in a variety of high-risk populations such as those with the highest BMI, in postmenopausal women taking HRT, and in diabetics who are not insulin dependent (Sonoda & Barakat, 2006). Data obtained from the Nurses' Health Study supports the risk-reducing benefits of smoking by demonstrating the relative risk of developing endometrial cancer among "never" smokers as being higher than nursing colleagues who were current or past smokers (Sonoda & Barakat, 2006). The nature of this benefit is related to the biologic effect that smoking has on lowering the endogenous levels of estrogen, possibly the alteration of liver metabolism of estrogen, and the effect smoking has on early onset of menopause. None of these benefits outweighs the many detrimental effects of smoking, particularly in women who are obese, diabetic, or hypertensive (Sonoda & Barakat).

The two most important risk reduction measures that women can practice are diet and physical activity. These measures have health maintenance benefits that extend beyond the prevention of endometrial cancer. A well-balanced, healthy diet and moderate physical activity could substantially mitigate the most common risk factors, such as those associated with metabolic syndrome. Studies have reached equivocal conclusions regarding the benefits of physical activity; for example, a Swedish study by Terry et al. (1999) supports the benefit of physical activity in reduction of risk, and data from the European Prospective Investigation Into Cancer and Nutrition reveal empirical evidence that physical activity reduces the risk of endometrial cancer especially among premenopausal women (Friedenreich et al., 2007). Diets high in fat and calories have shown an association with increased risk, and likewise, risks are decreased when diets are rich in fruits, vegetables, and complex carbohydrates (Sonoda & Barakat, 2006). There is some suggestion that isoflavones, lignans, and phytoestrogens have some protective benefit, as evidenced in the research of Goodman et al. (1997) and Horn-Ross, John, Canchola, Stewart, and Lee (2003). Based on these findings, additional larger randomized clinical trials will need to be conducted for confirmation.

Screening

No specific tests or exams are available for early detection of endometrial cancer for women at average risk; however, ACS recommends regular Pap tests for women for detection of other types of gynecologic cancers (ACS, 2008b). Screening for endometrial cancer is only considered beneficial in women who meet the highest at-risk categories already described (see Figure 6-1). In this subset of women, annual screening can begin at 35 years of age and would include transvaginal ultrasound and endometrial biopsy (ACS, 2008b).

Clinical Presentation and Diagnostic Evaluation

The glandular epithelial tissue lining the inside of the uterus is the functional layer of the endometrium that is responsive to hormonal influence, particularly the systemic abundance of unopposed estrogen that leads to a proliferative endometrium (Mutter et al., 2007). The proliferative endometrium leads to vaginal bleeding, the classic and most frequently reported symptom (Horn, Meinel, Handzel, & Einenkel, 2007). In an environment of chronically unopposed estrogen exposure, the endometrial layer undergoes a progression of abnormal cellular changes from benign endometrial hyperplasia to endometrial intraepithelial neoplasia (EIN) and to endometrial adenocarcinoma (Mutter et al.). EIN, described as a preinvasive glandular proliferation, may at some point become the replacement term in the classification system used to describe the precursor pathologic change that precedes endometrial cancer (Horn et al.). The usefulness of EIN may be in determining when, in the face of high morbidity risks that are encountered in some patients, nonsurgical interventions can be implemented (Horn et al.). Table 6-1 lists the classifications of endometrial hyperplasia.

The diagnostic evaluation of endometrial cancer includes a thorough history and physical examination followed by a pelvic examination. The simplest diagnostic test that may be done in the provider's office is an endometrial biopsy. This biopsy is obtained during the vaginal examination by inserting a Pipelle® (Cooper

Figure 6-1. Risk Factors of Types I and II Endometrial Cancer

Type I
- Age (younger than 50)
- Metabolic syndrome (obesity, diabetes mellitus)
- Nulliparity, infertility
- Irregular menstrual cycles
- Polycystic ovarian syndrome

Type II
- Postmenopause
- Metabolic syndrome (obesity, diabetes mellitus)
- Nulliparity
- Late menopause
- Unopposed exogenous estrogen; sequential use of oral contraceptives
- Tamoxifen therapy

Note. Based on information from Soliman et al., 2005.

Table 6-1. Classification of Endometrial Hyperplasia

Type	Risk of Progression to Endometrial Cancer
Simple	1%
Complex	3.5%
Simple with atypia	~ 8%–10%
Complex with atypia	~ 25%–30%

Note. From "Endometrial Hyperplasia," by S.G. Chudnoff, 2005, *Medscape Ob/Gyn and Women's Health, 10*(1). Retrieved April 25, 2009, from http://www.medscape.com/viewarticle/507187. Copyright 2005 by Medscape. Reprinted with permission.

Surgical, Inc.) through the cervical os and removing a sample of endometrial tissue by applying manual suction to the Pipelle. During the procedure, the provider may use a uterine sound to determine the depth of the uterine cavity. A tenaculum may be used to secure and stabilize the cervix if necessary. An endocervical curettage (ECC) is sometimes obtained if lower uterine segment involvement is a concern (Guido & Stoval, 2007). Once an adequate sampling is obtained and placed in a preservative, it is sent for pathologic examination. See Figure 6-2 for photo of instruments used for biopsy.

The pathologic results of the endometrial biopsy and ECC, if done, are integral in determining the treatment. National Comprehensive Cancer Network (NCCN, 2009) recommends supplementary testing, when endometrial cancer is suspected, to include a complete blood count including a platelet count, a chest x-ray, and a Pap test. If the pathologic finding is of the epithelial type, further treatment decisions are based on the grade and whether it is endometrioid, papillary serous, clear cell, or carcinosarcoma (once referred to as malignant mixed Müllerian cell type or mixed mesodermal tumors) (Wolfson et al., 2007). Endometrial stromal sarcomas and carcinosarcomas are covered in Chapter 9. If the endometrial biopsy is negative for either EIN or cancer, further diagnostic workup for the symptomatic or at-risk patient may include hysteroscopy, dilation and curettage, pelvic ultrasound, or further radiographic testing (e.g., computed tomography [CT], magnetic resonance imaging [MRI]) (NCCN).

Staging

Prior to 1988, endometrial cancer was clinically staged. However, with the improvement in surgical techniques and procedures, the International Federation of Gynecology and Obstetrics (FIGO) adopted a surgical staging system that is in effect today (FIGO, 1989). (Refer to the Appendix for staging and Figure 6-3 for poor prognostic risk factors.) As surgical techniques have advanced, efforts have been increasing toward using minimally invasive procedures such as laparoscopically assisted vaginal hysterectomy (LAVH) or robotic-assisted laparoscopic hysterectomy (RALH), perhaps in part because 75% of these tumors are confined to the uterus (Seamon et al., 2009). Currently, the role of minimally invasive surgery has yet to be defined, and NCCN (2009) recommends this approach be confined to clinical trial investigations until further data are available to adequately support the overall benefits.

Treatment

Surgery

Regardless of the surgical approach, it is highly recommended that women diagnosed with endometrial cancer be referred to a gynecologic oncologist for treatment. GOG conducted a 2,500-patient randomized clinical trial, GOG

Figure 6-2. Instruments Used in Endometrial Biopsy

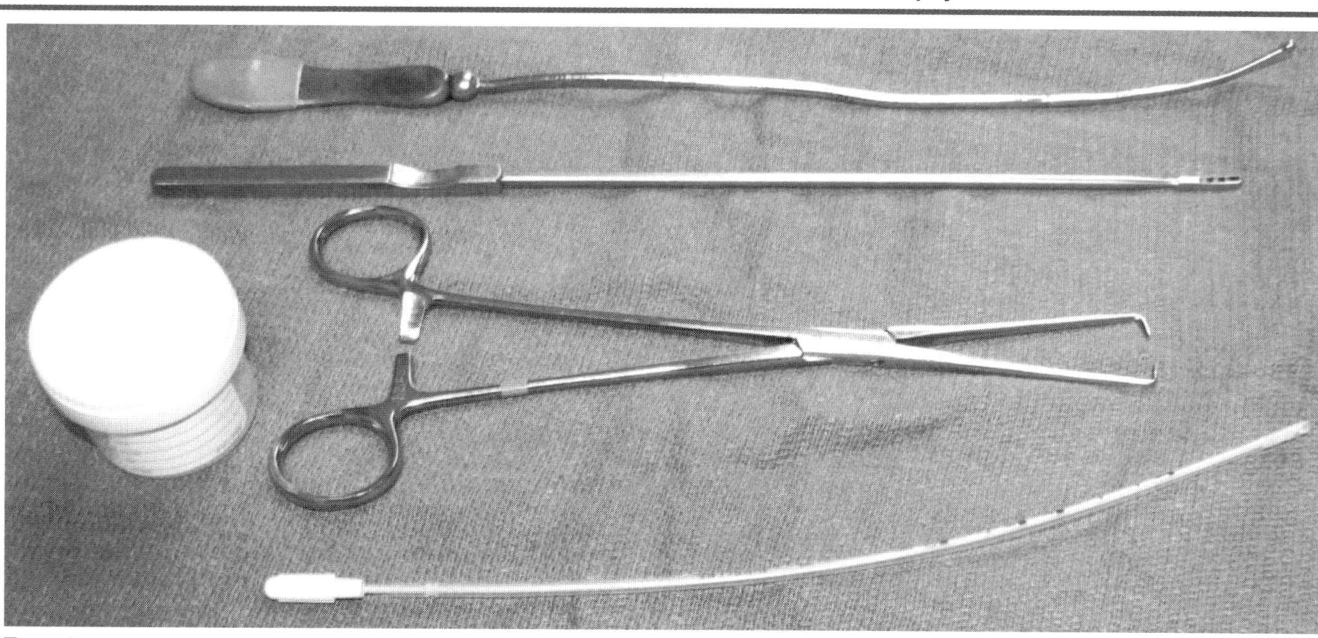

Top to bottom—uterine sound, endocervical curettage, specimen jar, tenaculum used to grasp the cervix for stabilization, and Pipelle® (Cooper Surgical, Inc.).

Note. Photo courtesy of Sheryl Redlin Frazier. Used with permission.

Figure 6-3. Poor Prognostic Predictors

- Advanced disease (stage IC–IV)
- Grade 3 or poorly differentiated histology
- Nonendometrioid cell type (e.g., papillary serous, clear cell)
  - Invasion of vascular space
  - Cervical stroma
  - Myometrium and proximity to serosa
- Positive peritoneal washings
- Lymph node metastases
- Age
- Race
- Obesity
- DNA (*TP53, ERBB2* [HER2/neu], *p53*]
- Recurrent disease

Note. Based on information from Amant et al., 2005; Ferguson et al., 2005; Ueda et al., 2008; Wright et al., 2009.

LAP 2, which compared a laparoscopic approach to an open laparotomy as the initial treatment to endometrial cancer surgery. Although the data from this concluded trial have yet to be published, ever-increasing evidence supports laparoscopy in some subsets of women with endometrial cancer such as early stage and the morbidly obese (Magrina, 2005; NCCN, 2009; Seamon et al., 2009). Results suggest that as many as 76% of a specific subset of women could successfully undergo a minimally invasive surgery, which includes a laparoscopically assisted vaginal hysterectomy, bilateral salpingo-oophorectomy, and exploration and sampling of abdominal lymph nodes (Seamon et al.). However, the length of surgery might be longer than the laparotomy, partly attributable to the learning curve of the surgeon (Holub, Jabor, Bartos, Hendl, & Urbanek, 2003); also, the women who receive laparoscopy have fewer postoperative complications, decreased morbidity, shortened hospital stay, and better quality of life with improved cosmesis (Barakat et al., 2007; Frederick & Straughn, 2009; McAlpine, Spirtos, & Chen, 2002). Minimally invasive surgery requires training and proficiency by the surgeon to obtain adequate lymph node sampling for staging and adequate inspection of the organs of the peritoneum while minimizing risk for injury.

Data suggest that occult cancer will be found during a pathologic examination of the uterus in 40% of women who, prior to surgery, appear to have only endometrial hyperplasia (NCCN, 2009). Based on these data, whenever possible and appropriate, recommended surgery should include a total hysterectomy, bilateral salpingo-oophorectomy, and abdominal staging that includes examination of abdominal organs, pelvic and para-aortic lymph node sampling, and lavage for cytologic examination to determine the presence of peritoneal metastasis (NCCN). The rationale for this thorough surgical staging is based on the most common pattern of spread, which is direct extension through the endometrium to the myometrium to the stroma. Additionally, lymphatic spread may occur to the pelvic and para-aortic lymph nodes via the lymphatic drainage pathways from the uterus. Finally, hematogenous spread can occur via the richly vascular uterine cavity.

Traditionally, a midline vertical incision most frequently is performed by the gynecologic oncologist. This incision is easy to perform; gains faster entry and access to the abdomen; provides for adequate visualization, exploration, and staging; and engenders less blood loss. However, "the midline approach is associated with a higher rate of wound dehiscence" (Berek, 2005, p. 747). In women with endocervical involvement, removal of the upper one-third of the vagina may be performed (NCCN, 2009).

In morbidly obese women, the abdominal approach may be modified based on the size and thickness of the abdominal wall and the size of the pannus (Higgins, Naumann, & Hall, 2007). In some cases, a panniculectomy, or removal of the pannus, is performed to minimize the risk of inadequate exposure of the operative field based on the depth of adipose tissue and limited length of instruments, even when using instruments specifically designed for surgery in the obese abdomen (Higgins et al.). Surgical incisions in the obese abdomen should be chosen above the folds of the pannus, when the panniculectomy is not performed, to improve wound healing and to prevent "button-holing" or going through the pannicular fold (Higgins et al.). In the past, low transverse incisions could be extended in a "J" or hockey-stick incision to gain access to the upper abdomen for exploration and lymph node sampling. Another approach to gain access to para-aortic lymph nodes for dissection is through a paramedian incision (Moore et al., 2008). Figure 6-4 diagrams types of surgical incisions. It is very important for nurses who are providing postoperative care to receive a report detailing the surgical procedure and the incisions made so that an appropriate assessment of the abdomen can be accomplished. Nurses should have an understanding of the risks associated with these incisions particularly in patients who are obese, are older, have comorbid conditions, or are malnourished.

The best technique to ensure adequacy of the surgery and staging is to have the uterus grossly examined in the operating room (see Figure 6-5). In this way, the surgeon and pathologist can determine the best course for the remaining surgery. The pathologist measures the depth of myometrial invasion in relationship to myometrial thickness and the size and location of the tumor and then makes a determination as to whether the disease is in the fundus, lower uterine segment, or cervix. The pathologist examines the specimen(s) microscopically, and the histologic subtype, grade, and presence of lymphovascular space invasion are determined (NCCN, 2009). The benefits of adequate surgical staging and pathologic examination are seen in the final analysis. Accuracy in staging combined with the best prognostic evidence determines the appropriateness of adjuvant therapy (Barakat et al., 2007).

Figure 6-4. Types of Surgical Incisions

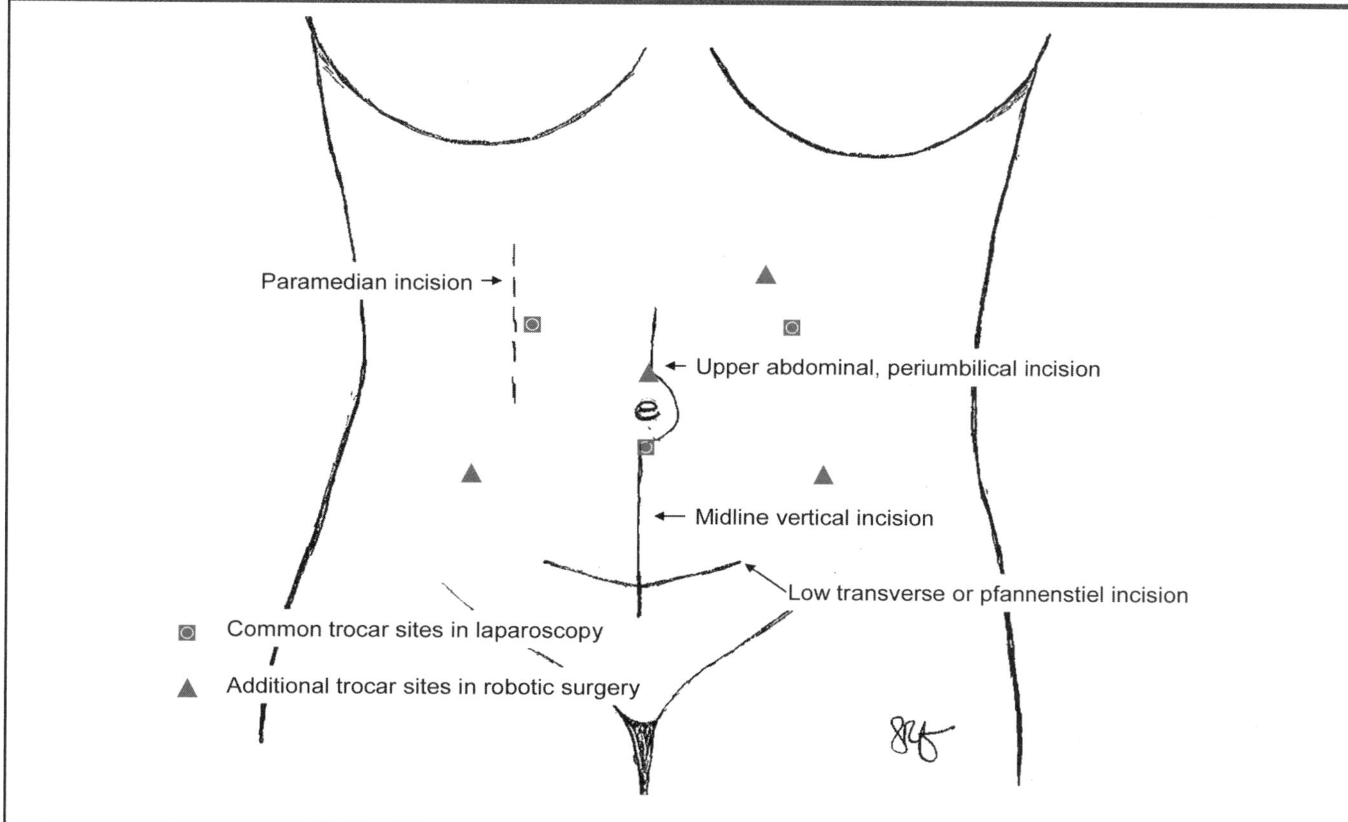

Alternatives to Surgery

When the patient wants to preserve fertility or if the surgical mortality risk is too high to consider surgery, alternative treatments can be considered. Bearing in mind that 25% of endometrial cancers occur in premenopausal women and that 14% of patients are younger than 40 years of age, issues related to the preservation of fertility should be anticipated (Rackow & Arici, 2006). Although not without risk of progression or occult metastases, high-dose progestin therapy, medroxyprogesterone acetate, and megestrol acetate can be used to regress the cancer with response rates ranging 51%–75% while preserving the potential for pregnancy afterward (Rackow & Arici; Shamshirsaz et al., 2007). Recommendations include a thorough evaluation for evidence of disease including examinations, biopsies, CT or MRI, and a surgical exploration with either laparoscopy or laparotomy to evaluate disease status and uncover any metastases (Rackow & Arici).

Hormone Therapy

Agents that have been used to treat advanced, recurrent endometrial cancers, such as tamoxifen, gonadotropin-releasing hormone agonists, and aromatase inhibitors, as yet have not been proven beneficial in the regression of early-stage endometrial cancer (Rackow & Arici). Gotlieb et al. (2003) performed a retrospective review of 13 cases of endometrial cancer in which progestins were used for tumor regression and fertility-sparing treatment. One of the patients who received an initial course of megestrol acetate 160 mg/day for 30 months recurred; then the megestrol dose was increased to 320 mg/day; subsequently, she received a progestin-secreting IUD and achieved another 39 months, remaining disease free at the time of publication (Gotlieb et al.). The use of a progestin-secreting IUD has been further explored in cases where surgical morbidity prevents traditional treatment. Montz, Bristow, Bovicelli, Tomacruz, and Kurman (2002) conducted a small trial of a progestin-secreting IUD in women diagnosed with early endometrial cancer who were poor surgical candidates, and the outcome was negative endometrial biopsy results ranging from three months to three years. Although this trial was small, it demonstrates that progestin-secreting IUD is a viable alternative to the morbidity of a staging surgery in high-risk surgical patients (Montz et al.).

Radiation

Radiation therapy is used as an adjunct to surgery with the goal being to target the radiation to the regions of the pelvic

Figure 6-5. Gross Specimen of Uterus Containing Endometrial Carcinoma

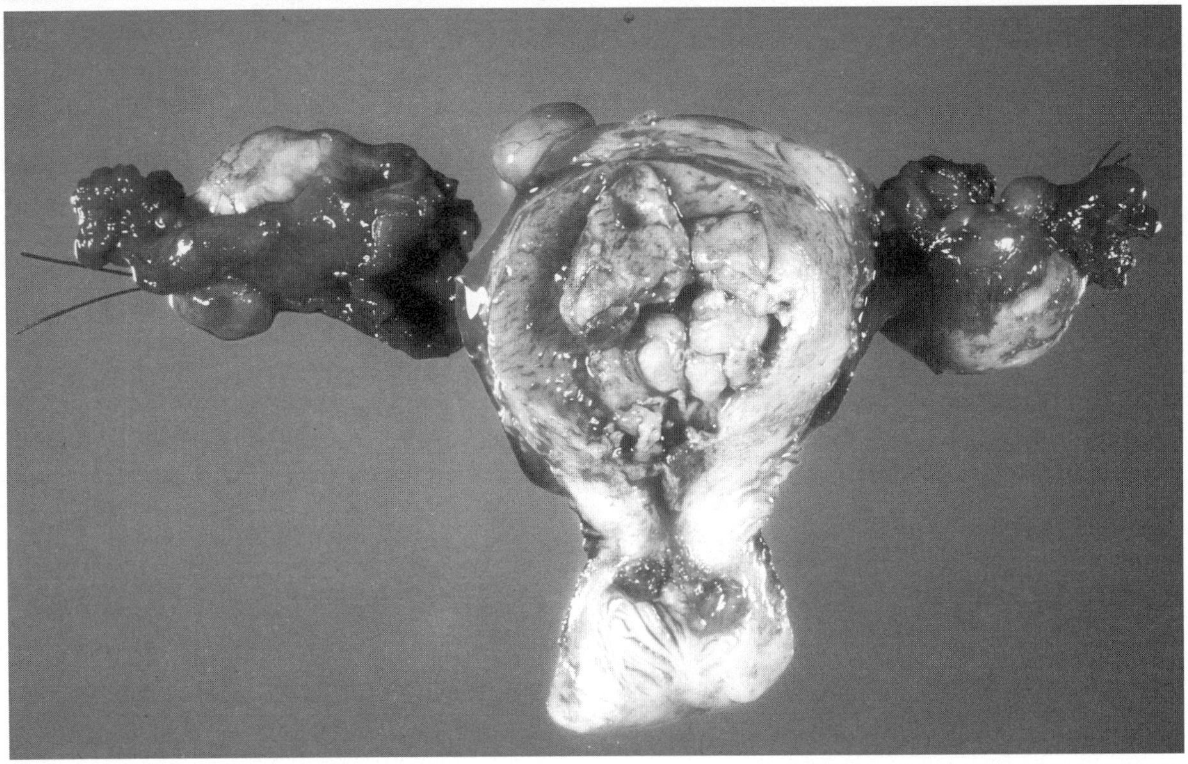

Note. Photo courtesy of Martha Ann Crispens, MD, FACOG, Assistant Professor, Vanderbilt University Medical Center, Division of Gynecologic Oncology. Used with permission.

lymph nodes, which has shown to be beneficial in the reduction of pelvic recurrences (Amant et al., 2005). The use of radiation therapy has been widely variable, but recent trials, the PORTEC (Postoperative Radiation Therapy in Endometrial Carcinoma) trial in particular, are beginning to demonstrate that following adequate staging surgery, recurrence rates may not be statistically significant between groups who receive radiation and those who do not (Creutzberg et al., 2003). Whole pelvic radiation usually is recommended in women who do not undergo adequate staging, meet poor prognostic criteria, are at increased risk for recurrence, and have Stage IC, grade 3 or greater disease (Amant et al., 2005) (see Figure 6-3), or perhaps when the area of recurrence is isolated. Intravaginal radiation therapy (IVRT) or vaginal brachytherapy with iridium or cesium isotopes in a high dose rate or low dose rate are used to prevent or treat recurrence at the vaginal cuff, the area of greatest risk of recurrence (Jolly et al., 2006). IVRT is used most commonly in stages IB–IIB with excellent treatment outcomes of 95% (Bakkum-Gamez, Gonzales-Bosquet, Laack, Mariani, & Dowdy, 2008). Nurses should not underestimate the physiologic and psychological effects of IVRT. Women who receive this treatment should be counseled carefully prior to treatment with a mindfulness that this may be humiliating, disturbing, and in cases of previous sexual abuse, an exceptionally difficult treatment. Women will be advised to use vaginal dilators to maintain vaginal patency and to prevent agglutination. Women who are sensitive or embarrassed about using dilators require frequent intervention and support.

Chemotherapy

The role of chemotherapy in the treatment of endometrial cancer is complex and evolving. At one time, whole abdominal irradiation (WAI) was the treatment of choice for advanced, para-aortic node-positive endometrial cancer. However, a randomized, phase III GOG trial found that when WAI was compared with combination cisplatin and doxorubicin chemotherapy, the chemotherapy arm demonstrated higher overall response rates and progression-free survival rates (Alvarez Secord et al., 2007). A second GOG trial demonstrated a benefit in the combination of doxorubicin and cisplatin in advanced endometrial cancer (Thigpen et al., 2004). In 1998, GOG 177 was opened for enrollment comparing cisplatin and doxorubicin to cisplatin, doxorubicin, and paclitaxel. The results of this trial showed superiority in the triplet regimen, and the NCCN guidelines (2009) list cisplatin and doxorubicin or cisplatin, doxorubicin, and paclitaxel as category 1 recommendations, indicating that these regimens have the highest quality of evidence to support their use as well as uniform level of committee consensus in favor of either regimen in this setting. Papillary serous type is a high-risk subtype of endometrial cancer that has a poor prognosis. It behaves more like ovarian cancer and consequently is typically treated in the same fashion with IV paclitaxel and carboplatin (Mariani, Webb, Keeney, Aletti, & Podratz, 2003).

Recurrent Disease

Most recurrences occur within the first three years following diagnosis (Amant et al., 2005). Symptoms associated with recurrence may include pain, weight loss, and vaginal bleeding. It is important that survivors be counseled on the signs and symptoms of recurrence and when to notify their provider. When the recurrence is in the vaginal vault, if brachytherapy has not previously been used, it can be used quite successfully approximately 87% of the time (Amant et al., 2005). Additional radiation is dependent upon previously given doses. The use of chemotherapy in the recurrent disease setting is only palliative, and participation in clinical trials should be encouraged. Except for vaginal cuff recurrences that might be cured with an upper vaginectomy where appropriate, other attempts at surgery are most often only aimed at relieving symptoms associated with the recurrence (Alvarez Secord et al., 2007; Amant et al., 2007).

Recommended follow-up with the gynecologic oncologist should be done every three months for three years, then every six months for two years. After five years of disease-free examinations, the woman may return to her general gynecologist for annual well-woman care.

Future Trends

The role of biologic therapies such as trastuzumab (Herceptin®, Genentech) and bevacizumab (Avastin®, Genentech) in endometrial cancer is yet to be determined. A new class of drugs called mTOR inhibitors that appear to have a very exciting effect on endometrial cancer cell pathways also currently are being studied. Traditional and novel chemotherapies, biotherapeutic agents, and radiation therapy will continue to be used to treat advanced and recurrent cancer (NCI, n.d.). Innovative surgical approaches such as the RALH, LAVH, and as-yet to be named procedures are being explored, investigated through clinical trials, and considered by gynecologic oncologists.

Methods aimed at cancer prevention in women at high risk will continue to be a priority (NCI, n.d.). Based on persistent evidence of survival differences among ethnic groups, work must continue to solve the problem of access to care and address the issue of variations in tumor biology in endometrial cancers (Wright et al., 2009). In doing so, treatment regimens could be tailored to the individual for more durable outcomes.

Summary

Endometrial cancer has a good prognostic outcome if diagnosed early, and it is particularly responsive to treatment. More than 500,000 U.S. women are survivors of endometrial cancer; therefore, the long-term effects of treatment are not to be minimized (ACS, 2008c). Women who are treated for endometrial cancer experience a variety of quality-of-life issues whose effects are not easily ameliorated by merely surviving the disease. The side effects range from persistent menopausal symptoms, including loss of femininity, sexual dysfunction, osteoporosis, and lymphedema, as well as bowel and bladder changes and fear of recurrence of this cancer or the chance of developing another cancer. The nurses who care for these women must remain sensitive to these long-term problems and needs, paying particular attention to health maintenance in the four domains of quality of life: physiologic, psychological, sociologic, and spiritual.

References

Alvarez Secord, A.A., Havrilesky, L.J., Bae-Jump, V., Chin, J., Calingarts, B., Bland, A., et al. (2007). The role of multi-modality adjuvant chemotherapy and radiation in women with advanced stage endometrial cancer. *Gynecologic Oncology, 107*(2), 285–291.

Amant, F., Moerman, P., Neven, P., Timmerman, D., Van Limbergen, E., & Vergote, I. (2007). Treatment modalities in endometrial cancer. *Current Opinion in Oncology, 19*(5), 479–485.

Amant, F., Moerman, P., Neven, P., Timmerman, D., Van Limbergen, E., & Vergote, I. (2005). Endometrial cancer. *Lancet, 366*(9484), 491–505.

American Cancer Society. (2008a). *Cancer facts and figures, 2008.* Atlanta, GA: American Cancer Society.

American Cancer Society. (2008b, July 26). *Detailed guide: Endometrial cancer: Can endometrial cancer be found early?* Retrieved March 27, 2009, from http://www.cancer.org/docroot/CRI/content/CRI_2_4_3X_Can_endometrial_cancer_be_found_early.asp?rnav=cri

American Cancer Society. (2008c, July 26). *Detailed guide: Endometrial Cancer—What are the key statistics about endometrial cancer?* Retrieved March 27, 2009, from http://www.cancer.org/docroot/CRI/content/CRI_2_4_1X_What_are_the_key_statistics_for_endometrial_cancer.asp?rnav=cri

Bakkum-Gamez, J.N., Gonzales-Bosquet, J., Laack, N.N., Mariani, A., & Dowdy, S.C. (2008). Current issues in the management of endometrial cancer. *Mayo Clinic Proceedings, 83*(1), 97–112.

Barakat, R.R., Lev, G., Hummer, A.J., Sonoda, Y., Chi, D.S., Alektiar, K.M., et al. (2007). Twelve-year experience in the management of endometrial cancer: A change in surgical and postoperative radiation approaches. *Gynecologic Oncology, 105*(1), 150–156.

Beral, V., Bull, D., & Reeves, G., (2005). Endometrial cancer and hormone-replacement therapy in the Million Women Study. *Lancet,* 365(9470), 1543–1551.

Berek, J.S. (2005). Surgical techniques. In J.S. Berek & N.F. Hacker (Eds.), *Practical gynecologic oncology* (4th ed., pp. 739–782). Philadelphia: Lippincott Williams & Wilkins.

Bokhman, J.V. (1983). Two pathogenetic types of endometrial carcinoma. *Gynecologic Oncology, 15*(1), 10–17.

Creutzberg, C.L., Van Putten, W.L., Koper, P.C., Lybeert, M.L., Jobsen, J.J., Warlam-Rodenhuis, C.C., et al. (2003). Survival after relapse in patients with endometrial cancer: Results from a randomized trial. *Gynecologic Oncology, 89*(2), 201–209.

Curtis, K.M., Marchbanks, P.A., & Peterson, H.B. (2007). Neoplasia with use of intrauterine devices. *Contraception, 75*(Suppl. 6), S60–S69.

Ferguson, S.E., Olshen, A.B., Viale, A., Barakat, R.R., & Boyd, J. (2005). Stratification of intermediate-risk endometrial cancer patients into groups at high risk or low risk for recurrence based on tumor gene expression profiles. *Clinical Cancer Research, 11*(6), 2252–2257.

Frederick, P.J., & Straughn, J.M. (2009). The role of comprehensive surgical staging in patients with endometrial cancer. *Cancer Control, 16*(1), 23–29.

Friedenreich, C., Cust, A., Lahmann, P.H., Steindorf, K., Boutron-Ruault, M.C., Clavel-Chapelon, F., et al. (2007). Physical activity and risk of endometrial cancer: The European prospective investigation into cancer and nutrition. *International Journal of Cancer, 121*(2), 347–355.

Gaudin, N., & Harding, R. (2003, April 3). Global cancer rates could increase by 50% to 15 million by 2020—World Cancer Report provides clear evidence that action on smoking, diet, and infections can prevent one third of cancers, another third can be cured [Press release]. Retrieved April 3, 2009, from http://www.who.int/mediacentre/news/releases/2003/pr27/en

Goodman, M.T., Wilkens, L.R., Hankin, J.H., Lyu, L., Wu, A.H., & Kolonel, L.N. (1997). Association of soy and fiber consumption with the risk of endometrial cancer. *American Journal of Epidemiology, 146*(4), 294–306.

Gotlieb, W.H., Beiner, M.E., Shalmon, B., Korach, Y., Segal, Y., Zmira, N., et al. (2003). Outcome of fertility-sparing treatment with progestins in young patients with endometrial cancer. *Obstetrics and Gynecology, 102*(4), 718–725.

Guido, R.S., & Stoval, D.W. (2007). *Dilation and curettage.* Retrieved May 4, 2009, from http://www.uptodate.com

Higgins, R.V., Naumann, R.W., & Hall, J. (2007, December). *Abdominal incisions and sutures in gynecologic oncological surgery.* Retrieved April 3, 2009, from http://emedicine.medscape.com/article/271349-overview

Holub, Z., Jabor, A., Bartos, P., Hendl, J., & Urbánek, S. (2003). Laparoscopic surgery in women with endometrial cancer the learning curve. *European Journal of Obstetrics, Gynecology, and Reproductive Biology, 107*(2), 195–200.

Horn, L.C., Meinel, A., Handzel, R., & Einenkel, J. (2007, August). Histopathology of endometrial hyperplasia and endometrial carcinoma. *Annals of Diagnostic Pathology, 11*(4), 297–311.

Horn-Ross, P.L., John, E.M., Canchola, A.J., Stewart, S.L., & Lee, M.M. (2003). Phytoestrogen intake and endometrial cancer risk. *Journal of the National Cancer Institute, 95*(15), 1158–1164.

International Federation of Gynecology and Oncology. (1989). Announcements. *Gynecologic Oncology, 35*(1), 125–127.

Jemal, A., Siegel, R., Ward, E., Hao, Y., Xu, J., Murray, T., & Thun, M.J. (2008). Cancer statistics, 2008. *CA: A Cancer Journal for Clinicians, 58*(2), 71–96.

Jolly, S., Vargas, C.E., Kumar, T., Weiner, S.A., Brabbins, D.S., Chen, P.Y., et al. (2006). The impact of age on long-term outcome in patients with endometrial cancer treated with postoperative radiation. *Gynecologic Oncology, 103*(1), 87–93.

Kaaks, R., Lukanova, A., & Kurzer, M.S. (2002). Obesity, endogenous hormones, and endometrial cancer risk: A synthetic review. *Cancer Epidemiology, Biomarkers and Prevention, 11*(12), 1531–1543.

Kosary, C.L. (n.d.). Cancer of the corpus uteri. In L.A. Gloeckler Ries, J.L. Young, G.E. Keel, M.P. Eisner, Y.D. Lin, & M.-J.D. Horner (Eds.), *SEER survival monograph: Cancer survival among adults: US SEER program, 1988–2001, patient and tumor characteristics* (pp. 123–132). Bethesda, MD: National Cancer Institute, SEER Program. Retrieved April 3, 2009, from http://seer.cancer.gov/publications/survival/surv_corpus_uteri.pdf

Lacey, J.V., Jr., Brinton, L.A., Lubin, J.H., Sherman, M.E., Schatzkin, A., & Schairer, C. (2005). Endometrial carcinoma risks among menopausal estrogen plus progestin and unopposed estrogen users in a cohort of postmenopausal women. *Cancer Epidemiology, Biomarkers and Prevention, 14*(7), 1724–1731.

Madison, T., Schottenfeld, D., James, S.A., Schwartz, A.G., & Gruber, S.B. (2004). Endometrial cancer: Socioeconomic status and racial/ethnic differences in stage at diagnosis, treatment, and survival. *American Journal of Public Health, 94*(4), 2104–2111.

Magrina, J.F., (2005). Outcomes of laparoscopic treatment for endometrial cancer. *Current Opinion in Obstetrics and Gynecology, 17*, 343–346.

Mariani, A., Webb, M.J., Keeney, G.L., Aletti, G., & Podratz, K.C. (2003). Endometrial cancer: Predictors of peritoneal failure. *Gynecologic Oncology, 89*(2), 236–242.

McAlpine, J.N., Spritos, N.M., & Chen, M.D., (2002). Surgical chores and approach in the management of endometrial cancer. *Current Opinion in Oncology, 14*(5), 512–518.

Montz, F.J., Bristow, R.E., Bovicelli, A., Tomacruz, R., & Kurman, R.J., (2002). Intrauterine progesterone treatment of early endometrial cancer. *American Journal of Obstetrics and Gynecology, 186*(4), 651–657.

Moore, K.N., Gold, M.A., McMeekin, D.S., Walker, J.L., Rutledge, T., & Zorn, K.K. (2008). Extraperitoneal para-aortic lymph node evaluation for cervical cancer via Pfannenstiel incision: Technique and perioperative outcomes. *Gynecologic Oncology, 108*(3), 466–471.

Mutter, G.L., Zaino, R.J., Baak, J.P., Bentley, R.C., & Robboy, S.J. (2007). Benign endometrial hyperplasia sequence and endometrial intraepithelial neoplasia. *International Journal of Gynecological Pathology, 26*(2), 103–114.

National Comprehensive Cancer Network. (2009). *NCCN Clinical Practice Guidelines in Oncology™: Uterine neoplasms* [v.2.2009]. Retrieved May 5, 2009, from http://www.nccn.org/professionals/physician_gls/PDF/uterine.pdf

National Cancer Institute. (2007). *SEER stat fact sheets: Cancer of the corpus and uterus, NOS.* Retrieved April 3, 2009, from http://www.seer.cancer.gov/statfacts/html/corp.html

Ogden, C.L., Carroll, M.D., Curtin, L.R., McDowell, M.A., Tabak, C.J., & Flegal, K.M. (2006). Prevalence of overweight and obesity in the United States, 1999–2004. *JAMA, 295*(13), 1549–1555. Retrieved April 25, 2009, from http://jama.ama-assn.org/cgi/reprint/295/13/1549

Parkin, D.M., Bray, F., Ferlay, J., & Pisani, P. (2005). Global cancer statistics, 2002. *CA: A Cancer Journal for Clinicians, 55*(2), 74–108.

Rackow, B.W., & Arici, A. (2006). Endometrial cancer and fertility. *Current Opinion in Obstetrics and Gynecology, 18*(3), 245–252.

Rossouw, J.E., Anderson, G.L., Prentice, R.L., LaCroix, A.Z., Kooperberg, C., Stefanick, M.L., et al. (2002). Risks and benefits of estrogen plus progestin in healthy postmenopausal women: Principal results from the Women's Health Initiative randomized controlled trial. *JAMA, 288*(3), 321–333.

Saltzman, B.S., Doherty, J.A., Hill, D.A., Beresford, S.A., Voigt, L.F., Chen, C., et al. (2008). Diabetes and endometrial cancer: An evaluation of the modifying effects of other known risk factors. *American Journal of Epidemiology, 167*(5), 607–614.

Seamon, L.G., Cohn, D.E., Henretta, M.S., Kim, K.H., Carlson, M.J., Phillips, G.S., et al. (2009). Minimally invasive comprehensive surgical staging for endometrial cancer: Robotics or laparoscopy? *Gynecologic Oncology, 113*(1), 36–41.

Shamshirsaz, A.A., Withiam-Leitch, M., Odunsi, K., Baker, T., Frederick, P.J., & Lele, S. (2007). Young patients with endometrial carcinoma selected for conservative treatment: A need for vigilance for synchronous ovarian carcinomas, case report and literature review. *Gynecologic Oncology*, *104*(3), 757–760.

Shelly, W., Draper, M.W., Krishnan, V., Wong, M., & Jaffe, R.B. (2008). Selective estrogen receptor modulators: An update on recent clinical findings. *Obstetrical and Gynecological Survey, 63*(3), 163–181.

Soliman, P.T., Oh, J.C., Schmeler, K.M., Sun, C.C., Slomovitz, B.M., Gershenson, D.M., et al. (2005). Risk factors for young premenopausal women with endometrial cancer. *Obstetrics and Gynecology, 105*(3), 575–580.

Sonoda, Y., & Barakat, R.R. (2006). Screening and the prevention of gynecologic cancer: Endometrial cancer. *Best Practice and Research Clinical Obstetrics and Gynaecology, 20*(2), 363–377.

Tao, M.H., Xu, W.H., Zheng, W., Zhang, Z.F., Gao, Y.T., Ruan, Z.X., et al. (2006). Oral contraceptive and IUD use and endometrial cancer: A population-based case-control study in Shanghai, China. *International Journal of Cancer, 119*(9), 2142–2147.

Terry, P., Baron, J.A., Weiderpass, E., Yuen, J., Lichtenstein, P., & Nyren, O. (1999). Lifestyle and endometrial cancer risk: A cohort study from the Swedish twin registry. *International Journal of Cancer, 82*(1), 38–42.

Thigpen , J.T., Brady, M.F., Homesley, H.D., Malfetano, J., DuBeshter, B., Burger, R.A., et al. (2004). Phase III trial of doxorubicin with or without cisplatin in advanced endometrial carcinoma: A gynecologic oncology group study. *Journal of Clinical Oncology, 22*(19), 3902–3908.

Tiffen, J.M., & Mahon, S.M. (2006). Educating women regarding the early detection of endometrial cancer—What is the evidence? *Clinical Journal of Oncology Nursing, 10*(1), 102–104.

Ueda, S.M., Kapp, D.S., Cheung, M.K., Shin, J.Y., Osann, K., Husain, A., et al. (2008). Trends in demographic and clinical characteristics in women diagnosed with corpus cancer and their potential impact on the increasing number of deaths. *American Journal of Obstetrics and Gynecology*, *198*(2), 218.e1–218.e6.

von Gruenigen, V.E., Tian, C., Frasure, H., Waggoner, S., Keys, H., & Barakat, R.R. (2006). Treatment effects, disease recurrence, and survival in obese women with early endometrial carcinoma: A Gynecologic Oncology Group Study. *Cancer, 107*(12), 2786–2791.

Weiderpass, E., Adami1, H., Baron, J. A., Magnusson, C., Lindgren, A., & Persson, I. (1999). Use of oral contraceptives and endometrial cancer risk (Sweden). *Cancer Causes and Control, 10*(4), 277–284.

Wolfson, A.H., Brady, M.F., Rocereto, T., Mannel, R.S., Lee, Y.C., Futoran, R.J., et al. (2007). A Gynecologic Oncology Group randomized phase III trial of whole abdominal irradiation (WAI) vs. cisplatin-ifosfamide and mesna (CIM) as post-surgical therapy in stage I–IV carcinosarcomas (CS) of the uterus. *Gynecologic Oncology, 107*(2), 177–185.

Wright, J.D., Fiorelli, J., Schiff, P.B., Burke, W.M., Kansler, A.L., Cohen, C.J., et al. (2009). Racial disparities for uterine corpus tumors: Changes in clinical characteristics and treatment over time. *Cancer, 115*(6), 1276–1285.

CHAPTER 7

Epithelial Ovarian Cancer, Fallopian Tube Carcinoma, and Primary Peritoneal Carcinoma

Paula J. Anastasia, RN, MN, AOCN®

Introduction

Ovarian cancer is the leading cause of death of all the gynecologic malignancies and the fourth most prevalent of all female cancers in the United States. The American Cancer Society (ACS, 2008) estimated 21,650 new ovarian diagnoses, or 3% of female cancers, in 2008. More than half, an estimated 15,520, will die of their disease because of the vague symptoms that are commonly overlooked until it is diagnosed in the advanced stage (ACS; Goff, Mandel, Muntz, & Melancon, 2000; National Cancer Institute [NCI], 2007a). The majority of ovarian malignancies are epithelial histopathologies, with less than 10% accounting for germ cell tumors, sex cord stromal tumors, and malignant mixed Müllerian tumors of the ovary (see Chapter 8). Epithelial ovarian cancer (EOC) develops from malignant transformation of the epithelial ovarian surface, which adjoins the peritoneal mesothelium, and then disseminates throughout the peritoneal cavity (Berek, 2005). The omentum is a frequent site for metastases, as is the lymphatic system. Despite being separate diagnoses and less common, fallopian tube carcinomas and primary peritoneal carcinomas are generally grouped in the EOC statistics because of similar biology, clinical presentation, and treatment protocol (Bloss et al., 2003; Cass & Karlan, 2003).

The survival rates for EOC have remained stable over the past 20 years and have shown a statistically significant improvement since the 1975–1977 Surveillance, Epidemiology and End Results (SEER) data were reported (Horner et al., 2009). The five-year survival rate for all stages reported in 1999–2005 was 45.9%, compared to 37.2% in the 1970s (Horner et al.). When EOC is diagnosed in the early stage, the five-year survival for all race and age groups is 92.4%. Less than 20% are diagnosed with early or localized disease, whereas 70% of women are diagnosed with distant metastasis, resulting in a 28.2% five-year survival rate for all races and age groups (ACS, 2008; Horner et al.). The five-year survival rate for African American women with stage III or IV EOC is only 19.6%, compared to 28.8% for Caucasian women (Horner et al.). The cause of this disparity is unknown, but African American women are less likely to receive aggressive therapy with surgery and chemotherapy (Winter et al., 2007). The majority of women with EOC are Caucasian, postmenopausal, and in the fifth or sixth decade of life (Berek, 2005). Women younger than 65 years have a twofold longer five-year relative survival rate than women older than age 65, regardless of race. The lifetime risk of EOC in the general population is 1.42%, with Hispanic and American Indian having the highest incidence after Caucasians (ACS, 2008).

Epidemiology and Risk Factors

Although the cause of EOC is not clearly understood, two general hypotheses have been proposed to explain its etiology. One hypothesis is incessant or uninterrupted ovulation, in which genetic and cellular alteration may occur from repeated trauma and healing with each monthly cycle (Berek, 2005; Martin & Cherry, 2006). Supporting this hypothesis are factors that decrease ovulation and protect against EOC (e.g., pregnancy, breastfeeding, oral contraceptive pills [OCPs]) (see Table 7-1). The use of OCPs for five years or longer has shown to decrease the risk of ovarian cancer by 50% for both the general population and carriers of *BRCA*-associated mutations, which have a hereditary propensity to EOC (Narod et al., 1998). Tubal ligation may protect against EOC, although the reason is unclear. It has been suggested that when the ovarian blood supply becomes impaired, the ability for carcinogens to travel through the vagina into the cervix and up to peritoneal cavity may predispose the woman to EOC. The second hypothesis of etiology suggests that increased gonadotropin secretion from increased estrogen proliferation leads to malignant alteration and EOC (Berek, 2005; Cass & Karlan, 2003; Whittemore, 1994). However, this second hypothesis lacks case controls to show that women who have twins or

Table 7-1. Ovarian Cancer Risks and Protective Factors

Category	Risk Factors	Protective Factors
Family/ genetics	*BRCA1* or *BRCA2* mutation Heriditary nonpolyposis colorectal cancer mutation Ashkenazi Jewish heritage	–
Reproductive	Early age of menarche Nulliparity Late menopause Female infertility Postmenopausal hormone replacement therapy Endometriosis	Oral contraceptives Multiparity Breast feeding Bilateral tubal ligation Bilateral salpingo-oophorectomy
Lifestyle	Use of talc Obesity	Normal body mass index Low-fat diet Exercise

Note. Based on information from Berek, 2005; Cass & Karlan, 2003; Martin & Cherry, 2006; Narod et al., 1998; Wong et al., 1990.

multiple births, and as a result, have a higher amount of gonadotropin, are at an increased risk for EOC. Whittemore, Harris, and Itnyre (1992) monitored 2,859 women with ovarian cancer and 7,434 women without ovarian cancer and reported no additional increase in EOC in women who had multiple births.

Risk factors identified by epidemiologic studies include older age, nulliparity, and infertility. In addition, women who begin menarche at an early age (before age 12) or experience a late menopause (after age 51) have an increased risk of EOC because of a longer life span of ovulation (Cannistra & McGuire, 2007; Heinz et al., 2001; Ryerson et al., 2007).

Primary female infertility (not exclusively fertility medication use) is a potential risk factor for EOC. A woman is not at increased risk if the inability to conceive is male factor related, such as decreased sperm count (Bankhead, Kehoe, & Austoker, 2005; Daly & Obrams, 1998; Eriksson & Frazier, 2000). Endometriosis is an independent risk factor and is associated with endometrioid and clear cell histology. The correlation between endometriosis and infertility may correspond to the risk factor (Cramer & Welch, 1983; Heaps, Nieberg, & Berek, 1990). Environmental factors such as talcum powder and obesity have been suspected as risk factors, but no clear relationships have been identified. In the past, talcum powder contained asbestos, a known carcinogen, but the risk has been alleviated with the elimination of this carcinogen from the talc (Cass & Karlan, 2003; Wong, Hempling, Piver, Natarajan, & Mettlin, 1990).

Hereditary Epithelial Ovarian Cancer

Most cancers, including EOC, are caused by random or sporadic cellular events, whereas less than 10% have a hereditary predisposition (Piver, 2002). Identified in 1994, the most common mutation in EOC is the *BRCA1*, a tumor suppressor gene located on chromosome 17, which occurs about twice as frequently as *BRCA2* (Karlan, Berchuck, & Mutch, 2007). The *BRCA2* gene, located on chromosome 13, was identified in 1995 and has less penetrance (or chance for development of cancer) for EOC than *BRCA1*. Both of these genes are associated primarily with breast and ovarian cancer; although, families with *BRCA1*-associated mutations may see an increase in other cancers such as prostate cancer (King, Marks, & Mandell, 2003) (see Table 7-2). *BRCA2* gene carriers also have a higher risk of male breast cancer, melanoma, and pancreatic cancer (Karlan et al., 2007; King et al.). The

Table 7-2. Characteristics Suggesting Genetic Testing for Hereditary Breast and Ovarian Cancer

- A three-generation pedigree, on both the paternal and maternal lineage, should be obtained from the patient.
- Personal or family history of breast cancer before age 50
- Personal history of ovarian cancer or one or more first-degree relatives at any age
- Ashkenazi Jewish ancestry with a personal or family history of breast cancer before age 50 or ovarian cancer at any age
- Two or more primary diagnoses of breast (i.e., two separate breast cancer primaries) and/or ovarian cancer
- Male breast cancer in family

Gene Mutation	Prevalence of Individual Cancer Risk
BRCA1	39%–46% lifetime risk for ovarian cancer; generally diagnosed 10 years younger than sporadic ovarian cancer 65%–74% risk for breast cancer Increased incidence of prostate cancer with this germ line mutation
BRCA2 mutation	12%–20% lifetime risk for ovarian cancer 65%–74% risk for breast cancer Increased incidence of melanoma and pancreatic cancer with this germ line mutation
HNPCC mutation	10%–12% lifetime risk for ovarian cancer 40%–71% lifetime risk for endometrial cancer 13% lifetime risk for stomach cancer 82% lifetime risk for colorectal cancer Increased incidence of ureter and renal pelvis, biliary tract, small bowel, pancreas, and brain cancer

Note. Based on information from Cass & Karlan, 2003; Chen et al., 2007; Karlan et al., 2007; Kauff & Barakat, 2007; King et al., 2003; Lu et al., 2009; National Cancer Institute, 2008b; National Comprehensive Cancer Network, 2009; Nelson et al., 2005; Piver, 2002.

median age of an EOC diagnosis for a *BRCA1* mutation carrier is the mid-40s and for a *BRCA2* mutation carrier, the early 60s. Because sporadic EOC generally occurs in the fifth or sixth decade of life, a woman with ovarian cancer in her 60s may not raise suspicion for genetic predisposition. The mutation is passed via autosomal dominance, which means that an offspring has a 50% chance of inheriting the gene from either the father or mother (Karlan, Markman, & Eifel, 2005; National Comprehensive Cancer Network [NCCN], 2009). Specific ethnic groups, especially Ashkenazi Jews, carry founder mutations, in that the same mutation is specific to their ancestry. As many as 60% of Ashkenazi Jewish women diagnosed with ovarian cancer are reported to have a mutation in either the *BRCA1* or *BRCA2* gene (Karlan et al., 2005). Three founder mutations have been identified in 2%–2.4% of the Ashkenazi Jewish population: 185delAG and 5382inC on *BRCA1* gene, and 6174delT on *BRCA2* gene (Berek, 2005). Other geographic populations with founder mutations and increased risks include people from the Netherlands, Sweden, Iceland, and Hungary (Arason et al., 1998; Einbeigi et al., 2001; Karlan et al., 2007; Peelen et al., 1997). Hereditary ovarian cancer generally is diagnosed at 10 years younger than those with sporadic ovarian cancer for *BRCA1* carriers (Martin & Cherry, 2006). Interestingly, several studies show a more favorable survival outcome in *BRCA*-associated gynecologic malignancies, possibly because of *BRCA* mutation carriers having an improved response in platinum-based chemotherapy compared to those in women with non-hereditary EOC (Cass et al., 2003).

Another mutation seen with EOC is hereditary nonpolyposis colorectal cancer (HNPCC), or Lynch syndrome, which also is associated with colon and endometrial carcinoma (Chen, Yang, Little, Cheung, & Caughey, 2007; Martin & Cherry, 2006). HNPCC is an autosomal dominant syndrome caused by the mutation of several DNA mismatch repair genes: *MLH1*, *MSH2*, *PMS1*, and *PMS2* (Karlan et al., 2005). Mismatch repair genes identify genes that do not belong together during replication and correct the errors. Individuals with HNPCC are at increased risk for colorectal carcinoma and extracolonic cancers such as gastrointestinal (GI), ovarian, and endometrial. The Amsterdam and the Bethesda criteria are used to identify family syndromes of colorectal and other cancers associated with HNPCC (Karlan et al., 2007).

Oncology nurses are in the ideal setting to identify patients with a potential risk for a genetic mutation, including but not limited to the *BRCA1, BRCA2,* and HNPCC mutations. Any women with hereditary cancer risk factors should be referred to a genetic counselor for further discussion regarding genetic testing (Martin & Cherry, 2006). Ideally, the family member with the cancer diagnosis should be tested. If a specific gene mutation is found, then other family members may request testing. Often family members do not want to know this information and may resist testing. Genetic testing and the ensuing results involve a psychological response of emotions and behaviors in addition to the medical implications for screening and surveillance. Therefore, a genetic counselor is the appropriate referral for an identified high-risk patient and her family (NCI, 2008b).

Prophylactic or risk-reducing surgery with a bilateral salpingo-oophorectomy (BSO) is the most effective way to reduce the risk for hereditary EOC, although a slight risk for primary peritoneal carcinoma still remains (Kauff & Barakat, 2007). In addition, the risk for breast cancer may be reduced by 50% in premenopausal women who undergo a BSO (Karlan et al., 2005). Risk-reducing surgery should be considered when a woman has completed childbearing, but generally by age 40, as most *BRCA*-associated cancers occur earlier than sporadic cancer. Surgery usually can be performed laparoscopically, which reduces recovery time (Karlan et al., 2005). Because most women undergoing risk reducing BSO will be premenopausal, the issue of surgically induced menopause and vasomotor side effects should be addressed preoperatively (Rebbeck et al., 2005). See Chapter 14 for menopausal management.

For women who are carriers of the *BRCA* or HNPCC mutations, current consensus recommendations include, beginning around age 30, at least an annual rectovaginal examination, CA-125 testing, and transvaginal ultrasonography (despite limited specificity and sensitivity) (NCCN, 2009). Breast health surveillance includes annual mammography and breast magnetic resonance imaging (MRI). Risk-reducing bilateral mastectomy is included in the genetic counseling and recommendation summary. Additional surveillance for HNPCC includes yearly colonoscopy and a yearly gastroscopy and urine cytology for families with GI cancer (Berek, 2005; Karlan et al., 2007).

Screening, Presentation of Symptoms, and Diagnostic Testing

An effective screening test for the early detection of ovarian cancer is not available. Symptoms for ovarian cancer are subtle, nonspecific, and vague; therefore, women have little motivation to seek early medical attention or reason to believe they have EOC because symptoms may appear to be nonurgent (Cannistra, 2004; Goff et al., 2000). For instance, women may experience variations of symptoms that mimic EOC, which in turn will not be cancer, and other women may present with cancer-related nongynecologic symptoms such as shortness of breath (caused by a pleural effusion) and are diagnosed on workup with stage IV EOC. Other less common presentations of EOC include paraneoplastic events such as humeral hypercalcemia associated with clear cell histology, Leser-Trélat sign evidenced by sudden appearance of multiple seborrheic keratoses, and Trousseau syndrome characterized by migratory thrombophlebitis (Cannistra, 2004; Evans, Mansi, & Bevan, 1996).

For years, EOC was called "the silent killer" because symptoms rarely manifested until the disease was advanced. We now know there *are* symptoms, often a classic cluster of symptoms (early satiety, bloating, and increased abdominal fullness), albeit insidious (Cannistra, 2004; Cass & Karlan, 2003; Martin & Cherry, 2006). A survey of 1,725 women with ovarian cancer reported that 95% of them did have symptoms prior to their diagnosis, including 89% with early-stage disease and 97% with advanced stage disease (Goff et al., 2004). The majority of these women went six months before being diagnosed correctly. Women who presented with gynecologic symptoms were more likely to be diagnosed earlier than women who presented with gastrointestinal symptoms (see Figure 7-1). National organizations such as the Society for Gynecologic Oncologists (SGO), Society of Gynecologic Nurse Oncologists, and the Gynecologic Cancer Foundation support more education and awareness to the public and medical community regarding symptoms of EOC.

The current recommendations for a woman with symptoms lasting longer than a couple weeks advocate seeking medical assessment from her primary care physician, nurse practitioner, or gynecologist (Goff et al., 2007; Karlan et al., 2005; NCCN, 2009; Whittemore, 1994). A routine physical and bimanual (vaginal and rectal) gynecologic examination rarely identifies an early-stage ovarian carcinoma because of the deep pelvic location of the ovaries. Palpation of an adnexal mass on examination is the usual finding, but this alone does not confirm malignancy (Cannistra, 2004; Ozols, Rubin, Thomas, & Robboy, 1997). A solid, irregular, and fixed pelvic mass is suspicious, especially if more concerning symptoms such as upper abdominal mass or ascites are present. A transvaginal pelvic ultrasonography is the least invasive and most inexpensive test to perform, although it is limited in its sensitivity and specificity to differentiate between benign and malignant ovarian masses (Berek, 2005). For women who are at high risk for EOC, annual screening with a CA-125 blood test, pelvic ultrasonography, and bimanual pelvic examination is recommended. A complex ovarian mass, with both solid and cystic components, is suggestive of malignancy and often has characteristics of septations and internal echoes (Karlan et al., 2005). Color flow Doppler imaging evaluates blood flow and abnormal neovascularization, helping to identify consistencies for EOC. The use of annual or biannual ultrasonography in high-risk women has not shown to contribute to early detection or a survival advantage (Kauff & Barakat, 2007). However, this surveillance is the only recommendation at this time for monitoring high-risk women (Karlan et al., 2007).

Figure 7-1. Symptoms of Epithelial Ovarian Cancer

Gastrointestinal
- Bloating
- Dyspepsia
- Early satiety
- Nausea
- Urinary symptoms
- Constipation
- Diarrhea
- Back pain
- Fatigue

Gynecologic
- Abdominal distension (caused by tumor or ascites)
- Increased abdominal girth (caused by tumor or ascites)
- Pelvic pain
- Menstrual irregularities
- Vaginal bleeding
- Watery vaginal discharge (associated with fallopian tube carcinoma)

Patient education and awareness should emphasize that one or more of these symptoms occurring for more than two weeks require medical assessment.

Note. Based on information from Cannistra, 2004; Goff et al., 2004; Martin & Cherry, 2006; Ryerson et al., 2007.

Computerized tomography (CT) may be beneficial in assessing involvement or abnormality in the liver, lymph nodes, omentum, and mesentery. MRI has not shown to have an advantage over a CT for EOC (Cass & Karlan, 2003). Positron emission tomography (PET) evaluates glucose metabolism by injecting a radioactive tracer, which releases positron-emitting isotopes or particles to measure metabolic activity, rather than CT assessment of anatomical abnormalities. The combination of PET/CT may provide more sensitive information at identifying small peritoneal recurrence using both metabolic and anatomical information (Soussan et al., 2008). Although not approved for evaluation in EOC, PET usefulness for metastatic or recurrent disease appears promising in clinical studies in this setting (Havrilesky, Kulasingam, Matchar, & Myers, 2005). A barium enema examination is not routinely performed unless a primary GU carcinoma is suspected. A chest x-ray and a full panel of laboratory studies, including complete blood count, chemistries, and a CA-125 blood test, also are included. However, only surgery can confirm a definitive diagnosis (Cannistra, 2004; Cass & Karlan, 2003).

CA-125

CA-125 is an antigen expressed by fetal, amniotic, and celomic epithelium (mesothelial cells of the pleura, pericardium, and peritoneum). In the adult female, the antigen is derived from the celomic epithelium and Müllerian epithelium (tubal, endometrial, and endocervical) (Bast et al., 1983; Menon & Jacobs, 2005). The serum CA-125 is a nonspecific tumor marker with variations in interpretation depending on the patient's medical history and age and therefore is not recommended as a mass screening modality. CA-125 levels may be elevated in a variety of benign and nongynecologic malignancies (Bast et al., 1998). It may be elevated in 50% of women with stage I EOC and 80% in late-stage disease. A serum CA-125 value of less than 35 U/ml is considered normal; however, in a premenopausal woman, the marker has less sensitivity and specificity. A serum level greater than 65 U/ml in a postmenopausal woman with a pelvic mass and ascites is cause for concern (Karlan et al., 2005). Combining a transvaginal ultrasound to correlate with an elevated CA-125 may provide useful information to suggest further testing (McIntosh et al., 2004). Preoperative consultation with a gynecologic oncologist is strongly recommended for any woman with a pelvic mass suspicious for a gynecologic malignancy (Schrag et al., 2006; SGO, 2000). If the CA -125 is elevated when a diagnosis of EOC is confirmed by pathology, the tumor marker becomes useful in assessing the patient's response to chemotherapy and remission status or perhaps detecting early recurrence (Saygili et al., 2002). During treatment, when the CA-125 nadir is less than or equal to 10 U/ml, a favorable prognosis and response is reported to result in a median progression-free survival of 24 months (Markman et al., 2006).

In the future, proteomics may be used as a more sensitive and specific tumor marker than CA-125. Protein patterns and characteristics are identified through surface-enhanced laser desorption ionization time-of-flight (SELDI-TOF) and matrix-associated laser desorption ionization time-of-flight (MALDI-TOF) technology. SELDI-TOF has shown to discriminate proteomic spectra patterns that differentiate serum proteins from patients with EOC and those with nonmalignant conditions (Boyce & Kohn, 2005; Menon & Jacobs, 2005). The sensitivity for predicting EOC has been reported at 100% with a specificity of 95% in early phase I trials (Petricoin et al., 2002). Larger population-based studies are being conducted by NCI (2008a).

Staging Surgery

Surgical staging is essential in women undergoing debulking or cytoreductive surgery for suspected EOC. The goal is to optimally debulk or remove all visible disease to less than 1 cm (Fader & Rose, 2007). Several studies have shown a direct correlation between small-volume residual disease and an improved response rate, longer disease-free interval, and overall survival (Bristow, Tomacruz, Armstrong, Trimble, & Montz, 2002).

An exploratory laparotomy through a midline vertical incision extending from above the umbilicus to above the symphysis pubis generally is performed to allow visualization of the upper abdomen for thorough tumor debulking. The surgery includes a total abdominal hysterectomy, BSO, omentectomy, para-aortic and pelvic lymph node assessment and biopsy, peritoneal surface biopsies, and peritoneal washings (Eisenkop, Friedman, & Wang, 1998). Women diagnosed with early-stage 1A disease may only require unilateral removal of the affected ovary, especially if fertility preservation is desired, although the contralateral ovary must be evaluated at the time of surgery (Cass & Karlan, 2003). Women with low-grade (1 or 2) stage 1A or 1B EOC often will not require adjuvant chemotherapy; and therefore, surgical staging is critical to confirm absence of metastatic spread (Berek, 2005).

In contrast, women who are unsuitable surgical candidates (e.g., patients with comorbid conditions, poor performance status) may be advised to undergo neoadjuvant chemotherapy. After three cycles of chemotherapy, if a tumor response is evident by imaging studies, physical examination, and/or CA-125 marker, the woman may be reevaluated for tumor debulking or interval cytoreduction surgery, after which chemotherapy would resume (Karlan et al., 2005).

If a woman was not completely staged at the time of surgery, a second surgery may be recommended prior to chemotherapy initiation, or surgical reassessment may be done at the completion of treatment (Fader & Rose, 2007). In some situations, a laparoscopic surgery can be performed for restaging. EOC spreads primarily by exfoliation of malignant cells from the surface of the ovary that implant along the surface of the peritoneal cavity. Metastases occurs through the circulatory path of the peritoneal fluid, often moving with the force of respirations, causing seeding along the intestinal mesenteries, right hemidiaphragm, liver capsule, and omentum (Cass & Karlan, 2003). Lymphatic spread to the pelvic and para-aortic lymph nodes is seen in advanced stage disease and in rare cases spreads to supraclavicular node (Karlan et al., 2005). Distant metastasis to brain, lungs, parenchymal liver, and supraclavicular node consistent with stage IV disease is rare. However, patients with disease above the diaphragm usually present with a cytology-positive right pleural effusion; this is the most common presentation of stage IV disease (Berek, 2005).

The staging system for ovarian cancer is based in accordance with the International Federation of Gynecology and Obstetrics (FIGO) (see Appendix I). Seventy-five percent of women with EOC are diagnosed with stage III or IV disease. The rates of long-term survival among patients with early-stage disease is as high as 90%, whereas survival rates decrease to 30% in women with advanced disease (NCI, 2007b).

Several nonrandomized studies (Bristow et al., 2002; Earle et al., 2006) suggest improved survival for women with EOC if surgery was performed by a gynecologic oncologist. Similarly, multiple retrospective studies confirm that the minimal amount of residual tumor correlates to increased survival, and patients are more likely to have optimal cytoreductive surgery under the care of a gynecologic oncologist (Earle et al.). In addition, Goff et al. (2007) attested that surgical practices for EOC showed colostomies were performed 23% of the time by general surgeons compared to 3% by gynecologic oncologists. In spite of these facts, less than 50% of women with EOC consult a gynecologic oncologist (Karlan et al., 2005). This has led to an awareness campaign to educate internists and general gynecologists about the symptoms of EOC so early referral to the specialist can be made. In addition, nurses are in an ideal position to educate the public about the warning signs and the need for appropriate referrals to a gynecologic oncologist for treatment.

Pathology

EOC has four predominant histology classifications (see Table 7-3) in addition to tumor grade, which provide information on the aggressiveness of the tumor (Ioffe, Simsir, & Silverberg, 2005). Histologic grade establishes how closely a cell has differentiated from a normal cell. Grades 1, 2 and 3, correlate with well, moderate, and poorly differentiated, respectively. A high-grade or poorly differentiated tumor has a worse prognosis than a well-differentiated, or grade 1, tumor (Berek, 2005).

The prognosis of EOC is affected by the stage of the cancer, the histologic subtype, volume of residual disease, performance status, and patient age. In a retrospective review of 1,895 women with stage IIIC EOC, Winter et al. (2007) identified four independent factors that equated to poor prognosis:

- Age
- Performance status
- Cell type
- Residual disease at the end of cytoreductive surgery.

Women younger than 40 had the best overall survival and women older than 70 had the shortest. Between ages 40 and 60, the progression-free and overall survival were similar. Patients with an Eastern Cooperative Oncology Group performance status of 2 also had a shorter overall survival and progression-free interval. Mucinous and clear cell histology had a worse prognosis compared to serous histology, but in this analysis, mucinous histology had twice the risk of death compared to clear cell. The amount of residual disease at the end of cytoreductive surgery is consistent with prognosis, with less than 1 cm being more favorable and less than 5 mm being most favorable (Fader & Rose, 2007).

Table 7-3. Pathology Classifications of Epithelial Ovarian Carcinoma

Histology	Incidence	Feature
Papillary serous carcinoma	Up to 50%	Bilateral; average age mid-50s Produced along tubal pathway Papillary structure; may see psammoma bodies on the surface of the cell in well-differentiated carcinoma
Endometrioid cell carcinoma	Up to 25%	Resulting from differentiation along the endometrial line Second most common cell type
Mucinous cell carcinoma	Up to 10%	Similar to a gastrointestinal primary Rule out appendiceal carcinoma
Clear cell carcinoma	5%–10%	Most aggressive histology and associated with endometriosis

Note. Based on information from Berek, 2005; Cass & Karlan, 2005; Ioffe et al., 2005; National Cancer Institute, 2007b.

Immunomarkers

More than 100 proto-oncogenes have been identified and are being studied as predictors of prognosis based on amplification and overexpression (Berek, 2005). HER2/neu is an oncogene, a member of the endothelial growth factor receptor family, and if overexpressed, may play a role in EOC pathogenesis. Early findings reported overexpression in 25%–30% of ovarian cancers (Rodriguez et al., 1993). The Gynecologic Oncology Group (GOG) conducted a phase I/II study in platinum-resistant recurrent disease and reported only a 12% overexpression and a 10% response rate to the anti-HER-2/neu monoclonal antibody, Herceptin® (Genentech) (Menon & Jacobs, 2005). FIGO stage and ploidy show a relationship to survival in EOC. Early-stage cancers most often are diploid and result in a longer median survival, whereas aneuploid tumors tend to be more advanced tumors associated with decreased survival (Karlan et al., 2005).

Ovarian tumors of low malignant potential (LMP) include serous, mucinous, and endometrioid and are by definition non-invasive, but they have more proliferation than other benign epithelial ovarian tumors (Berek, 2005). Overall, LMP tumors confined to the ovary have an excellent prognosis, although approximately 1.5% of these tumors may recur or progress to carcinoma. It is possible for serous LMP to have invasive implants, which may require chemotherapy. Mucinous LMP tumors generally are confined to the ovary, but if advanced, histologic assessment of the appendix is necessary to rule out occult appendiceal carcinoma (Karlan et al., 2005).

Adjuvant Chemotherapy

Early-Stage Epithelial Ovarian Cancer

Women diagnosed with grade 1 stage IA and IB have a greater than 90% survival when managed solely with surgery. However, women with early-stage EOC and with high-risk features (see Figure 7-2) have a relapse rate as high as 25%–40% and are recommended to have systemic chemotherapy (Cannistra, 2004). IV chemotherapy with carboplatin and paclitaxel is the standard of practice, but research continues to determine the adequate number of cycles to be administered (Bell et al., 2006).

Figure 7-2. Early-Stage Epithelial Ovarian Carcinoma

Low Risk	High Risk
• Stage 1A, 1B • Grade 1 • Intact capsule • Non–clear cell • No ascites • No surface tumor	• Stage 1C, stage II • Grade 2–3 • Ruptured tumor capsule • Clear cell histology • Ascites or positive washings • Tumor present on external surface of ovary

Note. Based on information from Berek, 2005; Cass & Karlan, 2005; Ioffe et al., 2005.

A GOG trial (175) designed for women with high-risk, early-stage EOC is closed to accrual and awaiting data evaluation. It consisted of three cycles of IV paclitaxel (175 mg/m^2) and IV carboplatin (AUC 6) followed by observation (control arm) versus the same chemotherapy regimen followed by weekly IV paclitaxel (40 mg/m^2) for 24 weeks (NCI, 2007c). The purpose of the additional weekly paclitaxel is to evaluate its antiangiogenic activity (Markman, 2007; Markman et al., 2006).

Advanced-Stage Epithelial Ovarian Cancer

For women with advanced (stage III–IV) EOC, chemotherapy with a platinum and taxane remains the mainstay, with up to a 75%–80% clinical remission for patients with optimally debulked tumors (Bookman, 2005; Ozols, 2002). The U.S. Food and Drug Administration's (FDA's) approval of paclitaxel in 1992 as a second-line regimen for ovarian cancer after initial relapse improved the clinical responses and overall survival outcomes for women with relapsed EOC (Berek, 2005; International Collaborative Ovarian Neoplasm Group, 2002; Ozols et al., 2003). Paclitaxel in combination with cisplatin replaced cyclophosphamide as first-line therapy in the mid-1990s (Piccart et al., 2000).

Three landmark randomized studies compared combination IV paclitaxel and IV carboplatin against IV paclitaxel and IV cisplatin to evaluate efficacy and toxicity (duBois, Luck, & Meir, 2003; Neijt et al., 2000; Ozols et al., 2003). All three studies used different doses of IV carboplatin and IV paclitaxel, in addition to different eligibility of disease stage. GOG #158 found similar efficacy and survival between IV paclitaxel/carboplatin and IV paclitaxel/cisplatin; however, the women reported better quality of life in the paclitaxel and carboplatin regimen, with documentation of less gastrointestinal and neurotoxic events (Ozols et al., 2003). Conclusions drawn from these studies support the use of either IV cisplatin (75 mg/m^2) or carboplatin (AUC 5–7.5) in combination with paclitaxel. The paclitaxel dose and infusion time may be modified depending on which platinum agent is used. It is believed that carboplatin is an easier tolerated regimen than cisplatin because patients report minimal, if any, nausea and vomiting, and do not require hydration to prevent nephrotoxicity. However, myelosuppression, defined as a decrease in red and white blood cell and platelet counts, required frequent laboratory assessment in those who received carboplatin (Martin & Cherry, 2006; Ozols et al., 2003).

Research determined the most effective dose and schedule for IV paclitaxel when used in combination with IV platinum. Paclitaxel initially was approved as a 24-hour IV infusion, but the 3-hour IV infusion has proven to be the most common, convenient, and cost-effective method (Eisenhauer, 1994; Ozols et al., 1997). Paradoxically, infusion durations affect toxicity profile. The IV paclitaxel 24-hour infusion has less neurotoxicity, but more neutropenia, and therefore is more appropriately paired with IV cisplatin (Eisenhauer). Because neurotoxicity is more frequent, and myelosuppression is less frequent with a three-hour infusion of paclitaxel, this dose schedule is more conducive with carboplatin to prevent overlapping of toxicities. Vasey et al. (2004) reported on the SCOTROC (Scottish Randomized Trial in Ovarian Cancer) trial, which randomized 1,077 women with stage IC–IV EOC to paclitaxel and carboplatin versus docetaxel and carboplatin. Although the efficacy appeared to be equal, neurotoxic and arthralgic effects decreased in the docetaxel arm, but gastrointestinal, neutropenia, and hypersensitivity reactions increased (Martin & Cherry, 2006; Vasey et al.).

High-dose chemotherapy and stem cell–supported high-dose chemotherapy has not proven to increase progression-free survival or overall survival over standard-dose chemotherapy (Mobus et al., 2007; NCCN, 2009). Platinum-sensitive patients had a better response than platinum-resistant patients, but in a phase III study of women with advanced, optimally debulked stage EOC, the four-year overall survival was equivalent between the two groups (Ledermann et al., 2005). In a similar study, but as consolidation, patients with less than 2 cm disease on second look were randomized to three cycles of standard chemotherapy or a single course of high-dose chemotherapy with stem cell transplant. This study also failed to show a difference in overall survival (Cure et al., 2004).

According to NCCN (2009), the recommended regimens for advanced EOC are IV paclitaxel (175 mg/m^2 over three hours) and IV carboplatin (AUC 5–7.5) every three weeks for six cycles. Alternative regimens for women with preexisting peripheral neuropathy or a paclitaxel allergy are IV docetaxel (60 mg/m^2–75 mg/mg over one hour) and IV carboplatin (AUC 5–6) every three weeks for six cycles. Intraperitoneal (IP) chemotherapy is another alternative front-line regimen. Armstrong et al. (2006) reported a 16-month overall survival advantage for women who were randomized to IP cisplatin over those who were randomized to receive IV cisplatin (see Table 7-4).

Table 7-4. Results of Gynecologic Oncology Group Trial 172: Intravenous Versus Intraperitoneal Chemotherapy for Postoperative Patients With Ovarian Cancer

Arm	Length of Treatment	Number of Subjects	Dosage and Administration	Overall Survival	Progression-Free Survival
Arm I: IV only	Every 21 days for 6 cycles	N = 210	Day 1: IV paclitaxel 135 mg/m^2 Day 2: IV cisplatin 100 mg/m^2	49.7 months	18.3 months
Arm II: IV and IP	Every 21 days for 6 cycles	N = 205	Day 1: IV paclitaxel 135 mg/m^2 over 24 hours Day 2: IP cisplatin 100 mg/m^2 Day 8: IP paclitaxel 60 mg/m^2	65.6 months	23.8 months

IP—intraperitoneal; IV—intravenous

Note. Based on information from Armstrong et al., 2006; Markman & Walker, 2006.

Intraperitoneal Chemotherapy

Since 1996, three randomized, phase III trials have demonstrated clinical benefit by using a combination of IV and IP chemotherapy versus IV alone in the treatment of EOC (Alberts et al., 1996; Armstrong et al., 2006; Markman et al., 2001). In 2006, after the results of GOG 172 were reported by Armstrong's group, NCI issued a clinical bulletin that all women with stage III EOC who have undergone optimal cytoreductive surgery should be considered for IP chemotherapy. The IP group showed a median overall survival of 65.6 months versus 49.7 months in the IV group, and the progression-free survival was 23.8 in the IP arm versus 18.3 months in the IV arm. These results were particularly impressive because only 42% of patients in the IP arm completed all six cycles of planned treatment (Markman & Walker, 2006; Rao, Crispens, & Rothenberg, 2007). The adoption of GOG 172 as the accepted standard of care, especially in the community setting, has been met with its own set of challenges. The IP protocol is time consuming and has a steep learning curve for nurses who are not experienced with this IP administration route (Almadrones, 2007). The IP regimen offers a distinctly different side effect profile from IV therapy. A quality-of-life evaluation in the Armstrong et al. trial resulted in a worse initial quality of life for the women who received the IP regimen. However, at one-year follow-up, the quality-of-life results for both arms were similar (Markman & Walker; Rao et al.).

The trial design of GOG 172 has been criticized because the drug, dose, and schedule differ from the standard of care of IV paclitaxel/carboplatin. Critics question whether the study can really answer if IP is better because the IP arm includes a dose-dense component of IV paclitaxel over 24 hours, IP cisplatin, and an additional IP paclitaxel on day 8 (Markman & Walker, 2006; Rao et al., 2007). Equally difficult to confirm is the use of two different cytotoxic drugs for IP administration, and IV and IP doses of paclitaxel. Paclitaxel administered into the peritoneal cavity has a greater than 1,000-fold increase in drug distribution and longer drug exposure than when administered via the IV route (Markman & Walker, 2006). Therefore, IP paclitaxel was administered on day 8, instead of day 1, to allow for clearance of the drug and to reduce possible toxicities if administered too closely with another chemotherapy agent.

Because the peritoneal cavity is the primary site of metastasis, administration of IP chemotherapy pharmacologically and clinically has an advantage over the IV route. Dedrick, Myers, Bungay, and DeVita (1978) demonstrated that IP chemotherapy administered in sizable volumes of fluid had higher concentration and longer half lives of drug level in the peritoneal cavity compared to IV administration. Cisplatin, when given IP, exhibits a concentration 10–20 times greater than plasma levels, especially in the woman with only microscopic residual disease following surgery (Howell et al., 1982; Markman et al., 2001; Markman & Walker, 2006). According to Howell et al. (1982), patients with the smallest amount of residual disease (less than 0.5 cm) after surgery had more impressive response rates to IP therapy than those with disease in the 0.5–2 cm range. In addition, the penetration of the IP chemotherapy is limited to 0.1–1 mm from the surface of the peritoneal tumor (Alberts et al., 1996); therefore, patients with bulky lymph nodes, or less than optimal cytoreductive surgery, may not receive the most favorable response if the drug is unable to penetrate the tumor.

Other conditions, such as catheter complications (e.g., improper placement, leakage, inability to infuse), comorbid diseases, and intolerable side effects such as nausea, vomiting, electrolyte imbalance, or persistent abdominal pain, may limit the use of IP chemotherapy (Almadrones, 2007; Hydzik, 2007). Not all patients are candidates for IP therapy, especially those with bulky or residual disease larger than 1 cm. If the diagnosis of stage IIIC EOC is probable, physicians should discuss placing an IP port at the time of surgery for possible IP chemotherapy treatment options. Women safely can have an IP port placed after optimal cytoreductive surgery, when the diagnosis of EOC was not expected or if they choose to wait, but they need to be counseled that this involves another surgical procedure (Armstrong et al., 2006; Markman & Walker, 2006).

Future research on IP therapy will answer lingering questions such as the role of IP chemotherapy in stage IIIA, IIIB, and IV disease; the minimal number of cycles needed; and other active IP agents such as carboplatin that may have equal efficacy and fewer side effects. It remains to be seen if IP therapy will become the standard of care over systemic IV therapy in first-line treatment for advanced EOC. More clinical trials are warranted to attempt to answer the unanswered questions. Oncology nurses have a pivotal role in side effect management and decreasing toxicity for women who receive IP therapy. More nursing research is needed in this area to maintain quality care for patients and to educate other nurses about the challenges and solutions for improving IP therapy.

Consolidation and Maintenance Therapy

More than 70% of women with EOC who are optimally debulked and receive combination IV platinum and taxane will have a complete clinical remission, defined as no evidence of disease on clinical examination and CT scan, and normal (ideally single digit) CA-125 (Berek, 2005). Unfortunately, the relapse rate even in those who achieve a complete clinical remission remains as high as 75% (Karlan et al., 2005). The question of whether to give additional chemotherapy or immunologic therapies sequentially to prevent or prolong relapse in these women remains unanswered. Therefore, consolidation regimens in a clinical trial setting are needed to further improve the outcomes (Markman et al., 2003).

A regimen currently being investigated is GOG 212, a three-arm randomized study that consists of observation with no treatment, monthly IV paclitaxel 135 mg/m^2 for 12 months, or 12 monthly cycles of Xylotax® (Cell Therapeutics, Inc.) 135 mg/m^2, a conjugation of paclitaxel (Martin, 2007).

Another type of consolidation treatment is anti-CA-125 monoclonal antibody–based therapy that binds with high affinity to circulating CA-125, resulting in the creation of immune complexes (Sabbatini & Odunsi, 2007). Other consolidation trials of interest for researchers include immunologic approaches with vaccines and cytokines (Sabbatini & Odunsi).

Second-Look Surgery

Clinical remission is determined by the absence or no evidence of disease on imaging scan, physical and recto-pelvic examination, and normalization of CA-125 (generally by the third cycle of chemotherapy) (Fader & Rose, 2007; Martin, 2007). A second-look surgery is used diagnostically, as it will only confirm disease status and is not used to gauge a patient's overall prognosis. Second-look surgeries can be performed as a laparotomy, using the same incision as the staging procedure, or as a laparoscopy (Karlan et al., 2005). Laparoscopy usually is preferred as it is less invasive, is more cost-effective, and offers reduced recovery time (Berek, 2005). The initial intent of second-look surgery was to prolong or improve survival by initiating more treatment to those who had positive disease. Unfortunately, survival benefits have not been proven, thus second-look surgery is recommended only in individual circumstances or under the directive of a clinical trial (Karlan et al., 2005).

Radiotherapy

The use of radiation therapy in EOC is limited, whether the treatment is for primary disease, relapse, or palliation. Research indicates that surgery and chemotherapy are more effective modalities in EOC; therefore, radiation generally is used only to treat localized disease (Bookman, 2005; NCI, 2007b). There have been small clinical trials of long-term disease-free outcomes with improved survival in patients who had less than 2 cm residual disease and who received abdominopelvic radiation versus pelvic radiation. Although the studies were small, there was improved survival in those who received abdominopelvic radiation (Dembo, 1992).

The GOG reported on the use of IP chromic phosphate, an isotope known as ^{32}P, in patients with early-stage disease who were randomized to receive the IP isotope versus chemotherapy, following optimal cytoreductive surgery. Although there was no difference in recurrence risk, there were significant bowel complications resulting in the abandonment of ^{32}P in treating women with early-stage EOC (Young et al., 2003).

The use of the standard combination platinum-based chemotherapy is advantageous in community-based populations who may not have geographically friendly radiation oncology facilities. Patients who have had previous radiation therapy may experience compromised wound healing if further surgery is required or limited bone marrow reserve for future chemotherapy (Karlan et al., 2005). In the palliative setting, to control pain or bleeding, radiation may be indicated to reduce symptoms. Patients with metastasis to bone or brain may also benefit from radiation to reduce the tumor size or lessen symptoms. Patients with localized brain metastasis may respond to cranial resection and postoperative radiation or gamma knife (Cass & Karlan, 2003; Karlan et al., 2005).

Surveillance

Most women are advised to receive follow-up with their gynecologic oncologist after the completion of standard care at three-month intervals for two years. Surveillance may be more frequent if the woman is part of a clinical trial or desires second-look surgery. Follow-up care should include a CA-125 test, especially if this has served as a response marker, and a clinical examination, including rectovaginal examination (Martin & Cherry, 2006). The rectovaginal exam is an important component of the pelvic examination, as thickening and early tumor nodularity may identify early disease progression. An imaging scan may be recommended (e.g., CT scan, MRI, combination PET/CT of chest, abdomen, and pelvis) every 6–12 months as indicated. As eager as women are to complete their treatment protocol, they often experience anxiety or vulnerability being independent and away from the treatment center and the healthcare team. Oncology nurses may have the opportunity to address these issues and to explore referral resources such as support groups, networking with other women who have completed their treatment, encouraging returning to the workplace, and future well-woman care.

Recurrent Disease

Although EOC is one of the most chemosensitive tumors, and the majority of women achieve a clinical remission with initial taxane/platinum treatment, approximately 50%–75% will relapse within two years (Karlan et al., 2005). Chemotherapy is the treatment of choice for recurrent EOC, with the goal to achieve another remission. Multiple approved chemotherapy agents to treat recurrent EOC are available (see Figure 7-3); however, most of them provide temporary remission. The use of novel molecular targeted agents is being studied in recurrent ovarian disease, either as a single agent or in combination with a cytoxic agent (Burger, 2007). Bevacizumab is a monoclonal antibody that targets vascular endothelial growth factor and currently is being used in clinical trials with paclitaxel and carboplatin in front-line treatment, as well as for recurrent disease (Cannistra & McGuire, 2007). Other molecular agents being studied are the nuclear enzyme poly(ADP-ribose) polymerase -1 and -2, also known as *PARP-1* and *PARP-2* inhibitors, which lead to DNA repair, specifically in patients with *BRCA1* and *BRCA2* mutations (Farmer et al., 2005).

Cytoreductive surgery may be an option if the patient has an isolated tumor mass or nodule and will benefit from surgery instead of only chemotherapy. The ideal candidate for a second cytoreductive surgery is a patient who was optimally debulked and had a greater than 12-month disease-free interval, and a focal or isolated tumor (Bristow et al., 2002; Karlan et al., 2005). Even if a second cytoreductive surgery is an option, chemotherapy would ensue as part of the treatment plan. At clinical relapse, the serum CA-125 usually is elevated, but this elevation may occur as early as four months before development of symptoms, including ascites (NCCN, 2009; Rustin, Marples, Nepstrop, Mahmoudi, & Meyer, 2001).

In early relapse, radiologic scans, such as the CT scan are often not diagnostic even if patients have small amounts of ascites or peritoneal deposits (Guppy & Rustin, 2002). Tumor measurement evaluation for relapse documentation needs to be

Figure 7-3. Chemotherapy Regimens for Recurrent Ovarian Cancer

Platinum-Sensitive Disease	Platinum-Resistant Disease
Greater than six months disease-free interval	Less than six months disease-free interval
Cytotoxics • Retreatment with platinum agent • Single or combination • Carboplatin/gemcitabine • Cisplatin/gemcitabine • Oxaliplatin	Cytotoxics • Should not retreat with platinum unless clinical trial using a platinum drug reversal agent
Retreatment with taxane • Taxane: paclitaxel or docetaxel • Single or in combination • Weekly or every 21 days	Retreatment with taxane • Taxane: paclitaxel or docetaxel • Single or in combination • Weekly or every 21 days
Ixabepilone	Ixabepilone
Liposomal doxorubicin • Topotecan daily for 3–5 days or weekly • Gemcitabine • Cyclophosphamide	Liposomal doxorubicin • Topotecan: daily for 3–5 days or weekly • Gemcitabine • Cyclophosphamide: oral or IV
Vinorelbine	Vinorelbine
Ifosfamide	Ifosfamide
Capecitabine: single or combination IV agent	Capecitabine: single or combination IV agent
Altretamine	Altretamine
Oral etoposide	Oral etoposide

The following are not U.S. Food and Drug Administration–approved for epithelial ovarian cancer (EOC) but are being studied in clinical trials for EOC.

Selective estrogen receptor modulators
- Tamoxifen
- Raloxifene

Aromatase inhibitors
- Anastrozole
- Exemestane
- Letrozole

Monoclonal antibody
- Trastuzumab

Anti-vascular endothelial growth factor
- Bevacizumab

TK1 inhibitors
- Erlotinib
- Sorafenib

Chemosensitizer for chemoresistance
- Phenoxodiol

Note. Based on information from Burger, 2007; Cannistra, 2004; Farmer et al., 2005; Karlan et al., 2005; National Cancer Institute, 2008b; National Comprehensive Cancer Network, 2009; Rao et al., 2007.

interpreted with universal consistency on radiographic scan, especially in the setting of clinical trials. The World Health Organization has the most commonly used system in the past three decades (Miller, Hoogstraten, Staquet, & Winkler, 1981; Therasse et al., 2000). In 1994, a panel of international investigators collaborated to develop new guidelines for tumor response. The Response Evaluation Criteria in Solid Tumors Group (RECIST) is a consistency system to evaluate radiographic responses for measurable disease, which is especially important in clinical research. Patients with one-dimensional measurements, instead of the traditional bidimensional measurements, are evaluated for response to treatment using complete response, which is absence of tumor, partial response, stable disease, and progressive disease. The RECIST criteria have limitations, including evaluating bone and bone marrow involvement. In addition, target lesions (measurable) and nontarget lesions, such as ascites, or serum CA-125 levels, are included in the response evaluation (Therasse et al.).

Rising levels of CA-125 have not been embraced universally as an accurate measurement of recurrence, although many physicians will begin treatment based on an elevated CA-125, before clinical or radiologic evidence of recurrence (Goonewardene, Hall, & Rustin, 2007). The Rustin criteria are a CA-125 response criteria often used as a secondary endpoint in clinical trial design (Rustin et al., 2006). Rustin, Marples, Nelstrop, and Mahmoudi (2001) and Rustin et al. (2006) concluded that patients who had normalization of CA-125 after chemotherapy (clinical remission) and who then had a gradual elevation of CA-125 were deemed to have progression of their cancer if the CA-125 doubled from the upper limit of normal (i.e., CA-125 level equal to or greater than 70 U/ml). However, the Rustin criteria have not been universally adopted into clinical trial protocols (Goonewardene et al.; Rustin, 2003).

Determining which drug to administer in the recurrent setting often depends on the toxicity and side effect profile from previously administered chemotherapy. Each agent has its own unique set of side effects when given as a single agent, which may be augmented in combination with an additional agent. Oncology nurses often are the most familiar with a woman's chemotherapy side effect profile and may serve as an advocate and the liaison between physician and patient when a new treatment is being considered. For instance, a patient with a persistent grade 2 peripheral neuropathy should avoid a neurotoxic agent if other choices with similar efficacy are available. Similarly, any persistent or difficult-to-manage side effects, such as myelosuppression, nausea, or even self-esteem adjustment because of alopecia, should be considered when determining the next treatment regimen (Almadrones, 2007; Martin & Cherry, 2006).

Oral cytotoxic agents are being used more frequently, but in order to be effective, patients require a functional GI system without symptoms of nausea and vomiting, diarrhea, or bowel obstruction (Moore, 2007). Oral medications require patient adherence, which requires taking the correct dose, on time, for the prescribed amount of days. Patients also need to be educated to report any side effects to their healthcare team. Scheduling monthly follow-up visits for the patient along with instructions to return with the empty medication bottles may assist in confirming the patient is taking the medication correctly. Patient education is important, as patients may have misconceptions that an oral cytotoxic agent is less effective or has less serious side effects compared to IV medications (Moore).

Once relapse occurs, the probability of cure is very low. The goals of treatment remain long-term progression-free intervals and prolonged survival with the maintenance of good quality of life. This can be accomplished by managing disease complications and the long-term treatment-related toxicities (see Chapter 14). It is not uncommon for a woman to have multiple relapses and to receive numerous regimens of chemotherapy, with or without surgery, in order to prolong survival. Small or large bowel obstruction often indicates tumor progression, and signs and symptoms reported are nausea, vomiting, abdominal distention, constipation, and abdominal discomfort. Diagnostic tests may reveal that bowel obstruction is caused by adhesions or scar tissue and not a malignant mass. Bowel obstructions are seen in 25%–50% of women with EOC because of extrinsic compression of the bowel from tumor or adhesions (Martin, 2007). Obstruction of the bowel can be complete or partial, and each is managed differently. A complete obstruction requires immediate surgical intervention. A partial obstruction usually is managed conservatively with bowel rest for several days including nothing by mouth, IV fluids, and bowel decompression with a nasogastric tube.

Other complications of disease progression commonly experienced are reaccumulation of abdominal ascites and/or pleural effusion. These may be managed with paracentesis, thoracentesis, or another chemotherapy or biologic agent. Bevacizumab, although not FDA approved for EOC, has shown to be effective in controlling ascites (Burger, 2007).

Future Outlook

Despite EOC remaining a serious and life-threatening disease, advances have been made in surgical techniques and active cytotoxic and biologic agents that allow longer survival outcomes. Many unanswered questions remain, such as the most effective chemotherapy regimen up front, which agents and what dose, and if a third agent should be added to the platinum and taxane combination. Women with advanced ovarian cancer will most likely receive numerous chemotherapy regimens in the recurrent and palliative setting. Current research is exploring the most effective use of targeted and receptor-specific agents. Molecular targeted pathways may hold promise as an adjunct to chemotherapy and offer longer survival and fewer side effects. In addition, as research focuses on early detection of EOC, clinician and patient awareness of early symptoms and risk factors must continue so women will seek medical attention sooner. Interventions that prevent the disease or provide a cure are the ultimate outcomes. Identification of families with high-risk gene mutations may result in early risk-reducing interventions and disease prevention. A screening test is essential if EOC is to be detected early when cure is within a 90% range. The future holds promise as incessant researchers and the multidisciplinary teams work together for the same goal on behalf of the women and families affected by ovarian cancer.

Summary

Most women with EOC will undergo cytoreductive surgery and either IV or IP chemotherapy. Because ovarian cancer tends to be a chemosensitive disease, every effort continues to be made for improving early diagnosis and for new drug development. Oncology nurses will continue to manage and coordinate patient care, and ideally improve outcomes of adherence to prescribed therapy by effectively minimizing treatment side effects. In addition, supportive care has improved quality of life and maintenance of treatment schedules with the use of growth factors, erythropoietin-stimulating factors, and new classifications of antiemetics such as 5-HT_3 receptor antagonists and substance P/NK1 antagonists. Oncology nurses are significant team members who make a difference in a woman's and her family's cancer experience and quality of life. The initial diagnosis and referral to the appropriate oncologist and oncology center can be aided by nursing education to the general public. Assessing the patients physical, emotional, spiritual, and financial needs are skills oncology nurses perform daily. Identifying personal support and referrals help women and their families to plan and organize care. Although oncology nurses occupy many roles, including inpatient, outpatient, infusion center, private practice office, advanced practice, and home health and hospice, the common denominator is assessment, education, and evaluation. Nurses provide the day-to-day care, including symptom management, education, and reassurance.

References

Alberts, D.S., Liu, P.Y., Hannigan, E.V., O'Toole, R., Williams, S.D., Young, J.A., et al. (1996). Intraperitoneal cisplatin plus intravenous cyclophosphamide versus cisplatin plus intravenous cyclophosphamide for stage III ovarian cancer. *New England Journal of Medicine, 335*(26), 1950–1955.

Almadrones, L. (2007). Evidence-based research for intraperitoneal chemotherapy in epithelial ovarian cancer. *Clinical Journal of Oncology Nursing, 11*(2), 211–216.

American Cancer Society. (2008). *Cancer facts and figures, 2008*. Atlanta, GA: Author.

Arason, A., Jonasdottir, A., Barkardottir, R.B., Bergthorsson, J.T., Teare, M.D., Easton, D.F., et al. (1998). A population study of mutations and LOH at breast cancer gene loci in tumours from sister pairs: Two recurrent mutations seem to account for all *BRCA1*/*BRCA2* linked breast cancer in Iceland. *Journal of Medical Genetics, 35*, 446–449.

Armstrong, D.K., Bundy, B., Wenzel, L., Huang, H.Q., Baergan, R., Lele, S., et al. (2006). Intraperitoneal cisplatin and paclitaxel in ovarian cancer. *New England Journal of Medicine, 354*(1), 34–43.

Bast, R.C., Jr., Xu, F.J., Yu, Y.H., Barnhill, S., Zhang, Z., & Mills, G.B. (1998). CA 125: The past and the future. *International Journal of Biological Markers, 13*(4), 179–187.

Bast, R.C., Jr., Klug, T.L., St. John, E., Jenison, J.E., Niloff, J.M., Lazarus H., et al. (1983). A radioimmunoassay using a monoclonal antibody to monitor the course of epithelial ovarian cancer. *New England Journal of Medicine, 309*(15), 883–887.

Bankhead, C.R., Kehoe, S.T., & Austoker, J. (2005). Symptoms associated with diagnosis of ovarian cancer: A systematic review. *British Journal of Obstetrics and Gynecology, 112*(7), 857–865.

Bell, J., Brady, M.F., Young, R.C., Lage, J., Walker, J.L., Look, K.Y., et al. (2006). Randomized phase III trials of three versus six cycles of adjuvant carboplatin and paclitaxel in early stage epithelial ovarian carcinoma: A Gynecologic Oncology Group study. *Gynecologic Oncology, 102*(3), 432–439.

Berek, J.S. (2005). Epithelial ovarian cancer. In N. Hacker & J.S. Berek (Eds.). *Practical gynecologic oncology* (pp. 443–510). Philadelphia: Lippincott Williams & Wilkins.

Bloss, J.D., Brady, M.F., Liao, S.Y., Rocereto, T., Partridge, E.E., & Clarke-Pearson, D.L. (2003). Extraovarian peritoneal serous papillary carcinoma: A phase II trial of cisplatin and cyclophosphamide with comparison to a cohort with papillary serous ovarian carcinoma—a Gynecologic Oncology Group study. *Gynecologic Oncology, 89*(1), 148–154.

Bookman, M.A. (2005). Standard treatment in advanced ovarian cancer in 2005: The state of the art. *International Journal of Gynecological Cancer, 15*(Suppl. 3), 212–220.

Boyce, E.A., & Kohn, E.C. (2005). Ovarian cancer in the proteomics era: Diagnosis, prognosis, and therapeutic targets. *International Journal of Gynecological Cancer, 15*(Suppl. 3), 266–273.

Bristow, R.E., Tomacruz, R.S., Armstrong, D.K., Trimble, E.L., & Montz, F.J. (2002). Survival effects of maximal cytoreductive surgery for advanced ovarian carcinoma during the platinum era: Meta-analysis. *Journal of Clinical Oncology, 20*(5), 1248–1259.

Burger, R. (2007). Experience with bevacizumab in the management of epithelial ovarian cancer. *Journal of Clinical Oncology, 25*(20), 2902–2908.

Cannistra, S.A., & McGuire, W.P. (2007). Progress in the management of gynecologic cancer. *Journal of Clinical Oncology, 25*(20), 2865–2866.

Cannistra, S.A. (2004). Cancer of the ovary. *New England Journal of Medicine, 351*(24), 2519 2529.

Cass, I., Baldwin, R.I., Varkey, T., Moslehi, R., Narod, S.A., & Karlan, B.Y. (2003). Improved survival in women with *BRCA*-associated ovarian carcinoma. *Cancer, 97*(9), 2187–2195.

Cass, I., & Karlan, B.Y. (2003). Neoplasms of the ovary and fallopian tube. In J.R. Scott, R.S. Gibbs, B.Y. Karlan, & A.F. Haney (Eds.), *Danforth's obstetrics and gynecology* (9th ed., pp. 971–1006). Philadelphia: Lippincott Williams & Wilkins.

Chen, L., Yang, K.Y., Little, S.E., Cheung, M.K., & Caughey, A.B. (2007). Gynecologic cancer prevention in lynch syndrome/hereditary nonpolyposis colorectal cancer families. *Obstetrics and Gynecology, 110*(1), 18–25.

Cramer, D.W., & Welch, W.R. (1983). Determinants of ovarian cancer risk. II. Inferences regarding pathogenesis. *Journal of the National Cancer Institute, 71*(4), 717–721.

Cure, H., Battista, C., Guastalla, J.P., Fabbro, N., Tubiana, H., Bourgeois, B., et al. (2004). Phase III randomized trial of high-dose chemotherapy (HDC) and peripheral blood stem cell (PBSC) support as consolidation in patients (pts) with advanced ovarian cancer (AOC): 5-year follow up of GINECO/FNCLCC/SFGM-TC study [Abstract]. *Journal of Clinical Oncology, 22*(14S), 5006.

Daly, M., & Obrams, G.I. (1998). Epidemiology and risk assessment for ovarian cancer. *Seminars in Oncology, 25*(3), 255–264.

Dedrick, R.L., Myers, C.E., Bungay, P.M., & DeVita, V.T., Jr. (1978). Pharmacokinetic drug administration in the treatment of ovarian cancer. *Cancer Treatment Reports*, *62*(1), 1–9.

Dembo, A.J. (1992). Epithelial ovarian cancer: The role of radiotherapy. *International Journal of Radiation Oncology, Biology, Physics, 22*(5), 835–845.

duBois, A., Luck, H.J., & Meir, W. (2003). A randomized clinical trial of cisplatin/paclitaxel versus carboplatin/paclitaxel as first-line treatment of ovarian cancer. *Journal of the National Cancer Institute, 95*(17), 1320–1329.

Earle, C.C., Schrag, D., Neville, B.A., Yabroff, K.R., Topor, M., Fahey, A., et al. (2006). Effect of surgeon specialty on processes of care and outcomes for ovarian cancer patients. *Journal of the National Cancer Institute, 98*(3), 172–180.

Einbeigi, Z., Bergman, A., Kindblom, L.-G., Martinsson, T., Meis-Kindbloom, J.M., Nordling, M., et al. (2001). A founder mutation of the BRCA gene in Western Sweden associated with a high incidence of breast and ovarian cancer. *European Journal of Cancer, 37*(15), 1904–1909.

Eisenhauer, E.A., ten Bokkel Huinink, W.W., Swenerton, K.D., Gianni, L., Myles, J., van der Burg, M.E., et al. (1994). European-Canadian randomized trial of paclitaxel in relapsed ovarian cancer: High-dose versus low-dose and long versus short infusion. *Journal of Clinical Oncology, 12*(12), 2654–2666.

Eisenkop, S.M., Friedman, R.I., & Wang, H.J. (1998). Complete cytoreductive surgery is feasible and maximizes survival in patients with advanced epithelial ovarian cancer: A prospective study. *Gynecologic Oncology, 69*(2), 103–108.

Eriksson, J.H., & Frazier, S.R. (2000). Epithelial cancers of the ovary and fallopian tube. In G.J. Moore-Higgs, L.A. Almadrones, L.M. Gossfield, J.H. Eriksson, & B. Colvin-Huff (Eds.), *Women and cancer: A gynecologic oncology nursing perspective* (2nd ed., pp. 186–233). Sudbury, MA: Jones and Bartlett.

Evans, T.R., Mansi, J.L., & Bevan, D.H. (1996). Trousseau's syndrome in association with ovarian carcinoma. *Cancer, 77*(12), 2544–2549.

Fader, A.N., & Rose, P.G. (2007). Role of surgery in ovarian carcinoma. *Journal of Clinical Oncology, 25*(20), 2873–2883.

Farmer, H., McCabe, N., Lord, C.J., Tutt, A.N.J., Johnson, D.A., Richardson, T.B., et al. (2005). Targeting the DNA repair defect in BRCA mutant cells as a therapeutic strategy. *Nature, 434*(7035), 917–921.

Goff, B.A., Mandel, L.S., Melancon, C.H., & Muntz, H.G. (2004). Frequency of symptoms of ovarian cancer in women presenting to primary care clinics. *JAMA, 291*(22), 2705–2712.

Goff, B.A., Mandel, L.S., Drescher, C.W., Urban, N., Gough, S., Schurman, K.M., et al. (2007). Development of an ovarian cancer symptom index: Possibilities for earlier detection. *Cancer, 109*(2), 221–227.

Goff, B.A., Mandel, L.S., Muntz, H.G., & Melancon, C.H. (2000). Ovarian carcinoma diagnosis. *Cancer, 89*(10), 2068–2075.

Goonewardene, T.I., Hall, M.R., & Rustin, G.J. (2007). Management of asymptomatic patients on follow-up for ovarian cancer with rising CA-125 concentrations. *Lancet Oncology, 8*(9), 813–821.

Guppy, A.E., & Rustin, G.J. (2002). CA-125 response: Can it replace the traditional response criteria in ovarian cancer? *Oncologist, 7*(5), 437–443.

Havrilesky, L.J., Kulasingam, S.L., Matchar, D.B., & Myers, E.R. (2005). FDR-PET for management of cervical and ovarian cancer. *Gynecologic Oncology, 97*(1), 183–191.

Heaps, J.M., Nieberg, R.K., & Berek, J.S. (1990). Malignant neoplasms arising in endometriosis. *Obstetrics and Gynecology, 75*(6), 1023–1028.

Heinz, A., Odicino, F., Maisonneuve, P., Beller, U., Benedet, J.L., Creasman, W.T., et al. (2001). Carcinoma of the ovary. *Journal of Epidemiology and Biostatistics, 6*(1), 107–138.

Horner, M.J., Ries, L.A.G., Krapcho, M., Neyman, N., Aminou, R., Howlader, N., et al. (Eds.). (2009). *SEER cancer statistics review, 1975–2006*. Bethesda, MD: National Cancer Institute. Retrieved April 25, 2009, from http://seer.cancer.gov/csr/1975_2006/index.html

Howell, S.B., Pfeifle, C.L., Wung, W.E., Olshen, R.A., Lucas, W.E., Yon, J.L., et al. (1982). Intraperitoneal cisplatin with systemic thiosulfate. *Annals of Internal Medicine*, *97*(6), 845–851.

Hydzik, C. (2007). Implementation of intraperitoneal chemotherapy for the treatment of ovarian cancer. *Clinical Journal of Oncology Nursing, 11*(2), 221–225.

Ioffe, O.B., Simsir, A., & Silverberg, S.G. (2005). Pathology. In J.S. Berek & N.F. Hacker (Eds.), *Practical gynecologic oncology* (4th ed., pp. 163–242). Philadelphia: Lippincott Williams & Wilkins.

International Collaborative Ovarian Neoplasm Group. (2002). Paclitaxel plus carboplatin versus standard chemotherapy with either single-agent carboplatin or cyclophosphamide, doxorubicin, and cisplatin in women with ovarian cancer: The ICON3 randomised trial. *Lancet, 360*(9332), 505–515.

Karlan, B., Berchuck, A., & Mutch, D. (2007). The role of genetic testing for cancer susceptibility in gynecologic practice. *Obstetrics and Gynecology, 110*(1), 155–167.

Karlan, B.Y., Markman, M.A., & Eifel, P.J. (2005). Ovarian cancer, peritoneal carcinoma, and fallopian tube carcinoma. In V.T. DeVita, S. Hellman, & S.A. Rosenberg (Eds.), *Cancer: Principles and practice of oncology* (7th ed., pp. 1364–1397). Philadelphia: Lippincott Williams & Wilkins.

Kauff, N.D., & Barakat, R. (2007). Risk-reducing salpingo-oophorectomy in patients with germ line mutations in *BRCA1* or *BRCA2*. *Journal of Clinical Oncology, 25*(20), 2921–2927.

King, M.C., Marks, J.H., & Mandell, J.B. (2003). Breast and ovarian cancer risks due to inherited mutations in *BRCA1* and *BRCA2*. *Science, 302*(5645), 643–646.

Ledermann, J.A., Frickhofen, N., Wandt, H., Bengala, K., Champion, A., & Hinke, V. (2005). A phase III randomised trial of sequential high dose chemotherapy (HDC) with peripheral stem cell support or standard dose chemotherapy (SDC) for first-line treatment of ovarian cancer [Abstract]. *Journal Clinical Oncology, 23*(16S), 5006.

Lu, K., Knauff, N., Powell, C.B., Chen, L.M., Cass, I., Lancaster, J., et al. (2009). ACOG practice bulletin no. 103: Hereditary breast and ovarian cancer syndrome. *Obstetrics and Gynecology, 113*(4), 957–966.

Markman, M. (2007). New, expanded, and modified use of approved antineoplastic agents in ovarian cancer. *Oncologist*, *12*(2), 186–190.

Markman, M., Blessing, J., Rubin, S.C., Connor, J., Hanjani, P., & Waggoner, S. (2006). Phase II trial of weekly paclitaxel (80 mg/m^2) in platinum and paclitaxel-resistant ovarian and primary peritoneal cancers: A Gynecologic Oncology Group study. *Gynecologic Oncology*, *101*(3), 436–440.

Markman, M., Bundy, B.N., Alberts, D.S., Fowler, J.M., Clark-Pearson, D.L., Carson, L.F., et al. (2001). Phase III trial of standard dose intravenous cisplatin plus paclitaxel versus moderately high-dose carboplatin followed by intravenous paclitaxel and intraperitoneal cisplatin in small volume stage II ovarian carcinoma: An intergroup study of the Gynecologic Oncology Group, Southwestern Oncology Group, and Eastern Cooperative Oncology Group. *Journal of Clinical Oncology, 19*(4), 1001–1007.

Markman, M., Liu, P.Y., Wilczynski, S., Monk, B., Copeland, L.J., Alvarez, R.D., et al. (2003). Phase III randomized trial of 12 versus 3 months of maintenance paclitaxel in patients with advanced ovarian cancer after complete response to platinum and paclitaxel-based chemotherapy: A Southwest Oncology Group and Gynecologic Oncology Group trial. *Journal of Clinical Oncology, 21*(13), 2460–2465.

Markman, M., & Walker, J.L. (2006). Intraperitoneal chemotherapy of ovarian cancer: A review, with a focus on practical aspects of treatment. *Journal of Clinical Oncology, 24*(6), 988–994.

Martin, V.R. (2007). Ovarian cancer: An overview of treatment options. *Clinical Journal of Oncology Nursing, 11*(2), 201–207.

Martin, V.R., & Cherry, C. (2006). Ovarian cancer. In K.H. Dow (Ed.), *Nursing care of women with cancer* (pp. 96–119). St. Louis, MO: Elsevier Mosby.

McIntosh, M.W., Drescher, C., Karlan, B., Scholler, N., Urban, N., Hellstrom, K.E., et al. (2004). Combining CA125 and SMR serum markers for diagnosis and early detection of ovarian carcinoma. *Gynecologic Oncology, 95*(1), 9–15.

Menon, U., & Jacobs, I.J. (2005). Tumor markers and screening. In J.S. Berek & N.F. Hacker (Eds.), *Practical gynecologic oncology* (4th ed., pp. 43–66). Philadelphia: Lippincott Williams & Wilkins.

Miller, A.B., Hoogstraten, B., Staquet, M., & Winkler, A. (1981). Reporting results of cancer treatment. *Cancer, 47*(1), 207–214.

Mobus, V., Wandt, H., Frickhofen, N., Bengala, C., Champion, K., Kimmig, R., et al. (2007). Phase III trial of high-dose sequential chemotherapy with peripheral blood stem cell support compared with standard dose chemotherapy for first line treatment of advanced ovarian cancer: Intergoup trial of the AGO-Ovar/AIO and EBMT. *Journal of Clinical Oncology, 25*(27), 4187–4193.

Moore, S. (2007). Facilitating oral chemotherapy treatment and compliance through patient/family-focused education. *Cancer Nursing, 30*(2), 112–122.

Narod, S.A., Risch, H., Moslehi, R., Dorum, A., Neuhausen, S., Olsson, H., et al. (1998). Oral contraceptives and the risk of hereditary ovarian cancer. *New England Journal of Medicine, 339*(7), 424–428.

National Cancer Institute. (2007a). *Cancer stat fact sheet: Cancer of the ovary*. Retrieved August 16, 2007, from http://seer.cancer.gov/statfacts/html/ovary.html

National Cancer Institute. (2007b). *Epithelial ovarian cancer: Recurrent or persistent ovarian epithelial cancer.* Retrieved August 16, 2007, from http://www.cancer.gov/cancertopics/pdq/treatment/html/ovary.html

National Cancer Institute. (2007c, February 13). *Phase III randomized study of carboplatin and paclitaxel with or without low-dose paclitaxel in patients with early stage ovarian epithelial cancer.* Retrieved May 6, 2009, from http://www.cancer.gov/clinicaltrials/GOG-175

National Cancer Institute. (2008a). *Clinical trials*. Retrieved May 21, 2008, from http://www.cancer.gov/clinicaltrials

National Cancer Institute. (2008b). *Cancer genetics: Risk assessment and counseling (PDQ®).* Retrieved April 12, 2008, from http://www.cancer.gov/cancertopics/pdq/genetics/risk-assessment-and-counseling

National Comprehensive Cancer Network. (2009). *NCCN Clinical Practice Guidelines in Oncology™: Ovarian cancer*. Retrieved April 25, 2009, from http://www.nccn.org/professionals/physician_gls/PDF/ovarian.pdf

Neijt, J.P., Engelholm, S.A., Tuxen, M.K., Sorensen, P.G., Hansen, M., Sessa, C., et al. (2000). Exploratory phase III study of paclitaxel and cisplatin versus paclitaxel and carboplatin in advanced ovarian cancer. *Journal of Clinical Oncology, 18*(17), 3084–3092.

Nelson, H.D., Huffman, L.H., Fu, R., & Harris, E.L. (2005). Genetic risk assessment and *BRCA* mutation testing for breast and ovarian cancer susceptibility: Systemic evidence review for the U.S. Preventive Services Task Force. *Annals of Internal Medicine, 143*(5), 362–379.

Ozols, R.F. (2002). Future directions in the treatment of ovarian cancer. *Seminars in Oncology, 29*(Suppl. 1), 32–42.

Ozols, R.F., Bundy, B.N., Greer, B.E., Fowler, J.M., Clarke-Pearson, D., Burger, R.A., et al. (2003). Phase III trial of carboplatin and paclitaxel compared with cisplatin and paclitaxel in patients with optimally resected stage III ovarian cancer: A Gynecologic Oncology Group study. *Journal of Clinical Oncology, 21*(17), 3194–3200.

Ozols, R.F., Rubin, S.C., Thomas, G., & Robboy, S. (1997). Epithelial ovarian cancer. In W.J. Hoskins, C.A. Perez, & R.C. Young (Eds.), *Principles and practice of gynecologic oncology* (2nd ed., pp. 919–986). Philadelphia: Lippincott-Raven.

Peelen, T., vanVliet, M., Petrij-Bosch, A., Miermet, R., Szabo, C., van den Ouweland, A.M., et al. (1997) .A high proportion of novel mutations in *BRCA1* with strong founder effect among Dutch and Belgian hereditary breast and ovarian families. *American Journal of Human Genetics, 60*(5), 1041–1049.

Petricoin, E.F., Ardekani, A.M., Hitt, B.A., Levine, P.J., Fusaro, V.A., Steinberg, S.M., et al. (2002). Use of proteomic patterns in serum to identify ovarian cancer. *Lancet, 359*(9306), 572–577.

Piccart, M.J., Bertelson, J., James, K., Cassidy, J., Mangioni, C., Simonsen, E., et al. (2000). Randomized intergroup trial of cisplatin-paclitaxel versus cisplatin-cyclophosphamide in women with advanced epithelial ovarian cancer: Three-year results. *Journal of the National Cancer Institute, 92*(9), 699–708.

Piver, M.S. (2002). Hereditary ovarian cancer. Lessons from the first twenty years of the Gilda Radner Familial Ovarian Cancer Registry. *Gynecologic Oncology, 85*(1), 9–17.

Rao, G., Crispens, M., & Rothenberg, M.L. (2007). Intraperitoneal chemotherapy for ovarian cancer: Overview and perspective. *Journal of Clinical Oncology, 25*(20), 2867–2872.

Rebbeck, T.R., Friebel, T., Wagner, T., Lynch, H.T., Garber, J.E., Daley, M.B., et al. (2005). Effect of short term hormone replacement therapy on breast cancer risk reduction after bilateral prophylactic oophorectomy in *BRCA1* and *BRCA2* mutation carriers: The PROSE Study Group. *Journal of Clinical Oncology, 23*(31), 7804–7810.

Rodriguez, G., Boente, M.P., Berchuck, A., Whitaker, R., O'Briant, K.C., Xu, F., et al. (1993). The effects of antibodies and immunotoxins reactive with HER-2/neu on growth of ovarian and breast cancer cell lines. *American Journal of Obstetrics and Gynecology, 168*(1, Pt. 1), 228–232.

Rustin, G.J. (2003). Use of CA-125 to assess response to new agents in ovarian cancer trials. *Journal of Clinical Oncology, 21*(Suppl. 10), 187s–193s.

Rustin, G.J., Marples, M., Nelstrop, A.E., Mahmoudi, M., & Meyer, T. (2001). Use of CA-125 to define progression of ovarian cancer in patients with persistently elevated levels. *Journal of Clinical Oncology, 19*(20), 4054–4057.

Rustin, G.J., Timmers, P., Nelstrop, A., Shreeves, G., Bentzen, S.M., Baron, B., et al. (2006). Comparison of CA-125 and standard definitions of progression of ovarian cancer in the intergroup trial of cisplatin and paclitaxel versus cisplatin and cyclophosphamide. *Journal of Clinical Oncology, 24*(1), 45–51.

Ryerson, A.B., Eheman, C., Burton, J., McCall, N., Blackman, D., Subramanian, S., et al. (2007). Symptoms, diagnoses, and time to key diagnostic procedures among older U.S. women with ovarian cancer. *Obstetrics and Gynecology, 109*(5), 1053–1061.

Sabbatini, P., & Odunsi, K. (2007). Immunologic approaches to ovarian cancer treatment. *Journal of Clinical Oncology, 25*(20), 2884–2893.

Saygili, U., Guclu, S., Uslu, T., Erten, O., Demir, N., & Onvural, A. (2002). Can serum CA-125 levels predict the optimal primary cytoreduction in patients with advanced ovarian carcinoma? *Gynecologic Oncology, 86*(1), 57–61.

Schrag, D., Earle, C., Xu, F., Panageas, K.S., Yabroff, K.R., Bristow, R.E., et al. (2006) Associations between hospital and surgeon procedure volumes and patient outcomes after ovarian cancer resection. *Journal of the National Cancer Institute, 98*(3), 163–171.

Society of Gynecologic Oncologists. (2000). Guidelines for referral to a gynecologic oncologist: Rationale and benefits. *Gynecologic Oncology, 78*(3, Pt. 2), S1–S13.

Soussan, M., Wartski, M., Cherel, P., Fourme, E., Goupil, A., Le Stanc, E.F., et al. (2008). Impact of FDG PET/CT imaging on the decision making in the biologic suspicion of ovarian carcinoma recurrence. *Gynecologic Oncology, 108*(1), 160–165.

Therasse, P., Arbuck, S.G., Eisenhauer, E.A., Wanders, J., Kaplan, R.S., Rubinstein, L., et al., (2000). New guidelines to evaluate the response to treatment in solid tumors. *Journal of the National Cancer Institute, 92*(3), 205–216.

Vasey, P.A., Jayson, G.C., Gordon, A., Gabra, H., Coleman, R., Atkinson, R., et al. (2004). Phase III randomized trial of docetaxel-carboplatin versus paclitaxel-carboplatin as first-line chemotherapy for ovarian carcinoma. *Journal of the National Cancer Institute, 96*(22), 1682–1691.

Whittemore, A.S. (1994). Characteristics relating to ovarian cancer risk: Implications for prevention and detection. *Gynecologic Oncology, 55*(3, Pt. 2), S15–S19.

Whittemore, A.S., Harris, R., & Itnyre, J. (1992). Characteristics relating to ovarian cancer risk: Collaborative analysis of 12 U.S. case-control studies. IV. The pathogenesis of epithelial ovarian cancer. *American Journal of Epidemiology, 136*(10), 1212–1220.

Winter, W.E., Maxwell, G.L., Tian, C., Carlson, J.W., Ozols, R.F., Rose, P.G., et al. (2007). Prognostic factors for stage III epithelial ovarian cancer: A Gynecologic Oncology Group Study. *Journal of Clinical Oncology, 25*(24), 3621–3627.

Wong, C., Hempling, R.E., Piver, M.S., Natarajan, N., & Mettlin, C.J. (1990). Perineal talc exposure and subsequent epithelial ovarian cancer: A case control study. *Obstetrics and Gynecology, 93*(3), 372–376.

Young, R.C., Brady, M.F., Nieberg, R.K., Long, H.J., Mayer, A.R., Lentz, S.S., et al. (2003). Adjuvant treatment for early ovarian cancer: A randomized phase III trial of intraperitoneal ^{32}P or intravenous cyclophosphamide and cisplatin: A Gynecologic Oncology Group study. *Journal of Clinical Oncology, 21*(23), 4350–4355.

CHAPTER 8

Nonepithelial Ovarian Cancer

Virginia R. Martin, RN, MSN, AOCN®

Introduction

Epithelial cell ovarian cancer (EOC) comprises the majority of the disease (more than 85%) and arises from the surface epithelium of the ovary (Chen & Berek, 2009).Tumors that arise from the sex cords, the ovarian stroma or mesenchyme, or from the primordial germ cells of the ovary are much rarer (see Figure 8-1). Sex-cord stromal cells secrete hormones and connect different components of the ovary together. The most common type of malignancy is called granulosa cell tumor. Germ cells are precursors of the ova, and the most common type of malignancy is called dysgerminoma. Within these two categories of nonepithelial ovarian cancer are many other histologic varieties of tumors. Additionally, a few extremely rare ovarian cancers exist, such as sarcomas, lipoid cell tumors, or small cell carcinomas of the ovary. Nonepithelial ovarian cancers have some similarities in their presentation and management, as well as other unique qualities that require understanding and a special approach (Berek & Sathima, 2007). This chapter will provide an overview of this infrequent but distinctive class of ovarian tumors.

Figure 8-1. Ovarian Tumor Types and Their Origins

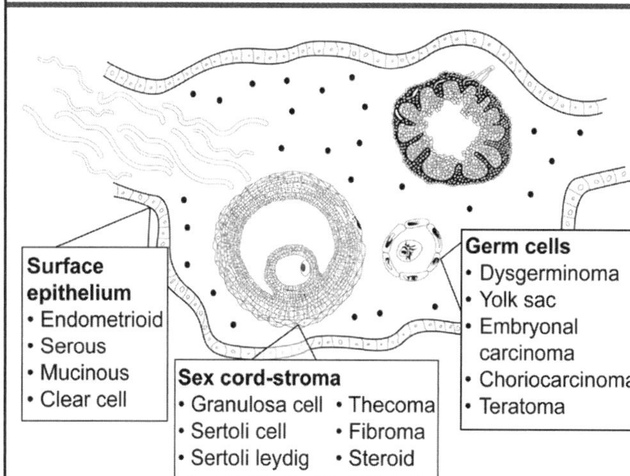

Note. From "Ovarian Cancer" (p. 99), by V.R. Martin and C. Cherry in K. Dow (Ed.), *Nursing Care of Women With Cancer,* 2006, St. Louis, MO: Elsevier Mosby. Copyright 2006 by Elsevier Mosby. Reprinted with permission. [Adapted from "Pathology and Classification of Ovarian Tumors," by V.W. Chen, B. Ruiz, J.L. Killeen, T.R. Cote, X.C. Wu, C.N. Correa, et al., 2003, Cancer, 97(Suppl. 10), p. 2632. Copyright 2003 by American Cancer Society. Used with permission of Wiley-Liss, Inc., a subsidiary of John Wiley & Sons, Inc.]

Ovarian Germ Cell Tumors

Malignant ovarian germ cell tumors (OGCT) make up about 5% of all ovarian cancers (Bekaii-Saab, Einhorn, &Williams, 1999; Dorigo & Berek, 2009). The age-adjusted incidence is 0.41 per 100,000, making it 40 times less common than epithelial tumors (Patterson & Rustin, 2006). OGCTs are rare but curable at most stages of the disease. These tumors arise from the primordial germ cells of the ovary and may be benign or malignant (Dorigo & Berek). They are the female equivalent of testicular cancer, arising in the gonad from undifferentiated germ cells. In fact, much of the treatment strategies come from the more frequently occurring testicular cancer. Dysgerminomas are the most common type of malignant OGCTs, accounting up to 40%; immature teratomas are the second most common (35.6%); and endodermal sinus tumors are the third most common type (14.5%) (Berek & Hacker, 2005; Dorigo & Berek). Also, other subtypes occur less frequently; these are listed in Figure 8-2.

Etiology and Epidemiology

OGCTs are seen most commonly in girls and young women between the ages of 10–30 years; the mean age is in the teenage years (Berek & Hacker, 2005; Dorigo & Berek, 2009; Gershenson, 2007). OGCTs represent about 70% of ovarian tumors found in this age group, and as many as one-third can

Figure 8-2. Histologic Typing of Ovarian Germ Cell Tumors

I. Primitive germ cell tumors
  A. Dysgerminoma
  B. Yolk sac tumor
  C. Embryonal carcinoma
  D. Polyembryoma
  E. Nongestational choriocarcinoma
  F. Mixed germ cell tumor

II. Biphasic or triphasic teratoma
  A. Immature teratoma
  B. Mature teratoma
    1. Solid
    2. Cystic, dermoid cyst
      a) Fetiform teratoma (homunculus)

III. Monodermal teratoma and somatic-type tumors associated with dermoid cysts
  A. Thyroid tumor
    1. Struma ovarii
      a) Benign
      b) Malignant
    2. Carcinoid
    3. Neuroectodermal tumor
    4. Carcinoma
    5. Melanocyte
    6. Sarcoma
    7. Sebaceous tumor
    8. Pituitary-type tumor
    9. Others

Note. From "WHO Histologic Classification of Tumors of the Ovary" (p. 1457), by J.S. Berek and N. Sathima in J.S. Berek (Ed.), *Berek and Novak's Gynecology* (14th ed.), 2006, Philadelphia: Lippincott Williams & Wilkins. Copyright 2006 by Lippincott Williams & Wilkins. Adapted with permission.

be malignant (Berek & Hacker; Zalel et al., 1996). For unclear reasons, malignant OGCTs occur more frequently in Asian and black women, which is in direct contrast to the incidence of epithelial ovarian cancer (Berek & Hacker; Dorgio & Berek). Malignant OGCTs are subdivided most practically into dysgerminoma (the most common type and the counterpart of the male seminoma) and nondysgerminoma tumors (e.g., endodermal sinus, yolk sac, immature teratoma, mixed germ cell) (Gershenson, 2007). An adaptation of the 2003 World Health Organization histologic classification of malignant germ cell tumors is presented in Figure 8-2 (Berek & Sathima, 2007). The histologic classification system divides the malignant OGCTs into three categories (Roth & Talerman, 2006):

- Primitive germ cell tumors
- Biphasic and triphasic teratomas
- Monodermal teratoma and somatic-type tumors associated with dermoid cysts.

Benign cystic mature teratomas (also called dermoid cysts) comprise the most common benign ovarian germ cell tumors.

Clinical Presentation and Diagnostic Evaluation

A pelvic mass is the most common presenting problem in a woman with an OGCT. Signs and symptoms may include acute abdominal pain mimicking appendicitis, which usually is caused by a rupture, hemorrhage, or torsion of the ovarian tumor. Eighty-five percent of women have both abdominal pain and an abdominal mass (Dorigo & Berek, 2009). Less commonly, women may present with distention of the abdomen, vaginal bleeding, precocious puberty, symptoms of pregnancy, or fever. Unlike epithelial tumors, these tumors can grow rapidly, with a large median size of 16 centimeters at diagnosis, but despite the size of the tumor, most patients present with stage IA disease.

Germ cell tumors produce hormonal or certain enzyme activity, which also occurs in testicular cancer. All women who present with a pelvic mass must have blood drawn for tumor markers alpha-feto protein (AFP) and human chorionic gonadotropin (HCG) because elevated tumor markers in the absence of pregnancy play a vital role in diagnosis. Besides aiding in diagnosis of the disease, the markers help to monitor response during treatment and for post-treatment surveillance. A summary of OGCTs and relevant circulating hormones is presented in Table 8-1. A small number of germ cell tumors commonly produce lactic dehydrogenase (LDH), and dysgerminoma tumors produce placental alkaline phosphatase and LDH. CA-125 may be elevated, but it is not reliable for diagnosis in premenopausal women. OCT-4 immunohistochemistry is a transcription factor expressed in pluripotent embryonic stem and germ cells (Patterson & Rustin, 2006). In two studies, OCT-4 immunohistochemistry demonstrated very high specificity for the diagnosis of embryonal tumors and dysgerminoma (Cheng et al., 2004; Looijenga et al., 2005). Another recent study of 30 cases of dysgerminoma found 87% expressed the tyrosine kinase receptor c-kit. This may become an additional marker for diagnosis and may lead to testing targeted therapies in this disease (Sever et al., 2005).

Staging

The OGCTs are staged surgically and according to the International Federation of Gynecology and Obstetrics (FIGO) surgical staging system for ovarian cancer (see Appendix). The disease spreads via the lymphatics, the bloodstream, or peritoneal surface dissemination. Nodal involvement is seen more commonly than in epithelial ovarian cancer. Prognostic factors include (Dorigo & Berek, 2009; Gershenson, 2007; Patterson & Rustin, 2006)

- Stage (FIGO)
- Presence of residual disease
- Histologic subtype
- Elevation of serum markers.

Lai et al. (2005) found that advanced stage and nondysgerminoma/immature teratoma histology were associated with

Table 8-1. Ovarian Germ Cell Tumors and Relevant Secreted Circulating Tumor Marker Substances

Germ Cell Tumor Type	Secreted Tumor Markers
Ovarian choriocarcinoma	– AFP + HCG
Immature teratoma	Rarely +AFP +/– LDH
Mixed germ cell (may contain embryonal, choriocarcinoma, endodermal sinus components)	+/– HCG +/– AFP +/– LDH
Dysgerminoma	Normal AFP + LDH Occasionally, small amounts hCG Placental alkaline phosphatase
Endodermal sinus tumor	+ AFP + LDH
Embryonal cancer	+/– AFP + HCG +/– LDH
Polyembryoma	+ HCG + AFP

AFP—alpha-fetoprotein; HCG—human chorionic gonadotropin; LDH—lactate dehydrogenase

Note. Based on information from Berek & Hacker, 2005; Dorigo & Berek, 2009; Gershenson, 2007.

increased risk of treatment failure, and nondysgerminoma/immature histology and bulky residual disease after salvage surgery were associated with a worse overall survival. Elevation of both HCG and AFP and a FIGO early stage are strong predictors of survival (Murugaesu et al., 2006).

Treatment

Malignant OGCT treatment generally follows the principles of EOC: surgery and postoperative chemotherapy. A few differences are as follows (Chalas, Valea, & Mann, 2009).

- Surgery often is able to be limited to the diseased ovary because many OGCTs present in early stages and in younger women.
- OGCTs are more sensitive to platinum-based therapy.
- The tumor marker C-125 is not useful in OGCTs, but the markers HCG, AFP, and LDH are very sensitive and may be used for monitoring the treatment response (see Table 8-1).

Surgery

Most gynecologic oncologists approach this disease similar to EOC and do a comprehensive surgical staging of the disease as the main approach to treatment. This surgical approach mostly has been extrapolated from experience with EOC and is both diagnostic and therapeutic. It provides information about the extent of the disease, assists in determining the prognosis, and helps to guide treatment postoperatively. The tumors tend to be quite large, and about 60% are confined to one ovary (Gershenson, 2007). Intraoperative frozen section of the ovarian mass is performed first during surgery to confirm the diagnosis. An expert gynecologic pathologist is crucial to diagnosing this rare ovarian neoplasm. After a frozen section diagnosis is made, the remaining surgical approach will be directed by the age of the woman and her desire for fertility preservation. Unilateral salpingo-oophorectomy with careful inspection of the contralateral ovary is the standard approach if fertility preservation is desired. Following 182 women whose disease was grossly confined to the one ovary, fertility-sparing surgery did not worsen the prognosis (Kurman & Norris, 1977). It is important to remove the corresponding fallopian tube of the ovarian tumor because of the lymphovascular connections between the tube and the ovary. Biopsy of the contralateral ovary is recommended if the ovary appears abnormal, but nothing further is done if on inspection it appears normal. Ovarian cystectomy may be adequate surgery in some patients but is not the recommended standard. The scope of the procedure in postmenopausal women or those who have completed childbearing includes (Gershenson, 2007)

- Bilateral salpingo-oophorectomy (BSO)
- Total abdominal hysterectomy (TAH)
- Peritoneal cytologic washings
- Careful and systematic abdominal exploration with inspection and palpation of all peritoneal surfaces
- Multiple biopsies of the pelvic and abdominal peritoneum, including
  - Posterior cul-de-sac
  - Bladder reflection
  - Bilateral pelvic sidewalls
  - Bilateral paracolic spaces
  - Diaphragmatic surfaces
  - Omentectomy
  - Retroperitoneal lymphadenectomy, including the bilateral pelvic and para-aortic lymph nodes.

These malignant tumors occur so rarely that beneficial extent of surgical reduction is difficult to establish because of the lack of ability to conduct randomized clinical trials. In a study conducted by Gynecologic Oncology Group (GOG), patients who received postoperative chemotherapy after complete resection fared better in overall survival than those who had not been completely resected (68% versus 28%) (Slayton et al., 1985). Two additional studies showed that nondysgerminoma tumors might in fact have a better outcome with optimal debulking surgery (Bafna et al., 2001; Williams, Blessing, Moore, Homesley, & Adcock, 1989). However, a 2004 study by the Pediatric Oncology Group and the Children's Study Group found that deviations from the standard surgical guidelines did not adversely affect survival (Billmire et al., 2004). As a result of this study, new surgical guidelines that are less comprehensive are being studied. Another dilemma seen with this diagnosis is the referral of a patient to a gynecologic oncologist after diagnosis; the question is posed as to whether additional surgical exploration is necessary if comprehensive surgical staging was not completed. The most recent study supports that further surgery is not necessary, but individual practitioners make the decision based typically on computed tomography (CT) scans and tumor markers (Billmire et al.; Gershenson, 2007). Second-look surgery is not recommended in general for women with malignant OGCT, and primary surgery remains the important component of management of OGCTs.

Chemotherapy

Chemotherapy for dysgerminoma: Following the advances made in the early 1970s with germ cell testicular tumors, cisplatin-based regimens have improved the overall prognosis of women with OGCTs. Even women with a very poor prognosis have been cured. At least 90% of early-stage and 75%–80% of advanced-stage disease are long-term survivors (Chalas et al., 2009; Gershenson et al., 1985, 1990; Williams et al., 1987, 1989). The first combination regimen used was vincristine, actinomycin-D, and cyclophosphamide (VAC) (Gershenson et al., 1985; Slayton et al., 1985). Vinblastine, bleomycin, and cisplatin (VBP) was the next platinum-based chemotherapy regimen to be implemented. In the largest trial, 89 stage II–IV patients demonstrated that 53% remained progression free following VBP chemotherapy (Gershenson et al., 1986). Based on the successful testicular cancer trials using etoposide, Williams et al. (1987) compared cisplatin, vinblastine, and bleomycin with bleomycin, etoposide, and cisplatin (BEP), which demonstrated equal efficacy with less toxicity. Four cycles of BEP postoperatively remains the standard treatment regimen today for dysgerminomas with occult metastatic disease, disease in the contralateral ovary, and metastatic disease. Disease confined to one or both ovaries with no evidence of metastatic disease does not require postoperative chemotherapy treatment; the patient is observed closely and evaluated with regular CT scans. Carboplatin can be the preferred substitution in the regimen if the patient has preexisting renal disease or peripheral neuropathy. The use of carboplatin as a replacement for cisplatin has been studied extensively in testicular and pediatric cancer, but cisplatin combination therapy is used more commonly (Chalas et al., 2009). The National Comprehensive Cancer Network (NCCN, 2009) guidelines recommend BEP. With current treatment regimens, the cure rates approach 100% for patients with early-stage disease and are at least 75% in patients with advanced stages (Gershenson, 2007).

Dysgerminomas often occur in young women and may coexist with pregnancy. Stage IA disease can be treated with surgical resection during pregnancy. If the disease is a higher stage, chemotherapy can be given in the second and third trimester without hurting the fetus (Berek & Hacker, 2005).

Chemotherapy for nondysgerminomatous tumors: Immature teratomas (stage IA, grade 1) require no adjuvant treatment. All other stages and grades require adjuvant chemotherapy. See Table 8-2 for an in-depth review of nondysgerminomatous tumor treatment. Endodermal sinus tumors require adjuvant treatment following surgery. Before the addition of combination chemotherapy, the two-year survival rate for this disease was 25% (Berek & Hacker, 2005). VBP became the preferred regimen over VAC based on results of a GOG trial with superior complete response rate (Williams et al., 1987). In the largest GOG trial using BEP in stages I, II, and III (Williams, Blessing, Liao, Ball, & Hanjani, 1994), 91 of 93 patients who received three postoperative courses of BEP after complete resection did not relapse; thus, BEP is the current the preferred regimen for both adjuvant and advanced disease. The optimal number of cycles has not been studied, but guidelines from NCCN (2009) recommend BEP for nondysgerminomatous tumors. Recurrence can occur rapidly after surgery, and chemotherapy is recommended to start postoperatively.

Long-Term Sequelae

Most of the information available regarding long-term sequelae is from the larger population of men being treated for testicular cancer with similar drug regimens. In men, renal and gonadal dysfunction, neurotoxicity, cardiovascular toxicity, and secondary malignancy have been found. In women, temporary ovarian dysfunction occurs with cisplatin-based therapy, but most women eventually resume normal ovarian functions (Kanazawa, Suzuki, & Sakumoto, 2000). Studies suggest that at least 80% of patients who were treated with fertility-sparing surgery followed by platinum-based chemotherapy had normal menstrual function and normal pregnancies (Brewer et al., 1999; Low, Perrin, Crandon, & Hacker, 2000; Tangir, Zelterman, Ma, & Schwartz, 2003; Zanetta et al., 2001). A second malignancy such as leukemia can occur in patients with testicular cancer treated with etoposide over a long period of time. This development is known to be dose related, and because BEP patients receive a limited number of cycles, second malignancies have not been seen in dysgerminoma patients (Nichols, Breeden, Loehrer, Williams, & Einhorn, 1993). GOG sponsored a study comparing survivors of germ cell tumors with a matched control group examining menstrual and reproductive outcomes, sexual functioning, and dyadic (ability to form close relationship) adjustment; 132 survivors and 137 controls completed the study questionnaires. The study results found that of the fertile survivors, 62 (87.3%) reported still having menstrual periods, and 24 had children (37 in total) after cancer treatment (Gershenson et al., 2007). The survivors reported more reproductive concerns and less sexual pleasure than the control group. The survivors

Table 8-2. Summary of the Treatment Approaches for Nondysgerminomatous Ovarian Tumors

Type	Characteristics	Treatment
Teratomas: Mature	Known as dermoid cysts Cystic or solid mass Benign Can contain tissues of ectoderm (skin, hair follicles, sebaceous cells)	Cystectomy 1% of mature teratomas malignant For those, treatment would be based on stage and include adjuvant chemotherapy with BEP.
Teratomas: Immature	Malignant teratoma, terablastoma, and embryonal teratoma Composed of tissue from all three germ cell layers: ectoderm, mesoderm, and endoderm The only ovarian germ cell tumor graded histologically	Surgery for all malignant tumors Unilateral salpingo-oophorectomy if future child-bearing desired or full surgical staging with total abdominal hysterectomy and bilateral-salpingo-oophorectomy Stage IA grade 1 tumors do not need further treatment. BEP chemotherapy for other stages
Monodermal	Most common: struma ovarii Thyroid tissue present in ovarian tumor Carcinoid: tissue gastrointestinal or respiratory epithelium; may have carcinoid syndrome	Surgery May use radioiodine therapy, and may need to treat for hyperthyroidism
Endodermal sinus tumors or yolk sac	Occurs in young girls and women, median age 18 years. Patients present most often with abdominal pain and a pelvic mass.	Unilateral salpingo-oophorectomy followed by chemotherapy, most often BEP for three cycles
Embryonal carcinoma	Aggressive ovarian malignancy, average age at diagnosis 15 years. Resembles embryonal carcinoma of the testes. Patients present with abdominal pain.	Surgery followed by chemotherapy, commonly BEP
Mixed germ cell tumor	Contain two or more ovarian germ cell types	Surgery and chemotherapy with BEP
Polyembryonic	Aggressive tumor composed of embryoid bodies that resemble normal embryos; occurs in young girls who may present with pseudo puberty	Surgery followed by chemotherapy with BEP or platinum-based regimen
Choriocarcinoma	Occurs very rarely Like the choriocarcinoma of the placenta; early hematogenous spread, more resistant to chemotherapy	Surgery followed by chemotherapy with BEP

BEP—bleomycin, etoposide, and cisplatin

Note. Based on information from Berek & Hacker, 2005; Chalas et al., 2009.

reported better dyadic consensus, dyadic satisfaction, and dyadic cohesion (Gershenson, 2007).

Radiation

Dysgerminoma stands apart from other germ cell tumors based on its radiosensitivity; the dose of 2,500–3,500 cGY is curative. Before the combination chemotherapy era, radiation therapy was the postoperative treatment for metastatic dysgerminomas with excellent outcomes (Chalas et al., 2009). However, ovarian failure after radiotherapy despite ovarian shielding during treatment was a problem. In the 1980s, combination platinum-based regimens replaced radiotherapy as the standard treatment for metastatic dysgerminomas thus enabling fertility preservation (Brewer et al., 1999; Gershenson et al., 1986; Williams, Blessing, Hatch, & Homesley, 1991; Williams et al., 2004). Today radiation therapy rarely is used as first-line treatment.

Recurrent Disease

Only a small percentage of women with OGCTs experience recurrence, and most (75%) occur within 12–24 months of primary diagnosis (Berek & Sathima, 2007). A standard approach for treatment after recurrence has not been determined, but women who had only initial surgery usually receive chemotherapy. If chemotherapy was given as primary therapy, radiation therapy may be given. Radiotherapy is effective in dysgerminomas and should be considered when disease recurs, although loss of fertility may result. If BEP was the primary therapy, POMB-ACE (cisplatin, vincristine, methotrexate, bleomycin, etoposide, actinomycin, and cyclophosphamide) may be used (Berek & Hacker, 2005). Other salvage regimens include vinblastine, ifosfamide, and cisplatin; etoposide, ifosfamide and cisplatin; and/or paclitaxel, ifosfamide, and cisplatin (Chalas et al., 2009). Consideration may also be given to the administration of high-dose chemotherapy utilizing carboplatin and etoposide (Berek & Sathima, 2007).

Sex Cord Stromal Tumors

Etiology and Epidemiology

Sex cord stromal tumors account for about 7% of all ovarian malignancies (Colombo, Parma, Zanagnolo, & Insinga, 2007). This group of tumors originates from the sex cords of the developing gonads and the ovarian stroma or mesenchyme. Sex cord cells may differentiate into granulosa cells or Sertoli cells, depending on the gonadal development going toward an ovarian or testicular pathway. Sex cord tumors are composed of various combinations of elements including the "female" cells (granulosa and theca cells) and "male" cells (Sertoli and Leydig cells). These sex cord cells surround the oocytes and include the cells that produce the ovarian hormones such as estradiol, or more infrequently, androgen. A clinical suspicion for this uncommon diagnosis may be excessive estrogen or androgen production. The exact etiology of these tumors in humans remains unknown. The tumors can be benign or malignant (Figure 8-3). Most are early stage, with low malignant potential, and the natural history is indolent, producing an overall favorable prognosis (Colombo et al.; Dorigo & Berek, 2009).

Figure 8-3. Classification of Sex Cord–Stromal Ovarian Tumors

Granulosa stromal cell tumors
- Granulosa
  - Adult type
  - Juvenile type
- Tumor in the thecoma-fibroma group
  - Thecoma
  - Fibroma-fibrosarcoma
  - Sclerosing stromal tumor

Sertoli-Leydig cell tumors, androblastomas
- Sertoli
- Leydig
- Sertoli-Leydig
  - Well differentiated
  - Intermediate differentiation
  - Poorly differentiated
  - With heterologous elements
  - Retiform
  - Mixed

Gynandroblastoma
Sex cord tumor with annular tubules
Unclassified

Note. From "Management of Ovarian Stromal Cell Tumors," by N. Colombo, G. Parma, V. Zanagnolo, and A. Insinga, 2007, *Journal of Clinical Oncology, 25*(20), p. 2945. Copyright 2007 by American Society of Clinical Oncology. Reprinted with permission.

Granulosa Stromal Cell Tumors

The granulosa stromal cell tumors' histologic types include granulosa cell tumors, thecomas, and fibromas and account for 70% of the ovarian sex cord tumors (Colombo et al., 2007). A granulosa cell tumor is a low-grade malignancy, whereas thecomas and fibromas rarely have features that resemble a malignancy but when malignant are referred to as fibrosarcomas. The granulosa cell tumor, although most commonly low grade, has the potential to recur and metastasize. Granulosa cell has two subtypes: adult, which is more frequently occurring (95%); and the juvenile granulosa cell tumor (5%) (Colombo et al.; Schumer & Cannistra 2003). The juvenile type usually is diagnosed in prepubertal girls and women younger than 30 (Calaminus, Wessalowski, Harms, & Gobel, 1997; Scully, 1988; Young, Dickersin, & Scully, 1984). The most common adult type of granulosa cell tumor is found in the perimenopausal or postmenopausal woman and diagnosed at a median age of 50–54 (Schumer & Cannistra). No inherited predisposition has been connected to the generation of granulosa cell tumors, and *BRCA1* and *BRCA2* mutations are not associated with it (Schumer & Cannistra). Adult granulosa cell tumors secrete excess estrogen. Most often the ovarian tumor is unilateral (95%), and 78%–91% of cases are stage I at diagnosis (Bjorkholm & Silfversward, 1981; Evans, Gaffey, Malkasian, & Annegers, 1980; Stenwig, Haczekamp, & Beecham, 1979). Slow growth, local spread, and late recurrence are all part of the disease's natural history, and this indolent growth pattern lends itself to late recurrence (Colombo et al.).

Clinical Presentation and Diagnostic Evaluation

The adult granulosa cell tumors' most common presentation is postmenopausal bleeding, and most women will have a palpable abdominal mass. This is often caused by prolonged exposure of the endometrium to tumor-derived estradiol resulting in hyperplasia or adenocarcinoma (Evans et al., 1980; Griffiths & Koelliker, 1995; Gusberg & Kardon, 1971; Schumer & Cannistra, 2003). Endometrial cancer occurs in association with granulosa cell tumors in at least 5% of cases, but 25%–50% are associated with endometrial hyperplasia (Aboud, 1997; Cronje, Niemand, Bam, & Woodruff, 1999; Segal, DePetrillo, & Thomas, 1995). Symptoms also may relate to endocrine abnormalities produced by the tumor such as menstrual irregularities in premenopausal women (Door, 2002). Nonspecific symptoms include ascites, increasing abdominal girth, or abdominal pain. A diagnosis of sex cord stromal tumor must be considered in someone who presents with signs of estrogen excess, including abnormal uterine bleeding, secondary amenorrhea, or endometrial hyperplasia/ carcinoma (Dorigo & Berek, 2009).

Juvenile granulosa cell tumors occur most frequently in prepubertal girls. Almost all prepubescent girls with these tumors present at stage I and are unilateral. The signs and symptoms include breast enlargement, development of pubic and axillary hair, irregular uterine bleeding, and other secondary sex characteristics. Infrequently, patients present with a virilization syndrome because the tumor is androgen-secreting (Colombo et al., 2007).

The size of the tumor can vary from a microscopic lesion not detectable at a pelvic exam to a very large mass; the average is around 12 centimeters (Colombo et al., 2007). Juvenile tumors developing in women after puberty present similar to the adult type with abdominal pain or swelling. Severe pain at diagnosis is usually from adnexal torsion, hemorrhage into the tumor, or rupture of a cystic component. Granulosa cell tumors tend to be hemorrhagic and occasionally rupture (Fox, Agrawal, & Langley, 1975; Schumer & Cannistra, 2003; Stenwig et al., 1979).

Granulosa cell tumors secrete protein, specifically inhibin. Inhibin is a heterodimeric polypeptide hormone that is produced by the ovaries in response to follicle-stimulating hormone and luteinizing hormone (Dorigo & Berek, 2009). It usually is undetectable after menopause. Inhibin levels can be used for tumor surveillance after treatment. Estradiol was used as a marker because it is secreted by granulosa cell tumors, but it is not a sensitive enough tumor marker for the disease. In fact, up to 30% of tumors do not produce estradiol (Dorgio & Berek). Müllerian inhibitory substance (MIS) is produced by granulosa cells and is a potential marker for the granulosa cell tumor (Matias-Guiu, Pons, & Prat, 1998), but its specific use is still being studied. These tumors are large and unilateral, are usually multicystic, and have a yellow coloration from accumulation of lipids. An ultrasound is recommended preoperatively along with an endometrial biopsy because of the correlation with endometrial hyperplasia and cancer (Schumer & Cannistra, 2007).

Histologic diagnosis is made by immunohistochemical staining for markers of granulosa cell tumors, including (Hildebrandt, Rouse, & Longacre, 1997; Matias-Guiu et al., 1998)

- Inhibin
- CD99
- MIS
- Vimentin
- Cytokeratin
- S-100 protein
- Smooth muscle actin.

The prognostic factor that is the most significant for granulosa cell tumor is the surgical stage. Other prognostic factors remain more controversial, including (Schumer & Cannistra, 2003)

- Tumor size (larger than 10–15 cm associated with inferior survival)
- Mitotic index (greater than or equal to 4–10 mitoses per 10 high-power fields worse prognosis in some series)
- Tumor rupture (some think it is worse, but equivocal)
- Age (younger than 40 worse prognosis).

Staging

Surgery is the cornerstone of management of this disease for definitive diagnosis, staging, and removing as much tumor as possible—the same as all ovarian cancers. The disease is staged surgically using the FIGO staging system as with EOC (see Appendix). Prognosis is presented by stage in Table 8-3.

Treatment

The treatment plan depends on the age of the patient and the extent of the disease. Surgery alone is sufficient treatment for most cases of granulosa cell tumors, with chemotherapy or radiation therapy reserved for those patients with recurrent or metastatic disease (Colombo et al., 2007; Dorigo & Berek, 2009; Schumer & Cannistra, 2003).

Surgery

A staging laparotomy procedure with careful inspection of the contralateral ovary and tube, as well as the pelvic and para-aortic lymph nodes, is needed (Dorigo & Berek 2009). If the opposite ovary appears enlarged or abnormal, it should be biopsied. A TAH and BSO are recommended for perimenopausal and postmenopausal women or if fertility is not a concern. The principle of surgery is the same as surgical management of EOC, and complete surgical staging is an important factor for prognosis. A vertical midline incision is

Table 8-3. Granulosa Cell Tumor Prognosis by Stage

FIGO Stage	5-Year Survival Percentage	10-Year Survival Percentage
I	90%–100%	84%–95%
II	55%–75%	50%–65%
III and IV	22%–50%	17%–33% (combined data)

Note. From "Granulosa Cell Tumor of the Ovary," by S.T. Schumer and S.A. Cannistra, 2003, *Journal of Clinical Oncology, 21*(6), p. 1181. Copyright 2003 by American Society of Clinical Oncology. Reprinted with permission.

the approach because the upper abdomen must be examined with inspection of the omentum, the diaphragm, the paracolic gutters, and the bowel to rule out metastases (Schumer & Cannistra, 2003). Unilateral salpingo-oophorectomy is appropriate for stage IA tumors in children or women of childbearing age. Retrospective studies show equal cure rates for unilateral versus bilateral salpingo-oophorectomy (Gershenson, 1994; Zhang et al., 2007). The long-term disease-free survival rates for women with stage I disease is approximately 90% (Dorigo & Berek). Positive outcomes are slightly less for women with higher stage disease or stage I disease with tumor larger than10 cm, if the tumor ruptures, or if the tumor has a high mitotic index (Dorigo & Berek).

Chemotherapy

The low number of women with sex cord stromal tumors makes randomized clinical trials difficult to conduct. No evidence exists that proves adjuvant chemotherapy will prevent recurrences in stage I disease because the disease has an overall good prognosis and the disease is indolent in nature. Postoperative chemotherapy must be part of the treatment plan for those women with advanced disease. Complete responses have been reported with single agents such as cyclophosphamide or melphalan, as well as combinations such as VAC, PAC (cisplatin, doxorubicin, and cyclophosphamide), EP (etoposide, cisplatin), or BEP (Briasoulis et al., 1997; Dorigo & Berek, 2009; Schumer & Cannistra, 2003). Retrospective analysis suggests that postoperative chemotherapy is associated with prolonged progression-free interval in stage III–IV disease (Uygun et al., 2003), with an overall response rate of 63%–80% (Colombo et al., 2007) but with no survival benefit (Al-Badawi et al., 2002). Despite convincing data, some experts recommend postoperative chemotherapy with BEP, PAC, or carboplatin or cisplatin alone for women with completely resected advanced-stage disease (Berek & Hacker, 2005). If patients are unable to achieve an optimal debulking at surgery, BEP combination chemotherapy produces response rates of 58% and 84% in selected studies (Gershenson et al., 1996; Homesley Bundy, Hurteau, & Roth, 1999). Most recently, platinum and paclitaxel therapy had favorable results and a better toxicity profile (Brown et al., 2005). In summary, women with stage I disease should have surgery (either fertility sparing or complete hysterectomy and BSO) with no further treatment but close surveillance. Patients with high-risk stage I disease and all disease stages greater than II should have postoperative platinum-based chemotherapy.

Radiation

No evidence supports the use of postoperative radiation for granulosa cell tumors. Palliative radiation may delay growth of isolated recurrent disease in the pelvis (Savage et al., 1998; Schumer & Cannistra, 2003; Wolf et al., 1999). Granulosa cell tumors are labeled as radioresponsive, and radiation can induce clinical responses and occasional long-term remissions (Wolf et al.). Overall, some patients may benefit from radiotherapy if their disease does not seem amenable to surgery; every case should be considered individually (Colombo et al).

Recurrent Disease

No standard approach exists for recurrent disease treatment. The most common site of recurrence is the pelvis or upper abdomen. If pelvic or intra-abdominal disease is present, consideration may be given to surgery followed by postoperative radiation. Median time to recurrence is four to six years after the initial diagnosis, but late recurrences have been reported as many as 40 years after diagnosis (Berek & Hacker, 2005; Wolf et al., 1999). Surveillance should include a pelvic examination and serum inhibin levels every three months for two years, then every four to six months for three to five years, and then annually (Dorigo & Berek, 2009; Schumer & Cannistra, 2003). Radiologic studies may be ordered if clinically indicated. Platinum-based chemotherapy is a reasonable choice for more widespread disease or disease that is suboptimally debulked. Use of hormonal agents or antiestrogens has been suggested, but no data support the effectiveness of this treatment approach (Schumer & Cannistra).

The more infrequently occurring sex-cord tumor characteristics and general treatment approaches are summarized in Table 8-4.

Rare Nonepithelial Ovarian Tumors

Small Cell Carcinoma

Ovarian small cell carcinoma usually presents with bilateral disease at an average age of 24 years (Young, Oliva, & Scully, 1994). A paraneoplastic syndrome of hypercalcemia may also present at diagnosis. More than half of women have disease spread beyond the pelvis at diagnosis, and similar to small cell carcinoma of the lung, it is very aggressive and often fatal. Treatment includes platinum-based chemotherapy and/or radiation (Berek & Hacker, 2005).

Lipoid Cell Tumors

Lipoid cell tumors are theorized to originate in adrenal cortical rests near the ovary (Berek & Hacker 2005). The tumor most often presents unilaterally, and at presentation the patient may exhibit virilization, obesity, hypertension, and/or glucose intolerance (Berek & Hacker). The tumor is mostly benign or low grade, and surgical removal of the primary lesion is the primary treatment (Berek & Hacker).

Sarcomas

Malignant mixed mesodermal sarcoma is a very rare ovarian tumor that occurs in postmenopausal women. It can be bio-

Table 8-4. Less Common Sex Cord Stromal Tumors Characteristics and Treatment

Tumor Type	Characteristics	Treatment
Juvenile granulosa cell	Less aggressive than adult 90% stage I	Surgery Platinum-based therapy in advanced tumors commonly BEP
Thecomas	Composed of theca cells Benign, solid fibromatous tumors. Usually unilateral. Found in postmenopausal women Present with abnormal bleeding	Surgery—TAH-BSO or unilateral oophorectomy Endometrial sampling
Fibromas	Benign solid tumors Unilateral Postmenopausal women Not hormonally active May have ascites	Unilateral salpingo-oophorectomy
Sertoli-Leydig Sertoli cells line the tubules Leydig cells are in the stroma 5 subtypes: well-differentiated, intermediate differentiated, poorly differentiated, retiform, and mixed	Occur in women under age of 40 Large, confined to one ovary May present with hormonal changes or abdominal pain or increasing abdominal girth. Pure Sertoli tumors—estrogenic and may lead to hyperkalemia or hypertension. Pure Leydig tumors—androgen secreting and cause virilization, oligomenorrhea, amenorrhea, breast atrophy, hirsutism, deepening voice, male pattern baldness, acne, clitoral enlargement. Combined Sertoli-Leydig tumors (androblastomas)	Unilateral and stage I Low grade usually Treatment usually TAH-BSO Poorly differentiated tumors and metastatic tumors are treated with chemotherapy BEP commonly used regimen
Gynandroblastoma Has Sertoli-Leydig cells and granulosa cells	Benign mixed tumor associated with androgen and estrogen	Unilateral salpingo-oophorectomy
Sex cord tumor with annular tubules	Can produce estradiol and progesterone Present with abnormal uterine bleeding	Surgery Advanced disease chemotherapy with BEP

BEP—bleomycin, etoposide, and cisplatin; BSO—bilateral salpingo-oophorectomy; TAH—total abdominal hysterectomy

Note. Based on information from Berek & Hacker, 2005; Dorigo & Berek, 2009.

logically aggressive with metastases at the time of diagnosis (Barakat et al., 1992; Berek & Hacker, 2005; Fowler, Nathan, Nieberg, & Berek, 1996). Surgery followed by platinum-based chemotherapy is the recommended treatment (Barakat et al.; Fowler et al.). For more specific details about gynecologic sarcomas, refer to Chapter 9.

Summary

The nonepithelial ovarian cancers occur much less frequently than EOC. Most have a good prognosis, are characterized by slow growth with local spread, and are treated with surgery. For the more aggressive late-stage tumors, postoperative chemotherapy is indicated, and the treatment is similar to the more common EOC. Because these tumors present in such a wide age range of women (from prepuberty to postmenopausal), the care of every patient must be individualized.

References

Aboud, E. (1997). A review of granulosa cell tumours and thecomas of the ovary. *Archives of Gynecology and Obstetrics, 259*(4), 161–165.

Al-Badawi, I.A., Brasher, P.M., Ghatage, P., Nation, J.G., Schepansky, A., & Stuart, G.C. (2002). Postoperative chemotherapy in advanced ovarian granulosa cell tumors. *International Journal of Gynecological Cancer, 12*(1), 119–123.

Bafna, U.D., Umadevi, K., Kumaran, C., Nagarathna, D.S., Shashikala, P., & Tanseem, R. (2001). Germ cell tumors of the ovary: Is there a role for aggressive cytoreductive surgery for nondysgerminomatous tumors? *International Journal of Gynecological Cancer, 11*(4), 300–304.

Barakat, R.R., Rubin, S.C., Wong, G., Saigo, P.E., Markman, M., & Hoskins, W.J. (1992). Mixed mesodermal tumor of the ovary: Analysis of prognostic factors in 31 cases. *Obstetrics and Gynecology, 80*(4), 660–664.

Bekaii-Saab, T., Einhorn, L.H., & Williams, S.D. (1999). Late relapse of ovarian dysgerminoma: Case report and literature review. *Gynecologic Oncology, 72*(1), 111–112.

Berek, J.S., & Hacker, N.F. (2005). Nonepithelial ovarian and fallopian tube cancers. In J.S. Berek & N.F. Hacker (Eds.), *Practical gynecologic oncology* (4th ed., pp. 511–540). Philadelphia: Lippincott Williams & Wilkins.

Berek, J.S., & Sathima, N. (2007). Ovarian and fallopian tube cancer. In J.S. Berek (Ed.), *Berek's and Novak's gynecology* (14th ed., 1504–1547). Philadelphia: Lippincott Williams & Wilkins.

Billmire, D., Vinocur, C., Rescorla, F., Cushing, B., London, W., Schlatter, M., et al. (2004). Outcome and staging evaluation in malignant germ cell tumors of the ovary in children and adolescents: An intergroup study. *Journal of Pediatric Surgery, 39*(3), 424–429.

Bjorkholm, E., & Silfversward, C. (1981). Prognostic factors in granulosa-cell tumors. *Gynecologic Oncology, 11*(3), 261–274.

Brewer, M., Gershendon, D.M., Herzog, C.E., Mitchell, M.F., Silva, E.C., & Wharton, J.T. (1999). Outcome and reproductive function after chemotherapy for ovarian dysgerminoma. *Journal of Clinical Oncology, 17*(9), 2670–2675.

Briasoulis, E., Karavasilis, V., & Pavlidis, N. (1997). Megestrol activity in recurrent adult type granulose cell tumour of the ovary. *Annals of Oncology, 8*(8), 811–812.

Brown, J., Shvartsman, H.S., Deavers, M.T., Ramondetta, L.M., Burke, T.W., Munsell, M.F., et al. (2005). The activity of taxanes compared with bleomycin, etoposide, and cisplatin in the treatment of sex-cord stromal ovarian tumors. *Gynecologic Oncology, 97*(2), 489–496.

Calaminus, G., Wessalowski, R., Harms, D., & Gobel, U. (1997). Juvenile granulosa cell tumor of the ovary in children and adolescents: Results from 33 patients registered in a prospective cooperative study. *Gynecology Oncology, 65*(3), 447–452.

Chalas, E., Valea, F.A., & Mann, W.J. (2009). T*reatment of malignant germ cell tumors of the ovary*. Retrieved April 21, 2009, from http://www.uptodate.com

Chen, L., & Berek, J.S. (2009) *Epithelial ovarian cancer: Clinical manifestations, diagnostic evaluation, staging, and histopathology.* Retrieved April 21, 2009, from http://www.uptodate.com

Cheng, L., Thomas, A., Roth, L.M., Zheng, W., Michael, H., & Karim, F.W. (2004). OCT4: A novel biomarker for dysgerminoma of the ovary. *American Journal of Surgical Pathology, 28*(10), 1341–1346.

Colombo, N., Parma, G., Zanagnolo, V., & Insinga, A. (2007). Management of ovarian stromal cell tumors. *Journal of Clinical Oncology, 25*(20), 2944–2951.

Cronje, H.S., Niemand, L., Bam, R.H., & Woodruff, J.D. (1999). Review of the granulosa-theca cell tumors from the Emil Novak ovarian tumor registry. *American Journal of Obstetrics and Gynecology, 180*(2, Pt. 1), 323–327.

Door, A. (2002). Less common gynecologic malignancies. *Seminars in Oncology Nursing, 18*(3), 207–222.

Dorigo, O., & Berek, J.S. (2009). *Sex cord-stromal tumors of the ovary*. Retrieved April 21, 2009, from http://www.uptodate.com

Evans, A.T., III, Gaffey, T.A., Malkasian, G.D., Jr., & Annegers, J.F. (1980). Clinicopathologic review of 118 granulosa and 82 theca cell tumors. *Obstetrics and Gynecology, 55*(2), 231–238.

Fowler, J.M., Nathan, L., Nieberg, R.K., & Berek, J.S. (1996). Mixed mesodermal sarcoma of the ovary in a young patient. *European Journal of Obstetrics, Gynecology, and Reproductive Biology, 65*(2), 249–253.

Fox, H., Agrawal, K, & Langley, F.A. (1975). A clinicopathologic study of 92 cases of granulosa cell tumor of the ovary with special reference to the factors influencing prognosis. *Cancer, 35*(1), 231–241.

Gershenson, D.M. (1994). Management of early ovarian cancer: Germ cell and sex cord-stromal tumors. *Gynecologic Oncology, 55*(3, Pt. 2), S62–S72.

Gershenson, D.M. (2007). Management of ovarian germ cell tumors. *Journal of Clinical Oncology, 25*(20), 2938–2943.

Gershenson, D.M., Copeland L.J., Kavanagh J.J., Cangir A., Del Junco G., Saul P.B., et al. (1985). Treatment of malignant nondysgerminomatous germ cell tumors of the ovary with vincristine, dactinomycin, and cyclophosphamide. *Cancer, 56*(12), 2756–2761.

Gershenson, D.M., Miller, A.M., Champion, V.L., Monahan, P.O., Zhao, Q., Cella, D., et al. (2007). Reproductive and sexual function after platinum-based chemotherapy in long-term ovarian germ cell tumor survivors: A Gynecologic Oncology Group study. *Journal of Clinical Oncology, 25*(19), 2792–2797.

Gershenson, D.M., Morris, M., Burke, T.W., Levenback, C., Matthews, C.M., & Wharton, J.T. (1996). Treatment of poor prognosis sex cord-stromal tumors of the ovary with the combination of bleomycin, etoposide, and cisplatin. *Obstetrics and Gynecology, 87*(4), 527–531.

Gershenson, D.M., Morris, M, Cangir, A., Kavanagh, J.J., Stringer, C.A., Edwards, C.L., et al. (1990). Treatment of malignant germ cell tumors of the ovary with bleomycin, etoposide, and cisplatin. *Journal of Clinical Oncology, 8*(4), 715–720.

Gershenson, D.M., Wharton, J.T., Kline, R.C., Larson, D.M., Kavanagh J.J., & Rutledge F.N. (1986). Chemotherapeutic complete remission in patients with metastatic ovarian dysgerminoma. Potential for cure and preservation of reproductive capacity. *Cancer, 58*(12), 2594–2599.

Griffiths, C.T., & Koelliker, D.D. (1995). Case 10-1995—A 56-year-old woman with abdominal pain, anemia, and a pelvic mass. *New England Journal of Medicine, 332*(13), 876–881.

Gusberg, S.B., & Kardon, P. (1971). Proliferative endometrial response to theca-granulosa cell tumors. *American Journal of Obstetrics and Gynecology, 111*(5), 633–643.

Hildebrandt, R.H., Rouse, R.V., & Longacre, T.A. (1997). Value of inhibin in the identification of granulosa cell tumors of the ovary. *Human Pathology, 28*(12), 1387–1397.

Homesley, H.D., Bundy, B.N., Hurteau, J.A., & Roth, L.M. (1999). Bleomycin, etoposide, and cisplatin combination therapy of ovarian granulosa cell tumors and other stromal malignancies: A Gynecologic Oncology Group study. *Gynecologic Oncology, 72*(2), 131–137.

Kanazawa, K., Suzuki, T., & Sakumoto, K. (2000). Treatment of malignant ovarian germ cell tumors with preservation of fertility: Reproductive performance after persistent remissions. *American Journal of Clinical Oncology, 23*(3), 244–248.

Kurman, R.J., & Norris, H.J. (1977). Malignant germ cell tumors of the ovary. *Human Pathology, 8*(5), 551–564.

Lai, C.H., Chang, T.C., Hsueh, S., Wu, T.I, Chao, A., Chou, H.H., et al. (2005). Outcome and prognostic factors in ovarian germ cell malignancies. *Gynecologic Oncology, 96*(3), 784–791.

Looijenga, L.H., Stoop, H., deLeeuw, H.P., de Gouveia Brazao, C.A., Gillis, A.J., van Roozendaal, K.E., et al. (2003). POU5F1 (OCT3/4) identifies cells with pluripotent potential in human germ cell tumors. *Cancer Research, 63*(9), 224–2250.

Low, J.J.H., Perrin, L.C., Crandon, A.J., & Hacker, N.F. (2000). Conservative surgery to preserve ovarian function in patients with malignant germ cell tumors: A review of 74 cases. *Cancer, 89*(2), 391–398.

Matias-Guiu, X., Pons, C., & Prat, J. (1998). Müllerian inhibiting substance, alpha-inhibin, and CD99 expression in sex cord-stromal tumors and endometrioid ovarian carcinomas resembling sex cord-stromal tumors. *Human Pathology, 29*(8), 840–845.

Murugaesu, N., Schmid, P., Dancey, G., Agarwal, R., Holden, L., McNeish, I., et al. (2006). Malignant germ cell tumors: Identification of novel prognostic markers and long-term outcome after multimodality treatment. *Journal of Clinical Oncology, 24*(30), 4862–4866.

National Comprehensive Cancer Network. (2009). *NCCN Clinical Practice Guidelines in Oncology™: Ovarian cancer including fallopian tube cancer and primary peritoneal cancer* [v.1.2009]. Retrieved April 7, 2009, from http://www.nccn.org/professionals/physician_gls/PDF/ovarian.pdf

Nichols, C.R., Breeden, E.S., Loehrer, P.J., Williams, S.D., & Einhorn, L.H. (1993). Secondary leukemia associated with a conventional dose of etoposide: Review of serial germ cell tumor protocols. *Journal of the National Cancer Institute, 85*(1), 36–40.

Patterson, D.M., & Rustin, G.J.S. (2006). Controversies in the management of germ cell tumours of the ovary. *Current Opinion in Oncology, 18*(5), 500–506.

Roth, L.M., & Talerman, A. (2006). Recent advances in the pathology and classification of ovarian germ cell tumors. *International Journal of Gynecological Pathology, 25*(4), 305–320.

Savage, P., Constenla, D., Fisher, C., Shepherd, J.H., Barton, D.P., Blake, P., et al. (1998). Granulosa cell tumors of the ovary; demographics, survival, and the management of advanced disease. *Clinical Oncology (Royal College of Radiologists, Great Britain), 10*(4), 242–245.

Schumer, S.T., & Cannistra, S.A. (2003). Granulosa cell tumor of the ovary. *Journal of Clinical Oncology, 21*(6), 1180–1189.

Scully, R.E. (1988). Juvenile granulosa cell tumor. *Pediatric Pathology, 8*(4), 423–427.

Segal, R., DePetrillo, A.D., & Thomas, G. (1995). Clinical review of adult granulosa cell tumors of the ovary. *Gynecologic Oncology, 56*(3), 338–344.

Sever, M., Jones, T.D., Roth, L.M., Karim, F.W.A., Zheng, W., Michael, H., et al. (2005) Expression of CD117 (c-kit) receptor in dysgerminoma of the ovary: Diagnostic and therapeutic implications. *Modern Pathology, 18*(11), 1411–1416.

Slayton, R.E., Park, R.C., Silverberg, S.C., Shingleton, H., Creasman, W.T., & Blessing, J.A. (1985). Vincristine, dactinomycin, and cyclophosphamide in the treatment of malignant germ cell tumors of the ovary: A Gynecologic Oncology Group study (a final report). *Cancer, 56*(2), 243–248.

Stenwig, J.T., Haczekamp, J.T., & Beecham, J.B. (1979). Granulosa cell tumors of the ovary. A clinicopathological study of 118 cases with long-term follow up. *Gynecologic Oncology, 7*(1), 136–152.

Tangir, J., Zelterman, D., Ma, W., & Schwartz, P.E. (2003). Reproductive function after conservative surgery and chemotherapy for malignant germ cell tumors of the ovary. *Obstetrics and Gynecology, 101*(2), 251–257.

Uygun, K., Aydiner, A., Saip, P., Kocak, Z., Basaran, M., Dincer, M., et al. (2003). Clinical parameters and treatment results in recurrent granulosa cell tumor of the ovary. *Gynecologic Oncology, 88*(3), 400–403.

Williams, S.D., Birch, R., Einhorn, L.H., Irwin, L., Greco, F.A., & Loehrer, P.J. (1987). Treatment of disseminated germ-cell tumors with cisplatin, bleomycin, and either vinblastine or etoposide. *New England Journal of Medicine, 316*(23), 1435–1440.

Williams, S.D., Blessing, J.A., Moore, D. H., Homesley, H.D., & Adcock, L. (1989). Cisplatin, vinblastine, and bleomycin in advanced and recurrent ovarian germ-cell tumors. A trial of the Gynecologic Oncology Group. *Annals of Internal Medicine, 111*(1), 22–27.

Williams, S.D., Blessing, J.A., Hatch, K.D., & Homesley, H.D. (1991). Chemotherapy of advanced dysgerminoma: Trials of the Gynecologic Oncology Group. *Journal of Clinical Oncology, 9*(11), 1950–1955.

Williams, S.D., Blessing, J.A., Liao, S., Ball, H.J., & Hanjani, P. (1994). Adjuvant therapy of ovarian germ cell tumors with cisplatin, etoposide, and bleomycin: A trial of the Gynecologic Oncology Group. *Journal of Clinical Oncology, 12*(4), 701–706.

Williams, S.D., Kauderer, J., Burnett, A.F., Lentz, S.S., Aghajanian, C., & Armstrong, D.K. (2004). Adjuvant therapy of completely resected dysgerminoma with carboplatin and etoposide: A trial of the Gynecologic, Oncology Group. *Gynecologic Oncology, 95*(3), 496–499.

Wolf, J.K., Mullen, J., Eifel, C., Burke, T.W., Levenback, C., & Gershenson, D.M. (1999). Radiation treatment of tumors of advanced or recurrent granulosa cell tumor of the ovary. *Gynecologic Oncology, 73*(1), 35–41.

Young, R.H., Dickersin, G.R., & Scully, R.E. (1984). Juvenile granulosa cell tumors of the ovary: A clinicopathologic analysis of 125 cases. *American Journal of Surgical Pathology, 8*(8), 575–596.

Young, R.H., Oliva, E., & Scully, R.E. (1994). Small cell carcinoma of the ovary, hypercalcemic type. A clinicopathologic analysis of 150 cases. *American Journal of Surgical Pathology, 18*(11), 1102–1116.

Zalel, Y., Piura, B., Elchalal, U., Czernobilsky, B., Antebi, S., & Dgani, R. (1996). Diagnosis and management of malignant germ cell ovarian tumors in young females. *International Journal of Gynaecology and Obstetrics, 55*(1), 1–10.

Zanetta, G., Bonazzi, C., Cantu, M.G., Bini, S., Locatelli, A., Bratina, G., et al. (2001). Survival and reproductive function after treatment of malignant germ cell ovarian tumors. *Journal of Clinical Oncology, 19*(4), 1015–1020.

Zhang, M., Cheung, M.K., Shin, J.Y., Kapp, D.S., Husain, A., Teng, N.N., et al. (2007). Prognostic factors responsible for survival in sex cord-stromal tumors of the ovary—an analysis of 376 women. *Gynecologic Oncology, 104*(2), 396–400.

CHAPTER 9

Gynecologic Sarcomas

Dorothy Dulko, PhD, RN, AOCNP®

Introduction

Gynecologic sarcomas are rare but devastating malignancies. Sarcomas arising from the uterine corpus comprise approximately 1% of all gynecologic cancers and less than 5% of all uterine malignancies (Hensley et al., 2002). Vulvar-vaginal sarcomas usually are classified as nonextremity soft tissue sarcomas and account for about 10% of nonextremity soft tissue malignancies (Hensley, 2000). Cervical and ovarian sarcomas are exceedingly rare, with most available data regarding these tumors being derived from case reports and small case series and limited data regarding optimal treatment or prognostic factors (Gari, Souhami, Arseneau, & Stanimir, 2006; Wright et al., 2005). The only identified risk factor in 10%–25% of these malignancies is prior pelvic radiation therapy administered for benign uterine bleeding 5–25 years earlier (Hensley, 2000; Robinson, Keus, Shasha, & Harrison, 1998).

Sarcomas arising from female genital tissues vary in (Chauveinc et al., 1999)

- Histology
- Sensitivity to cytotoxic chemotherapy
- Response to hormonal agents
- Prognosis, with prognosis depending on
  - Stage
  - Histology
  - Grade
  - Mitotic index.

Women with gynecologic sarcomas are at high risk for recurrence, even when diagnosed at an early stage (Look, Sandler, Blessing, Lucci, & Harrison, 2004). Although low-grade uterine sarcomas have an indolent course, high-grade uterine sarcomas commonly are associated with survival length of only one to two years (Hensley, 2000). Sarcomas of the vulva and vagina carry an especially poor prognosis and a high rate of recurrence, with a five-year survival rate of approximately 30% even in early-stage disease (Chauveinc et al., 1999). Surgery is the primary treatment for patients with uterine sarcoma and may be curative in cases where the tumor is confined to the uterus (Leitao et al., 2002). Radiation and chemotherapy are used in the adjuvant setting and as primary treatments in patients presenting with advanced disease (Denschlag, Masoud, Stanimir, & Gilbert, 2006).

Patients with recurrent or persistent disease are not curable with currently available treatments. Despite recent identification of new chemotherapy and novel agents for gynecologic sarcomas, outcome data regarding cost and quality of life are extremely scarce. With scant evidence available from prospective trials to guide management decisions, the review of current practice is needed continually. Traditional clinical trial end points such as disease control and overall survival are needed to establish best possible treatment strategies in this rare malignancy. Future research in patients with gynecologic sarcomas should incorporate surrogate end points and evaluate the effect of noncurative treatment on outcomes such as symptom experience and quality of life.

Etiology and Epidemiology

Uterine Sarcomas

The literature describing the epidemiology of uterine sarcomas is limited, with the most comprehensive reports describing these sarcomas published in 1989 and 1999 (Brooks, Zhan, Cote, & Baquet, 2004). Because of the relatively low incidence of this malignancy and its pathologic multiplicity, no overall consensus has been reached on the epidemiology of uterine sarcoma. Likewise, no consensus has been reached on the optimum management of these tumors, with considerable variation in the type of surgery and choices of adjuvant treatment offered to women with uterine sarcoma.

Harlow, Weiss, and Lofton (1986) described an increased incidence of leiomyosarcoma (LMS) and mixed mesodermal sarcoma for African American women when compared with Caucasian females; however, little data were available at that time regarding survival, stage distribution, and treatment.

Subsequent research by Platz and Benda (1995) indicated that Caucasian women were more likely to be diagnosed with localized disease when compared with African Americans. An age-specific, age-adjusted analysis of Surveillance, Epidemiology and End Results (SEER) program of the National Cancer Institute (NCI) of more than 2,500 women with uterine sarcomas over a 10-year period confirmed the prior findings of Harlow et al. (1986) that African Americans are at greater risk than Caucasians for the occurrence of uterine LMS and carcinosarcoma (Brooks et al., 2004). The etiology of this increased incidence remains unknown. Notably, the analysis by Brooks et al. reported no significant difference in survival when the treatment received by African-American and Caucasian women was similar. A few studies have correlated tamoxifen use with an increased incidence of uterine sarcomas (Wickerham et al., 2002; Wysowski, Honig, & Beitz, 2002). Also, isolated reports have determined that oral contraceptive use and noncontraceptive estrogens may be associated with a higher risk of LMS and mixed mesodermal tumor, respectively (Schwartz et al., 1996).

The histology of uterine sarcomas is subcharacterized by tissue of origin. Tumor stage is the most important prognostic factor for all histologic subtypes (Gadducci, Cosio, Romanini, & Genazzani, 2008). Uterine sarcomas are classified into four main histologic subtypes: carcinosarcomas, leiomyosarcomas, endometrial stromal sarcomas, and "other" sarcomas (Kempson & Bari, 1970). Table 9-1 presents SEER data for 1988–2001 outlining the distribution of uterine sarcoma cases by pathologic classification (Kosary, 2007). Table 9-2 summarizes the five-year relative survival rates by histology and stage.

Uterine sarcomas have aggressive clinical behavior, with a propensity to local recurrence and more frequently to distant spread (Gadducci et al., 2008). Median time to recurrence for uterine sarcoma, except low-grade endometrial stromal sarcoma, is less than two years, with this time interval being inversely related to tumor stage (Gadducci et al., 1996, 2008; Sartori et al., 1997). Conversely, low-grade endometrial stromal sarcoma can recur more than 20 years after diagnosis (Berchuck et al., 1990; Gadducci et al., 2008; Inayama et al., 2000). Most distant relapses of uterine sarcomas involve the lungs and upper abdomen, whereas brain metastases are less common (Gadducci et al., 2008). Recognizing the metastatic potential of uterine sarcomas is important, as distant lesions can be found everywhere (Falconi, Crippa, Sargenti, Capelli, & Pederzoli, 2006; Gadducci et al., 2008; Iwamoto et al., 2005; Yokoyama, Ono, Sakamoto, Fukuda, & Mizunuma, 2004).

Leiomyosarcoma

LMS is the most common uterine sarcoma (Acharya, Hensley, Montag, & Fleming, 2005). The median age at diagnosis is in the early 50s, with cases occurring more often in women aged 30–50 years, as compared to other uterine sarcomas, which have a much higher incidence in women older than 50 years (Brooks et al., 2004; Leitao, Sonoda, Brennan, Barakat, & Chi, 2003). Approximately 0.1% of uterine LMSs are diagnosed incidentally at the time of myomectomy or hysterectomy performed for presumed benign leiomyomas (Leitao et al., 2003). Five-year survival rates are 18.8%–65% for all stages of disease (Giuntolli et al., 2003; Mayerhofer et al., 2004), with the five-year overall survival being reported as 52%–85% in stage I disease (Wu et al., 2005). In women with stage I and II high-grade uterine LMS, recurrence rates at two years are 60%–70% (Acharya et al.).

Table 9-1. Pathologic Classification and Incidence of Uterine Sarcomas

Tissue of Origin	Classification	Percent of All Uterine Malignancies*
Myometrium	Leiomyosarcoma	1.9%
Endometrial epithelium	Endometrial stromal sarcoma	1.3%
Mixed epithelial and mesenchymal differentiation	Carcinosarcoma or malignant mixed Müllerian tumor	1.6%
Mixed epithelial and stromal differentiation	Müllerian adenosarcoma	2.6%

*Ages 20 and older, 12 SEER areas

Note. Based on information from Kosary, 2007.

Uterine LMS is composed of smooth muscle and typically is composed of large spindle cells with pleomorphic nuclei and numerous mitotic features, including atypical forms. Traditionally, mitotic activity was considered the most reliable indicator of malignancy (Gadducci et al., 1996). Whereas ordinary uterine LMSs almost always have high levels of mitotic activity, they invariably manifest hypercellularity and nuclear atypia of at least moderate degree, with most containing gross or microscopic areas of tumor cell necrosis (Prayson & Hart, 1992). Tumor grade, stage, and mitotic count have all been shown to be predictive of outcome (Leitao et al., 2004). The principle histologic parameters used to predict tumor behavior include moderate to severe cytologic atypia, mitotic index, and coagulative tumor cell necrosis (Levenback et al., 1996). As a result, the gold standard for diagnosing uterine LMS relies on the analysis of three criteria: mitotic count, atypia, and necrosis (Bell, Kempson, & Hendrickson, 1994).

The data vary regarding the immunohistochemical patterns of estrogen receptor (ER), progesterone receptor (PR), and androgen receptor (AR) in uterine LMS. Historically, the expression of hormone receptors in uterine LMS has been reported to range from 11% to 60% (Bodner, Bodner-Adler,

Table 9-2. Uterine Sarcoma Survival Rate by Stage and Histology

Histology	Number of Cases	5-Year Relative Survival Rate (%)†					
		Total	Stage I	Stage II	Stage III	Stage IV	Unstaged
Leiomyosarcoma	939	48.2	60.0	35.1	27.7	14.9	51.6
Carcinosarcoma	706	53.7	73.7	43.3	26.2	13.6	–
Endometrial stromal sarcoma	610	74.6	89.8	40.0	64.3	37.0	–
Müllerian adenosarcoma	1,264	45.3	66.7	45.7	34.8	18.2	19.4

† Ages 20 and older, 12 SEER areas
– Not displayed because less than 25 cases

Note. Based on information from Kosary, 2007.

Kimberger, Czerwenka, & Mayerhofer, 2004). Kelley, Borden, and Goldblum (2004) reported hormone receptor positivity in 70–80% of a small number of cases (N = 16) of uterine LMS. In contrast, Leitao et al. (2004) reported that the rate of ER and PR expression was significantly less in uterine LMS when compared with uterine leiomyoma, with ER, PR, and AR expression observed in 30%–40% of cases. The presence of hormone receptors does not correlate with any clinicopathologic parameters and has no prognostic impact on the outcome of disease (Bodner et al., 2004).

Endometrial Stromal Sarcoma

Endometrial stromal sarcoma (ESS) is a heterogeneous histopathologic entity that is considered less aggressive and has a better outcome than other uterine sarcomas (Blom, Malström, & Guerrieri, 1999). These tumors account for 7%–15% of all uterine sarcomas (Acharya et al., 2005). Although often indolent in behavior, ESS is malignant with as many as 30% of women with low-grade ESS having extrauterine disease at presentation (Ashraf-Ganjoei, Behtash, Shariat, & Mosavi, 2006). These tumors have usually an indolent clinical course with an 80%–100% five-year survival, but approximately 37%–60% of patients eventually recur, and 15%–25% of women die of the disease (Gaducci et al., 2008). The most powerful predictor of clinical outcome whether measured in terms of survival, number of relapses, or time to first relapse is surgical stage (Acharya et al., 2005; Chang, Crabtree, Lim-Tan, Kempson, & Hendrickson, 1990).

Endometrial stromal sarcomas are divided into two subtypes: low-grade and high-grade. The distinction between high- and low-grade ESS is made by the level of mitotic activity; more than 10 mitoses per high-power field are considered high-grade, and less than 10 are described as low-grade (Bodner et al., 2001). Low-grade ESS is composed of cells that replace proliferative endometrial stromal cells, thus infiltrating the myometrium (Scully et al., 1994). High-grade ESS is a poorly differentiated sarcoma without precise characteristics or heterologous features. However, ESS typically has an infiltrating pattern that depicts an origin from endometrial stromal cells (Scully et al.). High-grade ESS usually is termed *undifferentiated endometrial sarcoma* (Oliva, Clement, & Young, 2000). According to Chang et al. (1990), once the surgical stage is known, mitotic index provides no further predictive information for stage I patients but is an independent predictor of outcome in high-stage patients. When both stage and mitotic indexes are high, each is a univariate predictor of unfavorable prognosis. Although high-stage tumors have a higher incidence of lymphovascular invasion compared to low-stage tumors, lymphovascular invasion is not an independent predictor of outcome (Nordal, Kristensen, Stenwig, Trope, & Nesland, 1998).

Distinction of ESS from leiomyoma of the uterus can be challenging because both can show a high degree of architectural and cytologic similarity. The use of immunohistochemical staining, such as CD10, can be useful in differentiating ESS from leiomyoma, with ESS consistently staining positive for CD10 (Zhu, Shi, Cheng, Zhao, & Wu, 2004). Reich, Regauer, Urdl, Lahousen, and Winter (2000) studied 21 low-grade ESSs and found ER in 71% and PR in 95% of the sample. Steroid receptor expression may have implications for hormone therapy in the management of these tumors, and both should be routinely quantified in low-grade ESS by immunohistochemical methods (Gadducci et al., 2008).

Endometrial stromal nodule is a rare subtype of endometrial stromal tumor. Endometrial stromal nodules, similar to other uterine neoplasms of stromal origin, occur primarily in peri- and postmenopausal women. Because margin evaluation is required to distinguish between endometrial stromal nodule and low-grade ESS and because the majority of these patients are beyond childbearing years, conservative therapy to spare fertility usually is not recommended (Tavassoli & Norris,

1981). Although the receptor status of stromal nodules has not been studied, their similarity on a cellular level to low-grade stromal sarcomas suggests that a trial of hormonal therapy when fertility preservation is desired may be a therapeutic intervention (Hui & Fedoriw, 2005).

Uterine tumors resembling ovarian sex-cord tumors (UTROSCT) are very rare, usually benign uterine tumors and probably are derived from uterine mesenchymal stem cells (Biermann, Heukamp, Büttner, & Zhou, 2008). Although more than 30% of these tumors have infiltrating borders, almost all of them behave in a benign fashion (Gadducci et al., 2008).

Carcinosarcoma

Uterine carcinosarcomas, or mixed malignant Müllerian tumors, are highly aggressive cancers with a five-year survival rate reported as 18%–39% (Raspollini et al., 2005). Perhaps more disconcerting than the relatively poor outcome among patients with this disease is the lack of appreciable improvement in survival within the past four decades despite advances in adjuvant therapy strategies (Lin & Slomovitz, 2008).

Uterine carcinosarcomas, unlike uterine papillary serous carcinomas and clear cell carcinomas, usually arise in women older than 65 years and commonly present at an advanced stage (Dinh et al., 1989). The epidemiologic features of carcinosarcoma include obesity, nulliparity, use of estrogen-replacement therapy, and history of tamoxifen treatment (Acharya et al., 2005; Fotiuo, Hatjieleftheriou, Kyrousis, Kokka, & Apostolikas, 2000). Uterine carcinosarcoma displays both epithelial and stromal differentiation and is further subdivided into homologous and heterologous subtypes based on the sarcomatous component. The homologous stromal element may be represented by endometrial stromal sarcoma, LMS, undifferentiated endometrial sarcoma, or fibrosarcoma, whereas the heterologous stromal component may consist of rhabdomyosarcoma, chondrosarcoma, osteosarcoma, or liposarcoma (Gadducci et al., 2008). The carcinomatous component is usually a high-grade adenocarcinoma (e.g., endometrioid, serous, clear cell). This element has the greatest influence on tumor behavior with 75% of metastases and recurrences manifested as the carcinomatous component (Levenback et al., 1996).

Until recently, carcinosarcomas were thought to be a subtype of uterine sarcoma and were treated more as a sarcoma than as a carcinoma (Acharya et al., 2005). Current evidence suggests that these tumors are actually metaplastic carcinomas displaying a pattern of metastasis akin to aggressive endometrial carcinomas rather than to sarcomas (McCluggage, 2002). Uterine carcinosarcoma tends to spread by local extension to pelvic structures but may metastasize with the manner of spread being mainly through the lymphatic system rather than through the blood (McCluggage).

Data are conflicting in regard to the utility of immunohistochemical analysis in the diagnosis of uterine carcinosarcoma. Inconsistent results of c-kit staining have been reported in these tumors, ranging in previous studies from 0% to 100% of cases (Adams et al., 2007). C-kit and PDGFR-β are unlikely to represent primary treatment targets in uterine sarcomas. The strong expression of PDGFR-α in uterine sarcoma specimens suggests a role for this receptor in tumor development, although its potential as a therapeutic target requires further investigation (Adams et al.). A promising therapeutic opportunity may be found in the antiangiogenic agents, such as vascular endothelial growth factor, which has exhibited high expression in both the epithelial and spindle elements of uterine carcinosarcoma (Cimbaluk, Rotmensch, Scudiere, Gown, & Bitterman, 2007).

Müllerian Adenosarcoma

Uterine Müllerian adenosarcoma is a biphasic tumor exhibiting a malignant stromal and a benign epithelial component. These neoplasms occur in woman 14–89 years old with a median age of 58 years at diagnosis (Oliva, Clement, & Young, 2002). Müllerian adenosarcoma with sarcomatous overgrowth was first described by Clement and Scully (1974). Available data suggest that histologic sarcomatous overgrowth and myometrial invasion are associated with a high risk of recurrence (Kaku et al., 1992; Seidman, Wasserman, Aye, MacKoul, & O'Leary, 1999; Verschraegen et al., 1998). Additional features that have been reported as poor prognostic indicators include high mitotic index of the stromal component, presence of heterologous elements, necrosis, and extrauterine spread (Kaku et al.). Lymphatic or vascular space involvement and rhabdomyosarcomatous differentiation may be associated with poor outcome (Kaku et al.). These sarcomas can have a long interval between diagnosis and recurrence, and thus, these women require long-term follow-up.

Ovarian Sarcoma

Primary ovarian sarcomas are rare tumors constituting approximately 1% of all ovarian malignancies. These sarcomas commonly present at an advanced stage and have a poor prognosis. Because of the rarity of this malignancy, most treatment information has been derived from case reports and small series. The optimal treatment remains unknown (Sood et al., 1998).

Cervical Sarcoma

Cervical sarcoma of the uterine cervix is a rare disease that usually occurs in older women and at an advanced stage. Extracervical disease usually is associated with a poor prognosis. Data about adjuvant therapies are limited and mainly obtained from studies on sarcomas of the uterine corpus (Laterza et al., 2007).

Vulvar-Vaginal Sarcoma

LMS is the most common histology found in vulvar sarcomas. Other less common histologies include epithelioid sarcoma, malignant rhabdoid tumor, and malignant histiocytoma (Finan & Barre, 2003). The malignant potential of vulvar sarcoma is estimated by pathologic determination of nuclear atypia, mitotic count, infiltrating border, and margin status (Hensley, 2000). Vulvar sarcoma is associated with a greater than 50% recurrence and death rate (Finan & Barre).

Pediatric vaginal sarcomas most commonly are classified as smooth muscle tumors, LMSs, or rhabdomyosarcomas, 90% of which occur in children younger than five years old (Hensley, 2000). Adult vaginal sarcomas usually present in an advanced stage, with grade being the most important prognostic feature. The mainstay of treatment for vaginal sarcomas is surgery (Temkin, Hellmann, Lee, & Abulafia, 2007).

Clinical Presentation and Diagnostic Evaluation

The most common presenting symptom with any type of uterine sarcoma is abnormal vaginal bleeding. Pelvic pain and malodorous vaginal discharge may accompany vaginal bleeding or occur as isolated symptoms (Levenback et al., 1996). An enlarged uterus is palpated in about 50% of patients with uterine sarcomas, and tumor may be seen protruding from the cervix particularly in women with carcinosarcoma (Dinh et al., 1989). Endometrial stromal sarcomas are particularly prone to bleeding and thus are diagnosed more frequently in stage I than the other histologic types (Levenback et al.).

Women with a suspected gynecologic sarcoma require a thorough history and physical examination, including bimanual and vaginal speculum examination to evaluate for the presence of visible and palpable lesions. An endometrial biopsy or curettage should be obtained for pathologic diagnosis (Hensley, 2000). Endometrial sampling is useful in diagnosing sarcomas that involve the endometrium (e.g., carcinosarcomas) but does not reveal smooth muscle and stromal tumors, which do not involve the endometrium (Levenback et al., 1996).

If extrauterine disease is known or suspected, a chest radiograph or computed tomography (CT) scan of the chest is warranted to rule out pulmonary metastasis. A preoperative CT or magnetic resonance imaging of the abdomen and pelvis may be appropriate to determine local resectability and to rule out extrauterine spread (Hensley, 2000). The frequency of occult extrauterine metastases during surgical exploration makes optimal surgical staging imperative (Yamada et al., 2000).

Staging

The Committee on Gynecologic Oncology of the International Federation of Gynecology and Obstetrics (FIGO) is the internationally recognized official advisory body that defines the staging criteria of all gynecologic sarcomas (Benedet, Bender, Jones, Ngan, & Pecorelli, 2000). The FIGO staging for carcinoma of the uterus has been applied to uterine sarcomas (Sutton, Kavanagh, Wolfson, & Tornos, 2005). See Appendix for staging.

Treatment

Surgery

The initial therapy for nonmetastatic uterine sarcomas is exploratory laparotomy, total abdominal hysterectomy, and bilateral salpingo-oophorectomy. In uterine LMS, routine lymph node dissection usually is not performed when disease is confined to the uterus and lymph nodes appear healthy on inspection and palpation, as lymph node involvement is highly unlikely in the absence of extrauterine disease (Acharya et al., 2005). If the LMS is low-grade, noninvasive, and lacks nuclear atypia, conservative management can be considered in younger women who wish to preserve fertility (Hensley, 2000). Women with uterine LMS who have isolated pulmonary metastases may be considered for thoracotomy and resection (Hensley, 2000; Leitao et al., 2002). Unilateral versus bilateral disease is a significant predictor of survival after pulmonary resection ($P = 0.02$). No single risk factor is sufficiently accurate to exclude an individual patient from consideration for pulmonary resection (Levenback et al., 1992).

Carcinosarcomas and ESS should be fully staged in the same way as endometrial adenocarcinomas, with pelvic and para-aortic lymph node dissection (Riopel, Plante, Renaud, Roy, & Tetu, 2005). Lymphadenectomy is important in this histology in order to discover occult metastatic disease and potentially provide these women with a therapeutic benefit (Gadducci et al., 2008); peritoneal washings and omentectomy also are recommended. Low-grade ESS patients with extrauterine spread of disease should undergo complete surgical debulking whenever possible.

Vaginal and vulval LMS usually are treated with wide local excision or more radical excision for larger masses to obtain clear surgical margins (Hensley, 2000). Vulval and vaginal rhabdomyosarcomas are treated with local surgical excision, followed by brachytherapy and adjuvant chemotherapy (Flamant et al., 1990). Neoadjuvant chemotherapy followed by surgical resection results in a greater than 85% survival rate in children diagnosed with this malignancy (Hensley, 2000). Preoperative chemotherapy in patients with locally advanced vulvovaginal rhabdomyosarcoma can preclude the need for exenterative surgery (Hensley, 2000).

Chemotherapy

To date, the combination of an anthracycline plus ifosfamide is the most active systemic therapy for adult soft-tissue sarcomas. No single chemotherapeutic agent is considered standard in the treatment gynecologic sarcomas (Hensley, 2000), and data are scant and conflicting regarding the use of adjuvant chemotherapy in the treatment of uterine sarcomas. The two most active agents in adult soft-tissue sarcomas are doxorubicin and ifosfamide, both of which have a dose-response relationship with response rates of 20%–35% (Gadducci et al., 2008). A number of chemotherapeutic agents have been studied in advanced, unresectable disease, with single agent ifosfamide and doxorubicin showing moderate activity in uterine LMS (Hensley, 2006). Liposomal doxorubicin, gemcitabine, and temozolomide have been studied in advanced or recurrent uterine LMS with responses of 8% and 16% in pretreated patients receiving temozolomide and gemcitabine, respectively (Gadducci, 2008; Hensley, 2006). Liposomal doxorubicin has not shown advantage over historical results with doxorubicin in the treatment of uterine LMS (Sutton, Blessing, Hanjani, & Kramer, 2005). The use of temozolomide obtained objective response rates of 8%–14% and stabilization of disease of 33%–57% in patients with metastatic or unresectable uterine LMS (Gadducci et al., 2008). Reported response rates of 20% were found with gemcitabine in pretreated patients with LMS (Anderson & Aghajanian, 2005; Hensley et al., 2002; Sutton et al., 2005). The addition of docetaxel to gemcitabine has yielded a response rate of up to 53% in patients with unresectable LMS, but the median time to progression remains less than six months (Hensley et al., 2002). In a small series of chemotherapy-naïve patients, the combination of paclitaxel plus carboplatin obtained an 80% complete response rate with a median progression-free and overall survival of 18 and 25 months, respectively (Toyoshima, Akahira, Moriya, Hayakawa, & Yaegashi, 2004). A regimen of cisplatin plus ifosfamide, with or without an anthracycline, is recommended for patients with advanced carcinosarcoma (Gadducci et al., 2008).

Endocrine therapy can cause regression or stabilization of disease in women with recurrent low grade ESS. Schwartz et al. (1996) suggested adjuvant progestin use for two years in patients with completely resected low-grade ESS. Hormonal treatment should be planned on the basis of hormone receptor status (Gadducci et al., 2008).

Radiation

The role of adjuvant radiotherapy in nonmetastatic disease is controversial. Although this therapy reduces the rate of local recurrences, it has no significant impact on overall survival, as most patients with recurrent disease have distant failures (Gadducci et al., 2008). Adjuvant pelvic radiation for resected stage I and II uterine LMS or carcinosarcoma has not been adequately studied in prospective randomized trials (Hensley, 2006). Radiation therapy is most useful when used in palliative treatment to distant sites, such as bone or brain metastasis (Gadducci et al., 2008).

Recurrent Disease

The treatment of recurrent gynecologic sarcoma often requires the use of multiple therapeutic modalities. Except for rare cases of resectable, isolated pulmonary metastases, such patients are not considered curable (Hensley et al., 2002). Enrollment into clinical trials is strongly encouraged to facilitate the identification of new active agents for these malignancies. In women with poorer performance status or multiple comorbidities, palliative measures and supportive care should be the mainstay of treatment.

Summary

Uterine sarcomas are a group of rare gynecologic tumors that usually have an aggressive clinical course and poor prognosis. The rarity of these sarcomas and their aggressive behavior has resulted in a paucity of literature. Total abdominal hysterectomy and bilateral salpingo-oophorectomy remains the surgical standard of care. Lymph node dissection is indicated for carcinosarcomas because of their high incidence of nodal involvement. Adjuvant pelvic radiotherapy may improve local control but has no significant affect on survival. Evidence in the literature is scant to support the routine use of adjuvant chemotherapy, except in carcinosarcomas. Further evaluation of adjuvant treatment in prospective trials clearly is warranted.

Oncology nurses collaborating with medical and surgical oncologists is pivotal to ensuring quality care. Assessing patients' needs, triaging symptoms, and if necessary, making referrals for services such as nutrition and social work are all integral to optimizing outcomes. Patient and family education regarding the details of the sarcoma treatment plan provides support to women from time of initial diagnosis and at the time of recurrence.

References

Acharya, S., Hensley, M.L., Montag, A.C., & Fleming, G.F. (2005). Rare uterine cancers. *Lancet Oncology, 6*(12), 961–971.

Adams, S.F., Hickson, J.A., Hutto, J.Y., Montag, A.G., Lengyel, E., & Yamada, S.D. (2007). PDGFR-alpha as a potential therapeutic target in uterine sarcomas. *Gynecology Oncology, 104*(3), 524–528.

Anderson, S., & Aghajanian, C. (2005). Temozolomide in uterine leiomyosarcomas. *Gynecologic Oncology, 98*(1), 99–110.

Ashraf-Ganjoei, T., Behtash, N., Shariat, M., & Mosavi, A. (2006, August). Low grade endometrial stromal sarcoma of uterine corpus, a clinico-pathological and survey study in 14 cases. *World Journal of Surgical Oncology, 4*, 50.

Bell, S.W., Kempson, R.L., & Hendrickson, M.R. (1994). Problematic uterine smooth muscle neoplasm. A clinicopathologic study of 213 cases. *American Journal of Surgical Pathology, 18*(6), 535–558.

Benedet, J.L., Bender, H., Jones, H., Ngan, H.Y., & Pecorelli, S. (2000). FIGO staging classifications and clinical practice guidelines in the management of gynecologic cancers. FIGO Committee on Gynecologic Oncology. *International Journal of Gynaecology and Obstetrics, 70*(2), 209–62.

Berchuck, A., Rubin, S.C., Hoskins, W.J., Saigo, P.E., Pierce, V.K., & Lewis, J.L. (1990). Treatment of endometrial stromal tumors. *Gynecologic Oncology, 36*(1), 60–5.

Biermann, K., Heukamp, L.C., Büttner, R., & Zhou, H. (2008). Uterine tumor resembling an ovarian sex cord tumor associated with metastasis. *International Journal of Gynecological Pathology, 27*(1), 58–60.

Blom, R., Malmström, H., & Guerrieri, C. (1999). Endometrial stromal sarcoma of the uterus: A clinicopathologic, DNA flow cytometric, p53, and mdm-2 analysis of 17 cases. *International Journal of Gynecological Cancer, 9*(2), 98–104.

Bodner, K., Bodner-Adler, B., Kimberger, O., Czerwenka, K., & Mayerhofer, K. (2004). Estrogen and progesterone receptor expression in patients with uterine smooth muscle tumors. *Fertility and Sterility, 81*(4), 1062–1066.

Bodner, K., Bodner-Adler, B., Obermair, A., Windbichler, G., Petru, E., Mayerhofer, S., et al. (2001). Prognostic parameters in endometrial stromal sarcoma: A clinicopathologic study in 31 patients. *Gynecologic Oncology, 81*(2), 160–165.

Brooks, S.E., Zhan, M., Cote, T., & Baquet, C.R. (2004). Surveillance, epidemiology, and end results analysis of 2,677 cases of uterine sarcoma 1989–1999. *Gynecologic Oncology, 93*(1), 204–208.

Chang, K.L., Crabtree, G.S., Lim-Tan, S.K., Kempson, R.L., & Hendrickson, M.R. (1990). Primary uterine endometrial stromal neoplasms. A clinicopathologic study of 117 cases. *American Journal of Surgical Pathology, 14*(5), 415–438.

Chauveinc, L., Deniaud, E., Plancher, C., Sastre, X., Amsani, F., de la Rochefordiere, A., et al. (1999). Uterine sarcomas: The Curie Institut experience. Prognosis factors and adjuvant treatments. *Gynecologic Oncology, 72*(2), 232–237.

Cimbaluk, D., Rotmensch, J., Scudiere, J., Gown, A., & Bitterman, P. (2007). Uterine carcinosarcoma: Immunohistochemical studies on tissue microarrays with focus on potential therapeutic targets. *Gynecologic Oncology, 105*(1), 138–144.

Clement, P.B., & Scully, R.E. (1974). Müllerian adenosarcoma of the uterus. A clinicopathologic analysis of ten cases of a distinctive type of Müllerian mixed tumor. *Cancer, 34*(4), 1138–1149.

Denschlag, D., Masoud, I., Stanimir, G., & Gilbert, L. (2006). Prognostic factors and outcome in women with uterine sarcoma. *European Journal of Surgical Oncology, 33*(1), 91–95.

Dinh, T.V., Slavin, R.E., Bhagavan, B.S., Hannigan, E.V., Tiamson, E.M., & Yandell, R.B. (1989). Mixed Müllerian tumors of the uterus: A clincopathologic study. *Obstetrics and Gynecology, 74*(3), 388–392.

Falconi, M., Crippa, S., Sargenti, M., Capelli, P., & Pederzoli, P. (2006). Pancreatic metastasis from leiomyosarcoma of the broad ligament of the uterus. *Lancet Oncology, 7*(1), 94–95.

Finan, M.A, & Barre, G. (2003). Bartholin's gland carcinoma, malignant melanoma and other rare tumours of the vulva. *Best Practice and Research: Clinical Obstetrics and Gynaecology, 17*(4), 609–603.

Flamant, F., Gerbaulet, A., Nihoul-Fekete, C., Valteau-Couanet, D., Chassagne, D., & Lemerle, J. (1990). Long-term sequelae of conservative treatment by surgery, brachytherapy, and chemotherapy for vulval and vaginal rhabdomyosarcoma in children. *Journal of Clinical Oncology, 8*(11), 1847–1853.

Fotiou, S., Hatjieleftheriou, G., Kyrousis, G., Kokka, F., & Apostolikas, N. (2000). Long-term tamoxifen treatment: A possible aetiological factor in the development of uterine carcinosarcoma: Two case-reports and review of the literature. *Anticancer Research, 20*(3B), 2015–2020.

Gadducci, A., Cosio, S., Romanini, A., & Genazzani, A.R. (2008). The management of patients with uterine sarcoma: A debated clinical challenge. *Critical Reviews in Oncology/Hematology, 65*(2), 129–142.

Gadducci, A., Landoni, F., Sartori, E., Zola, P., Maggino, T., Lissoni, A., et al. (1996). Uterine leiomyosarcoma: Analysis of treatment failures and survival. *Gynecologic Oncology, 62*(1), 25–32.

Gari, A., Souhami, L., Arseneau, J., & Stanimir, G. (2006). Primary malignant mesodermal ovarian sarcomas. *International Journal of Gynecological Cancer, 16*(1), 106–109.

Giuntoli, R.L., Metzinger, D.S., DiMarco, C.S., Cha, S.S., Sloan, J.A., Keeney, G.L., et al. (2003). Retrospective review of 208 patients with leiomyosarcoma of the uterus: Prognostic indicators, surgical management, and adjuvant therapy. *Gynecologic Oncology, 89*(3), 460–469.

Harlow, B.L., Weiss, N.S., & Lofton, S. (1986). The epidemiology of sarcomas of the uterus. *Journal of the National Cancer Institute, 76*(3), 399–402.

Hensley, M.L. (2000). Uterine/female genital sarcomas. *Current Treatment Options in Oncology, 1*(2), 161–168.

Hensley, M.L. (2006). Uterine sarcomas and carcinosarcomas: Advances for advanced disease and updates for adjuvant therapy. *American Society of Clinical Oncology 2006 educational book* (pp. 301–304). Alexandria, VA: American Society of Clinical Oncology.

Hensley M.L., Maki, R., Venkatraman, E., Geller. G., Lovegren, M., Aghajanian, C., et al. (2002). Gemcitabine and docetaxel in patients with unresectable leiomyosarcoma: Results of a phase II trial. *Journal of Clinical Oncology, 20*(12), 2824–2831.

Hui, P., & Fedoriw, G. (2005). Recurrent endometrial stromal tumors with smooth-muscle differentiation and a protracted clinical course. *Nature Clinical Practice Oncology, 2*(11), 588–593.

Inayama, Y., Shoji, A., Odagiri, S., Hirahara, F., Ito, I., Kawano, N., et al. (2000). Detection of pulmonary metastasis 25 years after hysterectomy. *Pathology Research and Practice, 196*(2), 129–134.

Iwamoto, I., Fujino, T., Higashi, Y., Tsuji, T., Nakamura, N., Komokata, T., et al. (2005). Metastasis of uterine leiomyosarcoma to the pancreas. *Journal of Obstetrics and Gynaecology Research, 31*(6), 531–534.

Kaku, T., Silverberg, S.G., Major, F.J., Miller, A., Fetter, B., & Brady, M.F. (1992). Adenosarcoma of the uterus: A Gynecologic Oncology Group clinicopathologic study of 31 cases. *International Journal of Gynecological Pathology, 11*(2), 75–88.

Kelley, T.D., Borden, E.C., & Goldblum, J.R. (2004). Estrogen and progesterone receptor expression in uterine and extrauterine leiomyosarcomas: An immunohistochemical study. *Applied Immunohistochemistry and Molecular Morphology, 12*(4), 338–341.

Kempson, R.L., & Bari, W. (1970). Uterine sarcomas. Classification, diagnosis, and prognosis. *Human Pathology, 1*(3), 331–349.

Kosary, C.L. (2007). Cancer of the corpus uteri. In L.A.G. Ries, J.L. Young, G.E. Keel, M.P. Eisner, Y.D. Lin, & M.-J. Horner (Eds.), *SEER survival monograph: Cancer survival monograph: Cancer survival among adults. U.S. SEER Program, 1988–2001 patient and tumor characteristics* [NIH Pub. No. 07-6215]. Bethesda, MD: National Institutes of Health.

Laterza, R., Seveso, A., Zefiro, F., Formenti, G., Mellana, L., Dondadello, N., et al. (2007). Carcinosarcoma of the uterine cervix:

Case report and discussion. *Gynecologic Oncology, 107*(1, Suppl. 1), S98–S100.

Leitao, M.M., Brennan, M.F., Hensley, M., Sonoda, Y., Hummer, A., Bhaskaran, D., et al. (2002). Surgical resection of pulmonary and extrapulmonary recurrences of uterine leiomyosarcoma. *Gynecologic Oncology, 87*(3), 287–294.

Leitao, M.M., Sonoda, Y., Brennan, M.F., Barakat, R.R., & Chi, D.S. (2003). Incidence of lymph node and ovarian metastases in leiomyosarcoma of the uterus. *Gynecologic Oncology, 91*(1), 209–212.

Leitao, M.M., Soslow, R.A., Nonaka, D.D., Olshen, A.B., Aghajanian, C., Sabbatini, P., et al. (2004). Tissue microarray immunohistochemical expression of estrogen, progesterone, and androgen receptors in uterine leiomyomata and leiomyosarcoma. *Cancer, 101*(6), 1455–1462.

Levenback, C., Rubin, S.C., McCormack, P.M., Hoskins, W.J., Atkinson, E.N., & Lewis, J.L. (1992). Resection of pulmonary metastases from uterine sarcoma. *Gynecologic Oncology, 45*(2), 202–205.

Levenback, C.F., Tortolero-Luna, G., Pandey, D.K., Malpica, A., Baker, V.V., Whittaker, L., et al. (1996). Uterine sarcoma. *Obstetrics and Gynecology Clinics of North America, 23*(2), 457–473.

Lin, J.F., & Slomovitz, B.M. (2008). Uterine sarcoma 2008. *Current Oncology Reports, 10*(6), 512–518.

Look, K.Y., Sandler, A., Blessing, J.A., Lucci, J.A., & Rose, P.G. (2004). Phase II trial of gemcitabine as second-line chemotherapy of uterine leiomyosarcoma: A Gynecology Oncology Group (GOG) study. *Genecology Oncology, 92*(2), 644–647.

Mayerhofer, K., Lozanov, P., Bodner, K., Bodner-Adler, B., Obermair, A., Kimberger, O., et al. (2004). Ki67 and vascular endothelial growth factor expression in uterine leiomyosarcoma. *Gynecologic Oncology, 92*(1), 175–179.

McCluggage, W.G. (2002). Uterine carcinosarcomas (malignant mixed Müllerian tumors) are metaplastic carcinomas. *International Journal of Gynecological Cancer, 12*(6), 687–690.

Nordal, R.R., Kristensen, G.B., Stenwig, A.E., Trope, C.G., & Nesland, J.N. (1998). Immunohistochemical analysis of p53 proteins in uterine sarcomas. *Gynecologic Oncology, 70*(1), 45–48.

Oliva, E., Clement, P.B., & Young, R.H. (2000). Endometrial stromal tumor: An update on a group of tumors with a protean phenotype. *Advances in Anatomic Pathology, 7*(5), 257–281.

Oliva, E., Clement, P.B., & Young, R.H. (2002). Epithelioid endometrial and endometrioid stromal tumors: A report of four cases emphasizing their distinction from epithelioid smooth muscle tumors and other oxyphilic uterine and extrauterine tumors. *International Journal of Gynecological Pathology, 21*(1), 48–55.

Platz, C.E., & Benda, J.A. (1995). Female genital tract cancer. *Cancer, 75*(Suppl. 1), 270–294.

Prayson, R.A., & Hart, W.R. (1992). Mitotically active leiomyomas of the uterus. *American Journal of Clinical Pathology, 97*(1), 14–20.

Raspollini, M.R., Susini, T., Amunni, G., Paglierani, M., Taddei, A., Marchionni, M., et al. (2005). COX-2, c-KIT and HER-2/neu expression in uterine carcinosarcomas: Prognostic factors or potential markers for targeted therapies? *Gynecologic Oncology, 96*(1), 159–167.

Reich, O., Regauer, S., Urdl, W., Lahousen, M., & Winter, R. (2000). Expression of estrogen and progesterone receptors in low-grade endometrial stromal sarcomas. *British Journal of Cancer, 82*(5), 1030–1034.

Riopel, J., Plante, M., Renaud, M., Roy, M., & Tetu, B. (2005). Lymph node metastases in low-grade endometrial stromal sarcoma. *Gynecologic Oncology, 96*(2), 402–406.

Robinson, M.H., Keus, R.B., Shasha, D., & Harrison, L.B. (1998). Is pre-operative radiotherapy superior to postoperative radiotherapy in the treatment of soft tissue sarcoma? *European Journal of Cancer, 34*(9), 1309–1316.

Sartori, E., Bazzurini, L., Gadducci, A., Landoni, F., Lissoni, A., Maggino, T., et al. (1997). Carcinosarcoma of the uterus: A clinicopathological multicenter CTF study. *Gynecologic Oncology, 67*(1), 70–75.

Schwartz, S.M., Weiss, N.S., Daling, J.R., Gammon, M.D., Liff, J.M., Watt, J., et al. (1996). Exogenous sex hormone use, correlates of endogenous hormone levels, and the incidence of histologic types of sarcoma of the uterus. *Cancer, 77*(4), 717–724.

Scully, S.P., Oleson, J.R., Leopold, K.A., Samulski, T.V., Dodge, R., & Harrelson, J.M. (1994). Clinical outcome after neoadjuvant thermoradiotherapy in high grade soft tissue sarcomas. *Journal of Surgical Oncology, 57*(3), 143–151.

Seidman, J.D., Wasserman, C.S., Aye, L.M., MacKoul, P.J., & O'Leary, T.J. (1999). Cluster of uterine Müllerian adenosarcoma in the Washington, DC metropolitan area with high incidence of sarcomatous overgrowth. *American Journal of Surgical Pathology, 23*(7), 809–814.

Sood, A.K., Sorosky, J.I., Gelder, M.S., Buller, R.E., Anderson, B., Wilkinson, E.J., et al. (1998). Primary ovarian sarcoma: Analysis of prognostic variables and the role of surgical cytoreduction. *Cancer, 82*(9), 731–1737.

Sutton, G., Blessing, J., Hanjani, P., & Kramer, P. (2005). Phase II evaluation of liposomal doxorubicin (Doxil) in recurrent or advanced leiomyosarcoma of the uterus: A Gynecologic Oncology Group study. *Gynecology Oncology, 96*(3), 749–752.

Sutton, G., Kavanagh, J., Wolfson, A., & Tornos, C. (2005). Corpus: Mesenchymal tumors. In W. Hoskins, C. Perez, R. Young, R. Barakat, M. Markman, & M. Randall (Eds.), *Principles and practice of gynecologic oncology* (4th ed., pp. 873–894). Philadelphia: Lippincott Williams & Wilkins.

Tavassoli, F.A, & Norris H.J. (1981). Mesenchymal tumours of the uterus. VII. A clinicopathological study of 60 endometrial stromal nodules. *Histopathology 5*(1), 1–10.

Temkin, S.M., Hellmann, M., Lee, Y., & Abulafia, O. (2007). Primary spindle cell sarcoma of the vagina treated with neoadjuvant radiation and pelvic exenteration. *Journal of Lower Genital Tract Disease, 11*(2), 105–107

Toyoshima, M., Akahira, J., Moriya, T., Hayakawa, S., & Yaegashi, N. (2004). Primary vaginal adenosarcoma with sarcomatous overgrowth. *Gynecologic Oncology, 95*(3),759–761.

Verschraegen, C.F., Vasuratna, A., Edwards, C., Freedman, R., Kudelka, A.P., Tornos, C., et al. (1998). Clinicopathologic analysis of Müllerian adenosarcoma: The M.D. Anderson Cancer Center experience. *Oncology Reports, 5*(4), 939–944.

Wickerham, D.L., Fisher, B., Wolmark, N., Bryant, J., Costantino, J., Bernstein, L., et al. (2002). Association of tamoxifen and uterine sarcoma. *Journal of Clinical Oncology, 20*(11), 2758–2760.

Wright, J.D., Rosenblum, K., Huettner, P.C., Mutch, D.G., Rader, J.S., Powell, M.A., et al. (2005). Cervical sarcomas: An analysis of incidence and outcome. *Gynecologic Oncology, 99*(2), 348–351.

Wu, T, Chang, T.C., Heueh, S., Kwang-Hung, H., Hung-Hsueh, C., Huei-Jean, H., et al (2005). Prognostic factors and the impact of adjuvant chemotherapy for uterine leiomyosarcoma. *Gynecologic Oncology, 100*(1), 166–172.

Wysowski, D.K., Honig, S.F., & Beitz, J. (2002). Uterine sarcoma associated with tamoxifen use. *New England Journal of Medicine, 346*(23), 1832–1833.

Yamada, S.D., Burger, R.A., Brewster, W.R., Anton, D., Kohler, M.F., & Monk, B.J. (2000). Pathologic variables and adjuvant therapy as predictors of recurrence and survival for patients with surgically evaluated carcinosarcoma of the uterus. *Cancer, 88*(12), 2782–2786.

Yokoyama, Y., Ono, Y., Sakamoto, T., Fukuda, I., & Mizunuma, H. (2004). Asymptomatic intracardiac metastasis from a low-grade endometrial stromal sarcoma with successful surgical resection. *Gynecologic Oncology, 92*(3), 999–1001.

Zhu, X.Q., Shi, Y.F., Cheng, X.D., Zhao, C.L., & Wu, Y.Z. (2004). Immunohistochemical markers in differential diagnosis of endometrial stromal sarcoma and cellular leiomyoma. *Gynecologic Oncology, 92*(1), 71–79.

CHAPTER 10

Trophoblastic Disease

Karen A. Bess, RN, MaEd, MSN, and Terry L. Wood, PhD, RN

Introduction

Trophoblastic disease is a rare pregnancy-related disorder with potentially devastating consequences for a childbearing family. It encompasses a spectrum of interrelated neoplasms ranging from benign to metastatic. Although the etiology of trophoblastic disease is not definitive, a combination of defects in gametogenesis and fertilization, as well as certain risk factors such as personal or family history of trophoblastic disease, maternal age, use of oral contraceptives, history of infertility, or low parity, contribute to this group of pregnancy-related disorders (Smith, 2003). All variants of trophoblastic disease arise following a gestational event resulting in abnormal growth of placental trophoblastic cells.

Although trophoblastic neoplasms are interrelated, they are histologically distinct variants. The term *gestational trophoblastic disease* (GTD) applies to a benign neoplasm (hydatidiform mole). GTD, also known as a molar pregnancy, is classified as either complete or partial. Either type of mole may progress to the second variant known as *gestational trophoblastic neoplasia* (GTN). GTN is classified as either nonmetastatic or metastatic (International Federation of Gynecology and Obstetrics [FIGO], 2006 (see Figure 10-1).

Nonmetastatic trophoblastic neoplasia (invasive mole) is confined to the uterus. When a trophoblastic neoplasm metastasizes to sites outside of the uterus, it is known as metastatic GTN or choriocarcinoma (FIGO, 2006). Placental site trophoblastic tumor (PSTT) is a third variant of trophoblastic disease with a distinct clinical presentation, clinical course, and management (FIGO) (see Figure 10-1).

Epidemiology of Trophoblastic Variants

Historically, comparing epidemiologic data across geographic locations and among racial/ethnic groups in a meaningful manner has been complicated. This difficulty existed because of discrepancies in data collection methods and reporting. For example, estimates regarding incidence may differ as a result of using population-based versus hospital-based pregnancy data (Garner, Goldstein, Feltmate, & Berkowitz, 2007; Smith & Kim, 2003; Steigrad, 2003). Furthermore, incidence rates were based on diverse denominators such as woman years (adult female population at risk), live births, or pregnancies. However, over the last two to three decades, registries dedicated to the study of trophoblastic disease have been established throughout the world. Common to these registries is the use of population-based statistics, which enhances the worldwide comparison of epidemiologic data (Smith & Kim, 2003).

The incidence of molar pregnancy varies geographically ranging from 0.5–2.5 per 1,000 pregnancies worldwide. In

Figure 10-1. Variants of Trophoblastic Disease

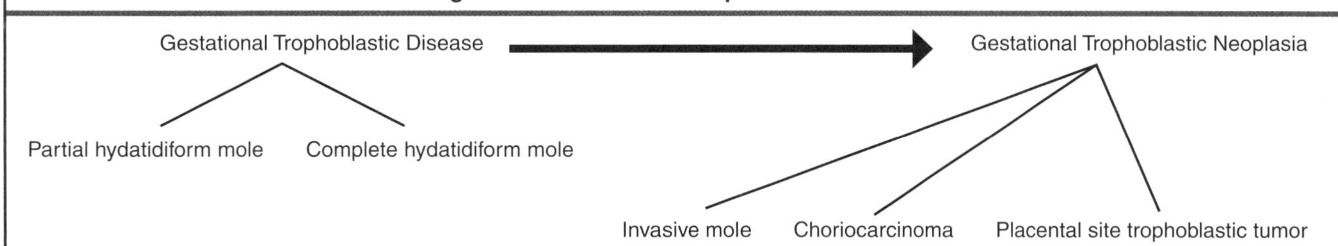

most parts of the world, the incidence is slightly less than 1.0 per 1,000 pregnancies with the exception of Japan, where it is closer to 2.0 per 1,000 pregnancies (Palmer, 1994). Invasive mole occurs in 15% of women with complete molar pregnancies (Berkowitz & Goldstein, 2003). Problems in estimating the incidence of choriocarcinoma are compounded by the rarity of the disease and by differences in data collection methods and reporting. In population-based studies, the incidence in the United States is reported as 0.05 per 1,000 live births (Brinton, Bracken, & Connelly, 1986). In contrast, when using woman years as the denominator, the reported incidence is 0.133 per 100,000 woman years (Smith et al., 2003). PSTT is a rare variant and constitutes 1%–2% of GTN cases (Ajithkumar, Abraham, Rejnishkumar & Minimole, 2003).

Ngan et al. (2006) reported that the total number of GTN cases decreased from 1,938 in 1979–1981 to 483 in 1999–2001. This decrease is postulated to be the result of decreased parity, more frequent use of ultrasound, improved socioeconomic conditions in many countries, and more stringent diagnostic criteria for GTN. Steigrad (2003) attributes the reduction of GTN to numerous factors, including improved contraceptive techniques, earlier diagnostic ultrasonography, and advances in suction curettage technique. In addition, advances in diagnostic imaging and biochemical testing has enabled earlier intervention, improved clinical outcomes, and systematic follow-up.

Gestational Trophoblastic Disease

Chromosomal Characteristics

Moles are genetically determined and the characteristic trophoblastic hyperplasia appears to be associated with more than one set of paternal chromosomes (Paradinas, Sebire, & Rees, 2003). Analysis of chromosomal differences between complete and partial moles enhances diagnostic accuracy. Complete hydatidiform mole results from the fertilization of an ovum that is without a nucleus. The sperm duplicates its own chromosomes creating embryonic tissue that is totally uniparental, in this case, paternally derived. The resulting karyotype is usually 46XX (Garner et al., 2007; Zivaljevic, Tesic, Vujkov, Rajovic, & Popovic, 2002). However, on occasion, a 46XY karyotype develops. Berkowitz and Goldstein (1996) and Soper (2006) theorized that it occurs when an anuclear ovum is fertilized by two sperm. In either circumstance, fetal development does not occur (Garner et al., 2007; Kurowski & Yakoub, 2003; Paradinas et al.; Soper). The fetus resorbs before the development of the circulatory system (Soper).

Partial molar pregnancy results from the fertilization of one ovum with two sperm resulting in three sets of chromosomes instead of the usual two sets (Kurowski & Yakoub, 2003; Smith, 2003). Embryonic tissue is composed of one set of chromosomes of maternal origin and two sets of chromosomes of paternal origin, with the karyotype equally likely to be 69XXX or 69XXY. This triploid karotype occurs in 90%–93% of partial moles (Berkowitz & Goldstein, 1996). A nonviable fetus may be present with identifiable multiple congenital anomalies and growth retardation (Berkowitz & Goldstein, 1996; Garner et al., 2007; Hui, Martel, & Parkash, 2005).

Etiology

Complete and partial molar pregnancies share several social, demographic, and physiologic risk factors. However, the role of each of these factors in the etiology of GTD is poorly understood. Risk factors include reproductive history, age, and socioeconomic status (see Figure 10-2). Race/ethnicity and geographic region also have been identified as risk factors. For example, there is a higher incidence of choriocarcinoma with lower survival rates among African Americans compared with Caucasians (Smith et al., 2003). Also, an increased incidence of hydatidiform mole in Asian countries is reported (Berman, DiSaia, & Tewari, 2004). Although these relationships are unclear, the variation in incidence may be attributed to nutritional and/or socioeconomic factors (Berkowitz & Goldstein, 2005; Hurteau, 2003) or genetics (Tham, Everard, Tidy, Drew, & Hancock, 2003). Researchers continue to explore role of genetics in the development and progression of trophoblastic variants, including the underlying explanation for racial/ethnic differences.

Clinical Presentation and Diagnostic Evaluation

Women with hydatidform mole initially have amenorrhea and may experience either characteristic or exaggerated signs or symptoms of pregnancy. First-trimester vaginal bleeding is the most common presenting symptom regardless of type of molar gestation (Berkowitz & Goldstein, 1996; Berman et al., 2004; Garner et al., 2007; Kurowski &Yakoub, 2003; Leiser & Aghajanian, 2006; Soper, 2006). Vaginal bleeding

Figure 10-2. Risk Factors for Gestational Trophoblastic Neoplasia

- Lower socioeconomic status (Hurteau, 2003)
- Nulliparous, low parity (Smith, 2003)
- Age extremes (Altman et al., 2008; Berman et al., 2004; Leiser & Aghajanian, 2006; Smith & Kim, 2003)
- Increased paternal age (Hurteau, 2003; Smith & Kim, 2003)
- Personal or family history of gestational trophoblastic disease (Hurteau, 2003; Smith, 2003)
- Previous spontaneous abortion (Berkowitz & Goldstein, 1996; Kurowski & Yakoub, 2003; Smith, 2003)
- History of infertility (Berkowitz & Goldstein, 2004; Smith, 2003)
- Use of oral contraceptives (Kurowski & Yakoub, 2003; Smith, 2003)

tends to be more severe with complete moles than with partial moles (Kurowski & Yakoub) and occurs when the molar villi separate from the deciduas with subsequent interruption of the maternal vessels. Bleeding may be intermittent or continuous and ranges from brisk hemorrhage to a dark-brown watery discharge resembling prune juice (Berkowitz & Goldstein, 2004; Berman et al.). The prune juice–like discharge is caused by liquefaction of intrauterine clots (Evans, Soper, & Hammond, 2003). Vaginal discharge may contain pieces of molar tissue (vesicles) that resemble grapelike clusters representing indisputable evidence of a molar pregnancy (Kurowski & Yakoub; Soper). In addition to vaginal bleeding, some individuals may present with fatigue and shortness of breath secondary to anemia from blood loss.

Classic manifestations of complete moles typically present in the second trimester (Kurowski & Yakoub, 2003). The traditional presentation results from extensive trophoblastic hyperplasia and elevated human chorionic gonadotropin (HCG) levels and includes excessive uterine size, theca lutein cysts, and medical complications of hyperemesis gravidarum, preeclampsia, and hyperthyroidism (Kurowski & Yakoub, 2003). However, clinical practice changes have allowed for the diagnosis of molar pregnancies and subsequent molar evacuations in the first trimester. These changes include (Tidy, 2003)

- The increased accuracy and use of HCG measurements
- The widespread use of sensitive ultrasound in prenatal screening
- Assessment of first-trimester vaginal bleeding
- Determination of gestational age.

Consequently, the classic presentation is less common at time of diagnosis (Berkowiz & Goldstein, 1996; Evans et al., 2003; Garner et al., 2007; Kurowski & Yakoub; Soto-Wright, Bernstein, Goldstein, & Berkowitz, 1995).

Although the current trend is for earlier diagnosis, some women may not be diagnosed with a molar pregnancy until the second trimester. They most likely will present with classic manifestations and subsequent medical complications at this stage (Kurowski & Yaloub, 2003). Women presenting with a uterus greater than 14–16 weeks gestational size also may present with classic manifestations (Soper, 2006). Moreover, the classic presentation of molar pregnancies may be more common in countries without well-developed health care (Evans et al., 2003).

Increased uterine size results from retained intrauterine clots, enlarged chorionic villi, and trophoblastic proliferation (Berkowitz & Goldstein, 2003; Leiser & Aghajanian, 2006). Theca lutein cysts result from hyperstimulation of the ovaries by HCG and may be palpable on pelvic exam. These fluid-filled cysts may be as large as 20 cm (Berkowitz & Goldstein) and usually are bilateral. Cysts greater than 6 cm may cause severe abdominal pain (Kurowski & Yakoub, 2003). In this case, Garner et al. (2007) suggested that ultrasound-directed or laproscopic decompression of the cysts be performed. Berman et al. (2004) noted that presentation with either an enlarged uterus beyond gestational date or a theca lutein cyst increases the likelihood of malignant sequelae. If both signs are present, more than 50% of complete molar pregnancies progress to GTN (Berman et al.).

Hyperemesis gravidarium, requiring antiemetics, may occur secondary to an enlarged uterus, elevated HCG levels (Evans et al., 2003), and high circulating levels of estrogen (Garner et al., 2007). The presentation of preeclampsia includes hypertension, edema, and proteinuria. These manifestations are related to increased uterine size and an elevation in HCG levels (Berkowitz & Goldstein, 2003).

Hyperthyroidism, although rare, is associated with markedly elevated HCG levels. Although the role of HCG is unclear, it may have properties similar to thyroid-stimulating hormone (Garner et al., 2007; Kurowski & Yakoub, 2003). Untreated or poorly controlled hyperthyroidism may precipitate development of thyroid storm, also known as thyrotoxic crisis, at the time of anesthesia induction for molar evacuation (Berkowitz & Goldstein, 2003; Berman et al., 2004). In thyroid storm, all hyperthyroid manifestations are heightened and may lead to heart failure or shock. This medical emergency may be prevented by treatment with beta adrenergic blocking agents. These agents aid in preventing or rapidly reversing many of the cardiovascular and metabolic complications of thyroid storm (Berkowitz & Goldstein; Garner et al.). Symptoms of hyperthyroidism disappear subsequent to evacuation of the molar pregnancy (Berkowitz & Goldstein; Berman et al.; Garner et al.).

The clinical presentation of a partial mole is considerably less dramatic than with a complete mole (Cunningham et al., 2005). Partial moles have less trophoblastic overgrowth than is characteristically found in complete moles and, in fact, trophoblastic excess may not be detected if the tissue is not thoroughly examined (Paradinas et al., 2003). Physical examination findings may include a nontender uterus that is generally small for gestational age, palpable fetal parts, and a fetal heart beat (Kurowski & Yakoub, 2003). Pathologic examination of an aborted conceptus is the only way to make a definitive diagnosis. An increasing number of spontaneous first-trimester abortions are recognized as partial moles after histologic review (FIGO, 2006; Garner et al., 2007; Kurowski & Yakoub).

Ultrasound examination in conjunction with HCG measurements is the gold standard for establishing a diagnosis of a molar pregnancy. Additionally, the use of immunohistochemical techniques as ancillary testing have proved invaluable in differentiating complete and partial moles based on genetic differences (Garner et al., 2007).

Classic complete moles have a characteristic sonographic pattern resulting from swelling of the chorionic villi. These edematous villi are commonly described as resembling a cluster of grapes and are associated with extensive trophoblastic proliferation. The average size of the villi is 1.5 centimeters in diameter, which is substantially larger than those found in normal gestations and in partial moles (Bently, 2003).

However, with the advent of advances in ultrasound technology, coupled with the routine use of ultrasound in the first trimester, the mean gestational age at diagnosis for complete moles is 8.5 weeks (Mosher, Goldstein, Berkowitz, Bernstein, & Genest, 1998). Consequently, the classic sonographic appearance is altered and is more subtle (Bently, 2003; Berkowitz & Goldstein, 1996; Garner et al., 2007; Wells, 2007) leading to the possible misclassification of an early complete mole as a partial mole (Fulop, Mok, Gati, & Berkowitz, 2002; Wells). Furthermore, Berkowitz and Goldstein cautioned that it may be difficult to distinguish an early mole from degenerating chorionic tissues. Leiser and Aghajanian (2006) indicated that this is also true for the identification of partial moles prior to the second trimester. Ultrasound has limited value in identification of partial moles (Royal College of Obstetricians and Gynaecologists [Royal College], 2004), although the placenta shows some hydatidiform changes, and fetal tissue may be identified.

In a normal pregnancy, HCG peaks at 100,000 mIU/ml and begins to decline by 10–12 weeks of gestation (Cunningham et al., 2005). Serum HCG measurements serve as a valuable diagnostic tool because they reflect trophoblastic volume (Berman et al., 2004; Garner et al., 2007). HCG levels greater than 100,000 mIU/ml suggest a diagnosis of a complete mole (Berkowitz & Goldstein, 2003). In contrast, with a partial mole, HCG is elevated over prenatal levels but is rarely elevated above the normal pregnancy range. Therefore, in partial mole, HCG may not be of diagnostic value (Bently, 2003; Garner et al., 2007).

The differential diagnosis of complete and partial moles has been refined since the availability of immunohistochemical staining for highly specific and sensitive markers such as p57kip2 and PHLDA2. *p57*, a cell cycle inhibitor protein, is a paternally imprinted, maternally expressed gene detectable in the placental villi of normal gestations, partial moles, and products of abortion but is absent in most villous cells of androgenetic complete moles (Akalin, Davidson, & Vang, 2006; Fisher et al., 2004; Garner et al., 2007; Hui et al., 2005; Wells, 2007). The absence of nuclear staining of *p57* confirms the diagnosis of a complete mole (Hui et al.). PHLDA2 is used in differentiating between a complete and partial mole. It is a product of a maternally expressed gene similar to *p57* and is undetectable in the villous cells of complete moles but is detectable via staining in partial moles (Fisher et al., 2004; Thaker et al., 2004).

Management

The cornerstone of GTD management encompasses uterine evacuation coupled with subsequent surveillance of quantitative serum HCG levels. Prior to molar evacuation, it is imperative to evaluate the woman closely for the presence of associated medical problems to avoid significant complications during and post evacuation. A pre-evacuation workup includes a chest x-ray, HCG levels, Rh status, complete blood cell count, electrolytes, along with renal, liver, and thyroid function tests.

Suction curettage is the method of choice for evacuation of complete molar pregnancies regardless of uterine size (Berkowitz & Goldstein, 2004; Berman et al., 2004; FIGO, 2006; Garner et al., 2007). Although IV oxytocin may be used to manage bleeding during evacuation, it should not be used prior to evacuation because of the resulting uterine stimulation. The increased pressure, caused by stimulation associated with uterine contractions, may cause embolization of trophoblastic tissue to the pulmonary system resulting in respiratory failure (Leiser & Aghajanian, 2006; Tidy et al., 2000). Embolization of molar tissue to the lung and other organs may be the genesis of metastasis and require chemotherapy post evacuation (Berman et al.; Tidy, 2003).

As an alternative to suction curettage, a hysterectomy without oophorectomy may be performed for those without childbearing plans. According to Berman et al. (2004), if theca lutein ovarian cysts are present, they will regress completely when serum HCG levels are negative. Although a hysterectomy eliminates trophoblastic tissue and limits the risk of local invasion (Garner et al., 2007), it does not prevent metastatic disease (Berkowitz & Goldstein, 1996; Garner et al., 2007; Soper, Mutch, & Schnik, 2004). Hysterectomy reduces the risk of post-molar GTN by 3%–5% when compared to evacuation by suction curettage but does not preclude post-evacuation follow-up (Hurteau, 2003; Leiser & Aghajanian, 2006; Soper et al.).

Medical termination methods through the use of prostaglandin, mifepristone, and oxytocin should be avoided because of the potential for incomplete molar evacuation and embolism along with dissemination of trophoblastic tissue through the venous system (Royal College, 2004; Tidy et al., 2000). Tidy et al. found that the mode of evacuation (e.g., spontaneous evacuation, surgical evacuation, medical evacuation) affects the incidence of GTN and the subsequent need for chemotherapy. In this study, spontaneous evacuation of molar pregnancy (2.3%) was associ ated with the lowest rate of chemotherapy treatment for GTN, followed by suction curettage (5.4%). With medical evacuation, 9.1% of women developed GTN and required chemotherapy post evacuation. However, medical evacuation may be indicated for treatment of partial moles when the size of fetal parts precludes the use of suction curettage (Royal College). It is recommended that all products of conception obtained after either medical or surgical evacuation undergo histologic examination to exclude GTN (Royal College). It is imperative that Rh-negative women receive Rh immune globulin following molar evacuation to prevent isoimmunization, thus protecting future pregnancies (FIGO, 2006).

Post-Evacuation Management

Following evacuation of molar pregnancies, a small percentage of women (1%–10%) will develop GTN as sequelae of complete moles or rarely, partial moles (Carney, 2003). Post-evacuation monitoring is crucial for early detection of GTN. Pelvic exams, serial HCG measurements, and hormonal contraceptive use are integral components of post-evacuation management.

Pelvic examinations are performed while HCG levels are elevated to monitor involution and to detect vaginal metastases. HCG is a valuable tumor marker (Pisal, Tidy, & Hancock, 2004) and is the mainstay for early detection of GTN following a molar pregnancy (Fong et al., 2005). Post-evacuation, HCG levels should decrease; therefore, an elevated plateau or a persistently elevated HCG titer suggests the development of GTN and treatment should be initiated (FIGO, 2006). Serum HCG levels should be obtained within 48 hours after evacuation (Hurteau, 2003; Soper et al., 2004). Guidelines include weekly HCG measurements until undetectable (FIGO, 2006). Once undetectable, the patient's HCG measurements should be monitored at the following intervals to ensure that HCG levels remain undetectable:

- Weekly for two weeks
- Monthly for six months
- Every two months for six additional months.

After completion of a documented remission for 6–12 months, HCG monitoring may be discontinued, and women who want to get pregnant may suspend contraceptive use (Soper et al., 2004).

Because post-evacuation HCG levels should decline, elevated levels are associated with a malignancy. If a pregnancy should occur during this time, HCG levels would naturally increase, and it would be impossible to attribute HCG increase to the development of GTN. This would result in delayed diagnosis and treatment. Therefore, the use of reliable hormonal contraception such as estrogen-progestin contraceptives or medroxyprogesterone is recommended while HCG values are being monitored (Cunningham et al., 2005; FIGO, 2006). The recommendation for oral contraceptive use during the post-treatment surveillance period is based on randomized control clinical trials. It was found that oral contraceptive use is safe and effective, as they do not increase the risk of GTN or alter HCG values (Curry et al., 1989; Morrow, Nakamura, Schlaerth, Gaddis, & Eddy, 1985).

Oral contraceptives were found to be more effective than no contraceptives or other contraceptive methods, such as barrier methods and intrauterine devices, in decreasing the risk of GTN (Deicas, Miller, Rademaker, & Lurain, 1991). The protective effect of oral contraceptives is unclear; however, Deicas et al. suggested that they suppress luteinizing hormone (LH) and inhibit trophoblastic tissue by suppressing gonadotropin production. Berkowitz and Goldstein (2005) recommended that an intrauterine device not be inserted until the HCG level is undetectable because of the possibility of uterine perforation if an invasive mole is present.

Noncompliance with the recommended gonadotropin regimen and oral contraceptive use is commonly related to myriad factors, including postponement of another pregnancy and financial and time commitments (Garner et al., 2007). Currently, research is being conducted to determine if the postmolar surveillance period can be shortened for women after complete or partial molar gestations. When a new pregnancy does occur, the woman is likely to have significant anxiety over the rising HCG levels (Carter, Lewin, Abu-Rustum, & Sonoda, 2007). Although most subsequent pregnancies progress normally, women with prior partial or complete mole have approximately a 1% risk for another molar gestation. This represents an increased incidence as compared with the general population (Garner et al., 2007). Repeat molar pregnancies increase the risk of malignant disease (Berkowitz & Goldstein, 2003; Berkowitz, Im, Bernstein, & Goldstein, 1998; Garner et al., 2007). Therefore, it is important that women who have had a molar pregnancy be aware of the increased risk of subsequent molar gestations. All future pregnancies should be evaluated by early ultrasound to confirm normal fetal development (Berkowitz & Goldstein, 2004; Garner et al.). Additionally, a post-pregnancy HCG level should be reviewed (Berkowitz & Goldstein, 2004).

Post-molar evacuation follow-up also will include sonography and Doppler imaging to aid in diagnosing the presence of invasive disease, detecting recurrent disease, and following effectiveness of chemotherapy (Jain, 2005). A magnetic resonance imaging (MRI) or computed tomography (CT) scan is indicated only when the ultrasound examination is inconclusive (FIGO, 2006). Additionally, the detection of *MCL-1*, an antiapoptotic gene, is significant, as it may be a marker used to predict GTN risk subsequent to a molar pregnancy (Fong et al., 2005). *Apoptosis*, or natural cell death, is necessary to prevent uncontrolled cell proliferation leading to neoplastic transformation. In GTN, the trophoblast evades naturally programmed cell death, and many chemotherapeutic agents used in treatment of GTN (e.g., etoposide, methotrexate, vincristine) are effective in the induction of apotosis (Fulop et al., 2002). Fong et al. (2005) demonstrated that moles progressing to GTN express higher levels of *MCL-1* compared to moles without malignant sequelae. They recommend further research to confirm these results.

Gestational Trophoblastic Neoplasia

GTN is the most curable gynecologic malignancy (Berman et al., 2004) with the highest percentage of GTN cases occurring between the ages of 25 and 29 years (Ngan et al., 2006). Garner et al. (2007) and Berman et al. (2004) related that GTN is more common following complete moles because of a greater trophoblastic volume and corresponding high HCG levels. Pre-evacuation signs that predict GTN development include HCG levels over 100,000 IU/L, significant uterine enlargement, and the presence of theca lutein cysts (Garner et al.). Hui et al. (2005) proposed that the reason GTN originates most often from complete moles is that they are closer to a neoplastic process, whereas partial moles, albeit anomalous gestational events, are closer to a normal pregnancy. Early detection and treatment of complete moles do not appear to alter the incidence of GTN (Garner et al., 2007; Hui et al.; Kurowski & Yakoub, 2003). Hui et al. proposed that the incidence of GTN relates to the innate biologic behavior of the neoplasm and not to the gestational age at evacuation.

Classification

Diagnosis of a post-molar GTN is based on persistently elevated HCG levels. GTN is subdivided into invasive mole and choriocarcinoma. The majority of GTN cases are nonmetastatic invasive moles (Leiser & Aghajanian, 2006). An invasive mole extends directly into the uterine muscle and is characterized by swollen chorionic villi and excessive trophoblastic overgrowth (Soper et al., 2004). It is generally confined to the uterus; however, occasionally it may perforate the uterus and metastasize to other organs (Paradinas et al., 2003). The most common symptom of an invasive mole is irregular bleeding following evacuation of a molar pregnancy. Because diagnosis requires histologic confirmation of myometrial invasion, it is usually confirmed after hysterectomy. Dilation and curretage should be avoided to prevent uterine perforation (Soper et al.).

Choriocarcinoma is the most aggressive form of GTN; however, even with metastases, it is highly curable because it is extremely responsive to chemotherapy (Fulop et al., 2002). The malignancy can occur after any term pregnancy, abortion, or ectopic pregnancy. Leiser and Aghajanian (2006) stressed that choriocarcinoma that does not develop following a known molar pregnancy may present several years post-gestational event. These women may have atypical symptoms such as cough, dyspnea, hemoptysis, and pulmonary metastases; headache and neurologic symptoms in brain metastases; and acute abdomen resulting from uterine perforation and bleeding, which makes diagnosis difficult (Zivaljevic et al., 2002). A diagnosis of choriocarcinoma should be considered in any woman of reproductive age with metastatic disease from an unknown primary site (Soper et al., 2004). In this case, an HCG level should be obtained to rule out GTN (Leiser & Aghajanian). Metastases often develop early and disseminate via the circulatory system because of the affinity of trophoblastic cells for blood vessels (Cunningham et al., 2005). Common sites of metastasis include the vagina, lung, liver, and brain, and presenting symptoms depend upon site of metastases.

The gestational or nongestational origin of choriocarcinoma can be distinguished using genetic analysis (Fisher, 2003). Fisher explained that if the tumor has both paternal and maternal genetic material, it developed from a gestational event such as a normal pregnancy or nonmolar abortion. However, if derived from a complete hydatidiform mole, it will be composed of paternal DNA. The precise molecular changes leading to choriocarcinoma are unknown. However, genetic analysis has demonstrated that epidermal growth factor receptors (EGFRs) present more commonly in a molar placenta as compared to a normal placenta of the same gestational age (Fulop et al., 2002). Cellular proliferation is mediated by the interaction of specific proto-oncogenes and tumor suppressor genes. Changes in the expression of suppressor genes such as *TP53*, *MDM2*, *p21*, and *RB* are implicated in trophoblastic proliferation and tumor development (Fulop et al.).

Staging

The current system for GTN staging and treatment includes a combination of anatomical staging and the World Health Organization prognostic scoring system as modified by FIGO (2006). According to this system, gestational trophoblastic neoplasms are classified as nonmetastatic, metastatic low risk, and metastatic high risk. The prognostic score includes the variables of age, antecedent pregnancy, tumor volume (e.g., HCG level, size and number of metastases), site of involvement, prior chemotherapy exposure, and duration of disease. The total score is obtained by adding the individual scores for each prognostic factor (see Table 10-1). This score along with anatomical staging aids in determining low- or high-risk disease categories.

Anatomic staging consists of four stages (see Appendix). Stage 1 disease is confined to the uterus and is classified as nonmetastatic low-risk disease. On the other end of the spectrum, stage IV indicates extensive metastatic disease involving the brain, liver, kidneys, or gastrointestinal tract and is considered high-risk disease. Stage II GTN extends outside the uterus but is limited to the genital structures, whereas Stage III GTN extends to the lungs with or without genital tract involvement. Stages II and III GTN are determined as low or high risk based on the prognostic score. For example, anyone with a prognostic score of 0–6 is at low risk and has a good prognosis regardless of how far the cancer has spread (anatomical stage). Women with a prognostic score of 7 or greater are classified as high risk; they tend to not respond as well to treatment and have a poorer prognosis than women with lower scores, even if the cancer has not spread as widely (FIGO, 2006).

Chemotherapeutic Management

The early identification of GTN and treatment with appropriate chemotherapy is crucial not only to reduce mortality but also to preserve reproductive function. However, it is recommended that women wait 12 months after completion of chemotherapy before attempting conception (FIGO, 2006).

Table 10-1. Modified World Health Organization Prognostic Scoring System as Adapted by International Federation of Gynecology and Obstetrics

Scores	0	1	2	4
Age	< 40	> 40	–	–
Antecedent pregnancy	Mole	Abortion	Term	
Interval months from index pregnancy	< 4	4–< 7	7 –< 13	> 13
Pretreatment serum HCG (IU/L)	< 10^3	10^3–<10^4	10^4–<10^5	> 10^5
Largest tumor size (including uterus)	< 3 cm	3 cm–< 5 cm	> 5 cm	–
Site of metastases	Lung	Spleen, kidney	Gastrointestinal	Liver, brain
Number of metastases	0	1–4	5–8	> 8
Previous failed chemotherapy	–	–	Single drug	2 or more drugs

Note. From *Staging Classifications and Clinical Practice Guidelines for Gynaecological Cancers* (p. 130), by International Federation of Gynecology and Obstetrics, 2006, London: Author. Copyright 2006 by International Federation of Gynecology and Obstetrics. Reprinted with permission.

GTN responds favorably to chemotherapy with an overall five-year survival rate estimate of 97.3% and 83–85% respectively for women with stage I or low-risk stage II and III disease and women with high-risk stage II and III disease. However, the five-year survival rate estimate for stage IV is lower at 62% (Ngan et al., 2006). At this time, there is no Cochrane level I or II evidence on which to base the management of GTN; therefore, the recommendations of FIGO are based on level III evidence.

Treatment guidelines for GTN were initially established by FIGO in 2000. According to FIGO, women with low-risk GTN (stages I, II, and III with a prognostic score of 6 or less) should initially receive a single chemotherapeutic agent such as methotrexate or actinomycin-D. Hysterectomy, in conjunction with a single agent, is recommended for women with stage I GTN who no longer desire to retain fertility (Berkowitz & Goldstein, 2003; Lurain, 2002). Adjunctive chemotherapy can reduce the dissemination of tumor cells at the time of surgery and provides a cytotoxic level of chemotherapy if this occurs. In addition, adjunctive chemotherapy will treat any occult metastases (Berkowitz & Goldstein, 2003). See Table 10-2 for single-agent protocols. If the initial single agent is not effective, FIGO suggested a schedule change, that is, give the same agent over a five-day course. If this does not produce a favorable response, the next step is to use the alternative agent. If resistance to both single-agent regimens occurs, multi-agent combination chemotherapy is then indicated. FIGO (2006) suggested that multi-agent chemotherapy can be avoided in 50%–60% of women when the aforementioned protocol sequence is followed.

For treatment of high-risk GTN (stage I, II, or III with a prognostic score 7 or greater or stage IV) multi-agent chemotherapy is required. The general consensus is that a combination of etoposide, methotrexate, actinomycin D, cyclophosphamide, and vincristine (EMA-CO) is the primary choice (Deng, Yan, Zhang, & Wu, 2006; FIGO, 2006). See Table 10-3 for the EMA-CO protocol and Figure 10-3 for administration criteria. When GTN does not respond to EMA-CO therapy, cyclophosphamide and vincristine are replaced by etoposide and platinum

Table 10-2. Single-Agent Chemotherapy Protocols for Low-Risk Gestational Trophoblastic Neoplasia

Drug	Dose and Time	Route	Comments
MTX	0.4 mg/kg daily x 5 days	IM	–
MTX with CF rescue	Days 1, 3, 5, 7–MTX: 1 mg/kg Days 2, 4, 6, 8–CF: 0.1 mg/kg	IM	On day 1, also perform CBC, platelet count, and SGOT
MTX	50 mg/kg weekly	IM	–
Actinomycin D	12 mcg/kg daily x 15 days	IV	–
Actinomycin D	1.25 mg/m² every 2 weeks	IV	Used as an alternative to pulsed weekly MTX protocol
MTX	250 mg	IV	Administer over 12-hour infusion

CBC—complete blood count; CF—citrovorum factor; IM—intramuscular; IV—intravenous; MTX—methotrexate; SGOT—serum glutamic-oxaloacetic transaminase

Note. From *Staging Classifications and Clinical Practice Guidelines for Gynaecological Cancers* (p. 137), by International Federation of Gynecology and Obstetrics, 2006, London: Author. Copyright 2006 by International Federation of Gynecology and Obstetrics. Adapted with permission.

Table 10-3. Multi-Agent Chemotherapy (EMA-CO) Protocol for High-Risk Gestational Trophoblastic Neoplasia

Day	Drug	Dose, Route, and Time
Day 1 (course A)	Actinomycin D	500 mcg IV push
	Etoposide	100 mg/m² IV infusion over 30–50 minutes
	Methotrexate	100 mg/m² IV infusion over 1 hour*
		200 mg/m² IV infusion over 12 hours
Day 2 (course A)	Actinomycin D	500 mcg IV push
	Etoposide	100 mg/m² IV infusion over 30–50 minutes
	Leucovorin	15 mg IV push every 6 hours for 8 doses –OR– PO every 12 hours for 4 doses
Day 8 (course B)†	Oncovin® (vincristine)	1 mg/m² IV
	Cyclophosphamide	600 mg/m² IV infusion
Day 15 (repeat cycle)		

(A)—Course A; (B)—Course B; EMA-CO—etoposide (VP-16), methotrexate, actinomycin-D, cyclophosphamide, Oncovin® (vincristine, Mayne Pharmaceuticals, USA)
*Begin leucovorin 24 hours after methotrexate bolus.
†If toxicity necessitates a delay in course B, course A is recycled.

Note. If filgrastim is administered, start 24 hours after day 2 and stop 24 hours before Cyclophosphamide and Oncovin. If creatinine is greater than 2 mg/dl, creatinine clearance should be greater than 50 mg/dl.

Note. From *Staging Classifications and Clinical Practice Guidelines for Gynaecological Cancers* (p. 138), by International Federation of Gynecology and Obstetrics, 2006, London: Author. Copyright 2006 by International Federation of Gynecology and Obstetrics. Adapted with permission.

(cisplatin) (EP-EMA) as shown in Table 10-4. This regimen is more rigorous and toxic than EMA-CO. A second alternative, BEP, includes bleomycin, etoposide, and platinum (cisplatin) as shown in Table 10-5.

Surgical Management

Surgery, as an adjunctive therapy, may be indicated when the patient has metastases to the lung, liver, brain, or other sites (FIGO, 2006). Adjunctive surgery may be indicated to (Lurain, Singh, & Schink, 2006)

- Remove resistant or persistent disease in the uterus or at metastatic sites
- Decrease tumor burden in the uterus in women when metastatic disease is limited
- Control tumor hemorrhage
- Treat complications such as bowel or urinary obstruction or infection.

In a review of women with choriocarcinoma, Lurain et al. found that high-risk women with uterine disease but no extrauterine disease (stage I) benefited from hysterectomy with an 86% survival rate. Additionally, the cure rate was 80% in women with drug-resistant disease and lung metastasis following a pulmonary resection.

Radiation Therapy Management

Although radiation therapy does not play a significant role in controlling GTN, it may be used to control hemorrhage from metastases (FIGO, 2006).When central nervous system metastases are present, whole brain irradiation is administered concurrently with chemotherapy to control tumor size and hemorrhage. In this case, the EMA-CO protocol is adjusted and the methotrexate dose is increased to 1,000 mg/m², and 30 mg of folinic acid is given every 12 hours for 3 days starting 32 hours after the methotrexate infusion begins (Lurain, 2002).

Post-Treatment Follow-Up

Post-treatment follow-up is imperative. Regardless of the stage of disease, women need weekly HCG levels until no detectable amount is found for three consecutive weeks, followed by monthly levels until no detectable HCG is found for 12 months for those with stage I, II, or III disease and 24 months for those with stage IV (Berkowitz & Goldstein, 2004).

Figure 10-3. Criteria for Administering Multi-Agent Chemotherapy for High-Risk Gestational Trophoblastic Neoplasia

- WBC > 3,000 μ
- Granulocytes > 1,500/ml
- Platelets > 100,000 μ
- Grade 3 GI infection has cleared
- Grade 3 mucositis morbidity has cleared

Note. From *Staging Classifications and Clinical Practice Guidelines for Gynaecological Cancers* (p.139), by International Federation of Gynecology and Obstetrics, 2006, London: Author. Copyright 2006 by International Federation of Gynecology and Obstetrics. Adapted with permission.

Table 10-4. Alternative 1—Multi-Agent Chemotherapy (EP-EMA) Protocol for EMA-CO Failure in High-Risk Gestational Trophoblastic Neoplasia

Day	Drug	Dose, Route, and Time
1 (course A)	Cisplatin	80 mgm/kg IV infusion over 12 hours
	Etoposide	100 mg/m² IV infusion over 1 hour
8 (course B)	Actinomycin D	500 mcg IV push
	Etoposide	100 mg/m² IV infusion over 30–50 minutes
	Methotrexate	100 mg/m² IV infusion over 1 hour; then 200 mg/m² IV infusion over 12 hours
9 (course B)	Leucovorin*	15 mg IV push every 6 hours for 8 doses
	-OR- Leucovorin acid†	15 mg PO every 12 hours for 4 doses

*Begin leucovorin 24 hours after methotrexate bolus.
† If a toxicity necessitates a delay in course B, course A is recycled.
P—platinum; PO—orally

Note. If filgrastim is administered, must start 24 hrs after 1st methotrexate and be stopped 24 hrs before next dose of platinum. It is recommended 24 hrs after platinum and stopped 24 hrs before next EMA.

Note. From *Staging Classifications and Clinical Practice Guidelines for Gynaecological Cancers* (p. 139), by International Federation of Gynecology and Obstetrics, 2006, London: Author. Copyright 2006 by International Federation of Gynecology and Obstetrics. Adapted with permission.

Placental Site Trophoblastic Tumor

PSTT is a rare variant of trophoblastic disease that is classified separately from GTN because of its unique and unpredictable clinical course (FIGO, 2006). It follows a gestational event; however, unlike choriocarcinoma, PSTT is more likely to follow a normal-term pregnancy than a molar pregnancy (Ajithkumar et al., 2005; Hassadia et al., 2005; Newlands, Hancock, Cole, & Berkowitz, 2003). Also, it may occur long after the gestational event (Dainty, Winter, & Maxwell, 2003). Baergen, Rutgers, Young, Osann, & Scully (2006) reported the antecedent pregnancy to be an average of 34 months (range 5–131 months) before diagnosis, whereas Hassadia et al. reported a median interval of 18 months (range 6–22 years).

These tumors are composed of intermediate trophoblast cells that contain only small amounts of HCG. The tumor invades the myometrium at the placental implantation site (Kim, 2003; Jain, 2005). Most cases are clinically benign; however, 15% of cases persist and metastasize (Hui et al., 2005).

Clinical Presentation and Diagnostic Evaluation

Most commonly, a woman presents with irregular bleeding or amenorrhea (Behtash, Ghaemmaghami, & Hasanzedeh, 2005; Kim, 2003); however, occasionally nephritic syndrome, sepsis, and erythrocytosis, or indications of metastasis, are presenting symptoms (Behtash et al., 2005). The uterus is often enlarged and asymmetrical. Human placental lactogen may be elevated; the HCG level is normal or marginally elevated and does not reflect the extensiveness of the tumor (Kim). However, Cole et al. (2006) found that the presence of greater than 35% HCG-free B-subunit could differentiate PSTT from choriocarcinoma. In addition, Machtinger et al. (2005) suggested that a Ki-67 index that exceeds 5% is indictive of PSTT. Diagnostic imaging is used to clarify tumor vascularity and evaluate tumor size (Machtinger et al.). A CT scan may reveal a uterine mass as well as detect metastases. Furthermore, MRI can assist in accurate localization of PSTT

Table 10-5. Alternative 2—Multi-Agent Chemotherapy BEP Protocol for EMA-CO Failure in High-Risk Gestational Trophoblastic Neoplasia

Day	Drug	Dose, Route, and Time
Day 1	Etoposide	100 mg in 500 ml NS over 1 hour prior to cisplatin
	Cisplatin	100 mg/m² IV continuous x 24 hours with NS x 6 at 250 ml/hour Add potassium chloride 20 mEq and magnesium sulfate to last 2 L of NS
Day 2	Etoposide	100 mg in 500 ml NS as part of day 1 cisplatin post-hydration. Complete post-hydration with D5NS at 150 ml/hr for 11 hours concurrent with bleomycin 10 u/m² IV infusion per day; continue IV fluids for 96 hours
Day 3	Etoposide	100 mg in 500 ml NS over 1 hour prior to bleomycin
	Bleomycin	10 u/m² IV infusion per day
Day 4	Etoposide	100 mg in 500 ml NS over 1 hour prior to bleomycin
	Bleomycin	10 u/m² IV infusion per day

NS—normal saline

Note. Granisetron, prochlorperazine, and diphenhydramine are given with these medications.

Note. From *Staging Classifications and Clinical Practice Guidelines for Gynaecological Cancers* (pp. 140–141), by International Federation of Gynecology and Obstetrics, 2006, London: Author. Copyright 2006 by International Federation of Gynecology and Obstetrics. Adapted with permission.

(Ajithkumar et al., 2003). A positron emission tomography scan may be used to evaluate the depth of invasion and the scope of metastasis. Definitive diagnosis often is made on the pathologic examination of either a dilation and curettage or hysterectomy specimen (Kim, 2003).

Management

Unlike choriocarcinoma, PSTT is resistant to chemotherapy (Baergen et al., 2006; Jain, 2005; Kim, 2003). Hysterectomy, with ovary preservation, is the primary mode of therapy when PSTT is limited to the uterus (Alazzam, Hancock, & Tidy, 2009; Dainty et al., 2003; Hassadia et al., 2005). When metastases are present, surgery alone is not sufficient. Following the protocols for high-risk metastatic GTN, combination chemotherapy with EMA-CO or EMA-EP should be initiated (FIGO, 2006; Kim). The majority of women are cured following surgery when PSTT is confined to the uterus (Behtash et al., 2005) and it is less than two years since last pregnancy; however, the prognosis is poorer as the interval between the gestational event and treatment lengthens and if metastases are present (Baergen et al.; Kim). In addition, the mitotic index may be important as a prognostic indicator. For example, a high mitotic index (greater than 5 per 10 high-power field) is reported to be associated with increased incidence of metastatic disease (Parul, Kriplani, & Vijayaraghavan, 2002). Radiation therapy is not a primary modality of treatment; however, it may be used to treat recurrent disease (Feltmate et al., 2001) and for palliative care (Hassadia et al., 2005).

Evidence-Based Practice

A paucity of randomized controlled trials and nonrandomized control experimental studies exists related to all aspects of trophoblastic disease. Currently, the diagnosis and treatment of trophoblastic disease is based almost entirely on level III evidence, that is, evidence obtained from well-designed nonexperimental descriptive studies, such as comparative studies, correlation studies, and case studies (Royal College, 2004). However, recommendations for oral contraceptive use during post treatment monitoring are based on randomized control studies.

Current chemotherapy protocols used for GTN management have not undergone the rigor of prospective randomized trials. No research currently fulfills Cochrane I or II levels of evidence for clinical studies. Deng et al. (2006) performed a Cochrane review to develop recommendations related to a combination chemotherapy regimen for managing high-risk GTN. Only one prospective randomized study was available in the literature and was dated 1989. However, the reviewers concluded that methodologic limitations prevented any firm conclusion about the most effective regimen. Thus, the evidence on which management of GTN is presently based fulfills Cochrane level III (FIGO, 2006).

Several clinical trials are currently in progress; information on clinical trials may be found at www.clinicaltrials.gov. Other suggested areas for research include (Newlands et al., 2003)

- New chemotherapeutic agents with improved long-term safety and effectiveness against variants that are resistant to current agents
- Cost-effectiveness of specialist centers to monitor and treat trophoblastic disease
- Understanding of the profile of HCG and degradation products related to different forms of trophoblastic disease.

EGFR inhibitors and antiangiogenesis agents for use in women with drug-resistant GTN are under investigation (Newlands, 2003).

Ongoing research in the area of molecular genetics continues to both discover and refine knowledge of highly specific and sensitive markers for each trophoblastic variant. Future research in this area includes determination of a common genetic event responsible for the development of all variants. Additionally, although trophoblastic disease is unequivocally a pregnancy-related disorder, the defect that exists in the ovum that permits abnormal fertilization and subsequent development of a molar pregnancy remains unclear (Newlands et al., 2003). Investigation continues to elucidate the relationship among various oncogenes and growth factors in the development of trophoblastic tumors (Berkowitz & Goldstein, 2004; Fulop et al., 2002).

Efforts to centralize research related to trophoblastic disease are ongoing through the establishment of specialized regional and national centers. Dissemination of research findings is facilitated by the efforts of the International Society for the Study of Trophoblastic Disease via a biannual World Congress and through the Society's informational Web site found at www.isstd.org.

Psychosocial Impact of Trophoblastic Disease

Psychosocial issues including reproductive concerns are integral to this diagnosis extending beyond initial diagnosis and persisting into survivorship. Inherent psychosocial stressors, including a loss of pregnancy, a potentially life-threatening diagnosis, and delay of future pregnancy may accompany this diagnosis. The couple must shift their sense of hopefulness and happiness related to the pregnancy to one of loss and uncertainty as well as being fearful of a potential malignancy (Wenzel, 2003).

Despite inherent emotional issues and concerns, survivors of trophoblastic disease reported an overall satisfaction with quality of life (physical, social, and emotion domains) 5–10 years after diagnosis and treatment (Wenzel et al., 2002). Results suggested that the women who reported the highest quality of life also were significantly more likely to have a successful pregnancy after trophoblastic disease. Forty percent of the women reported feelings of powerlessness over their reproductive future, whereas 35% were unsatisfied with their family size, and 17% expressed feelings of anger because their ability to have children had been compromised. Additionally, 74% of women indicated that if a support group had been available at the time of initial diagnosis, they most likely would have participated.

Proactive psychosocial care may be provided via support groups facilitated by nurses. These groups could be resources for the couple to process reproductive and other issues related to trophoblastic disease and treatment. However, because of the rarity of the disorder, access to these groups may be limited unless women are referred to large medical centers specializing in the treatment of trophoblastic disease. On the other hand, support groups related to pregnancy loss are available in many communities and may assist individuals and families in resolving grief issues. Additionally, referral to a mental health professional may be indicated for individual and family counseling for reproductive and sexuality issues. Internet resources available to the public include

- www.cancer.org
- www.cancer.gov
- www.mskcc.org
- www.obgyn.net.

Summary

Trophoblastic disease is highly curable, and reproductive function usually can be preserved. Early detection, diagnosis, treatment, and follow-up care are integral components of the management of trophoblastic disease and the achievement of positive outcomes. It is important for healthcare professionals to understand that trophoblastic disease is a multidimensional diagnosis with interrelated physical and emotional consequences. Members of the healthcare team have a unique opportunity to educate, facilitate communication, enhance coping, and provide support as families navigate through the crisis of this diagnosis (Bess & Wood, 2006).

References

Ajithkumar, T.V., Abraham, E.K., Rejnishkumar, R., & Minimole, A.L. (2003). Placental site trophoblastic tumor. *Obstetrics and Gynecology Surveillance, 58*(7), 484–488.

Akalin, A., Davidson, S.A., & Vang, R.R.S. (2006). Does this woman have gestational trophoblastic disease? *Oncology, 20*(13), 1699–1703.

Alazaam, M., Hancock, B.W., & Tidy, J. (2009). Role of hysterectomy in managing persistent gestational trophoblastic disease. *Journal of Reproductive Medicine, 53*(7), 519–524.

Altman, A.D., Bentley, B., Murray, S., & Bentley, J.R. (2008). Maternal age-related rates of gestational trophoblastic disease. *Obstetrics and Gynecology, 112*(2), 244–250.

Baergen, R.N., Rutgers, J.L., Young, R.H., Osann, K., & Scully, R.E. (2006). Placental site trophoblastic tumor: A study of 55 cases and review of the literature emphasizing factors of prognostic significance, *Gynecologic Oncology, 100*(3), 511–520.

Behtash, N., Ghaemmaghami, F., & Hasanzadeh, M. (2005). Long term remission of metastatic placental site trophoblastic tumor (PSTT): Case report and review of literature. *World Journal of Surgical Oncology, 3*(1), 34. Retrieved June 5, 2007, from http://www.wjso.com/content/3/1/34

Bently, R.C. (2003). Pathology of gestational trophoblastic disease. *Clinical Obstetrics and Gynecology, 46*(3), 513–522.

Berkowitz, R.S., & Goldstein, D.P. (1996). Chorionic tumors. *New England Journal of Medicine, 335*(3), 1740-1748.

Berkowitz, R.S., & Goldstein, D.P. (2003). Presentation and management of persistent gestational trophoblastic tumors in the USA. In B.W. Hancock, E.S. Newlands, R.S. Berkowitz, & L.A. Cole (Eds.), *Gestational trophoblastic disease* (2nd ed., pp. 248–267). Orange, CT: International Society for the Study of Trophoblastic Diseases. Retrieved June 20, 2007, from http://www.isstd.org/gtd.html

Berkowitz, R.S., & Goldstein, D.P. (2004). Gestational trophoblastic diseases. In W.J. Hoskins, C.A. Perex, R.C. Young, R.R. Batakat, M. Markmann, & M.E. Randall (Eds.), *Principles and practice of gynecologic oncology* (4th ed., pp. 1005–1075). Philadelphia: Lippincott Williams & Wilkins.

Berkowitz, R.S., & Goldstein, D.P. (2005). Gestational trophoblastic disease. In W.J. Hoskins, C.A. Peres, R.C. Young, R.R. Barakat, M. Markman, & M.E. Randall (Eds.), *Principles and practice of gynecologic oncology* (4th ed., pp. 1005–1075). Philadelphia: Lippincott Williams & Wilkins.

Berkowitz, R.S., Im, S.S., Bernstein, M.R., & Goldstein, D.P. (1998). Gestational trophoblastic disease: Subsequent pregnancy outcome, including repeat molar pregnancy. *Journal of Reproductive Medicine, 43*(1), 81–86.

Berman, M.L., DiSaia, P.J., & Tewari, K.S. (2004). Pelvic malignancies, gestational trophoblastic neoplasia, and nonpelvic malignancies. In R.K. Creasy & R. Resnik (Eds.), *Maternal-fetal medicine: Principles and practice* (pp. 1213–1242). Philadelphia: Elsevier Saunders.

Bess, K.A., & Wood, T.L. (2006). Understanding gestational trophoblastic disease. *Lifelines, 10*(4), 321–326.

Brinton, L.A., Bracken, M.B., & Connelly, R.R. (1986). Chroiocarcinoma incidence in the United States. *American Journal of Epidemiology, 123*(6), 1094–1100.

Carney, M.E. (2003). Treatment of low risk gestational trophoblastic disease, *Clinical Obstetrics and Gynecology, 46*(3), 579–592.

Carter. J., Lewin, S., Abu-Rustum, N., & Sonoda, Y. (2007). Reproductive issues in the gynecologic cancer patient. *Oncology, 21*(5), 598–606.

Cole, L.A., Khanlian, S.A., Muller, C.Y., Giddings, A., Kohorn, E., & Berkowitz, R. (2006) Gestational trophoblastic disease: 3. Human chorionic gonadotropin-free beta subunit, a reliable marker of placental site trophoblastic tumors, *Gynecologic Oncology, 102*(2), 160–164.

Cunningham, F.G., Hauth, J.C., Leveno, K.J., Gilstrap, L., Bloom, S.L., & Wenstron, K.D. (Eds.). (2005). *Williams obstetrics* (22nd ed.). New York: McGraw-Hill.

Curry, S.L., Schlaeth, J.B., Kohorn, E.L., Boyce, J.B., Gore, H., Twiggs, L.B., et al. (1989). Hormonal contraception and trophoblastic sequelae after hydatidiform mole. A Gynecologic Oncology Group study. *American Journal of Obstetrics and Gynecology, 43*(4), 906–914.

Dainty, L.A., Winter, W.E., & Maxwell, G.L. (2003). The clinical behavior of placental site trophoblastic tumor and contemporary methods of management. *Clinical Obstetrics and Gynecology, 46*(3), 607–611.

Deicas, R.E., Miller, D.S., Rademaker, A.W., & Lurain, J.R. (1991). The role of contraception in the development of postmolar gestational trophoblastic tumor. *Obstetrics and Gynecology, 78*(2), 221–226.

Deng, L., Yan, X., Zhang, J. & Wu, T. (2006). Combination chemotherapy for high-risk gestational trophoblastic tumour [Review]. *Cochrane Database of Systematic Reviews 2006,* Issue 3. Art. No.: CD005196. DOI: 10.1002/14651858.CD005196.pub2.

Evans, A.C., Soper, J.T., & Hammond, C.B. (2003). Clinical features of molar pregnancies and gestational trophoblastic tumors. In B.W. Hancock, E.S. Newlands, R.S. Berkowitz, & L.A. Cole (Eds.), *Gestational trophoblastic disease* (2nd ed., pp. 182–225). Orange, CT: International Society for the Study of Trophoblastic Diseases. Retrieved June 20, 2007, from http://www.isstd.org/gtd.html

Feltmate, C.M., Genest, D.R., Wise, L., Bernstein, M.R., Goldstein, D.P., & Berkowitz, R.S. (2001). Placental site trophoblastic tumor: A 17 year experience at the New England trophoblastic disease center. *Gynecologic Oncology, 82*(3), 415–419.

Fisher, R. (2003). Genetics. In B.W. Hancock, E.S. Newlands, R.S. Berkowitz, & L.A. Cole (Eds.), *Gestational trophoblastic disease* (2nd ed., pp. 6–29). Orange, CT: International Society for the Study of Trophoblastic Diseases. Retrieved June 20, 2007, from http://www.isstd.org/gtd.html

Fisher, R.A., Nucci, M.R., Thaker, H.M., Weremowicz, S., Genst, D.R., & Castrillon, D.H. (2004). Complete hydatidiform mole retaining a chromosome 11 of maternal origin: Molecular genetic analysis of a case. *Modern Pathology, 17*(9), 1155–1160.

Fong, P., Xue, W., Ngan, H.Y., Chan, K.Y., Khoo, U., Tsao, S., et al. (2005). Mcl-1 expression in gestational trophoblastic disease correlates with clinical outcome. *Cancer, 103*(2), 268–276.

Fulop, V., Mok, S.C., Gati, I., & Berkowitz, R.S. (2002). Recent advances in molecular biology of gestational trophoblastic disease. *Journal of Reproductive Medicine, 47*(5), 369–379.

Garner, E.I., Goldstein, D.P., Feltmate, C.M., & Berkowitz, R.S. (2007). Gestational trophoblastic disease. *Clinical Obstetrics and Gynecology, 50*(1), 112–122.

Hassadia, A., Gillespie, A., Tidy, J., Everard, R.G.N.J., Wells, M., Coleman, R., et al. (2005). Placental site trophoblastic tumour: Clinical features and management. *Gynecologic Oncology, 99*(3), 603–607.

Hui, P., Martel, M., & Parkash, V. (2005). Gestational trophoblastic diseases: Recent advances in histopathologic diagnosis and related genetic aspects. *Advances in Anatomic Pathology, 12*(3), 116–225.

Hurteau, J.A. (2003). Gestational trophoblastic disease: Management of hydatidiform mole. *Clinical Obstetrics and Gynecology, 46*(3), 557–569.

International Federation of Gynecology and Obstetrics. (2006). *Staging classifications and clinical practice guidelines for gynaecological cancers.* London: Author.

Jain, K.A. (2005). Gestational trophoblastic disease: Pictorial review. *Untrasound Quarterly, 21*(4), 245–253.

Kim, S.J. (2003). Placental site trophoblastic tumour. *Best Practice and Research Clinical Obstetrics and Gyneacology, 17*(6), 969–984.

Kurowski, K., & Yakoub, N. (2003). Staying alert for gestational trophoblastic disease: Implication for primary care clinicians. *Women's Health in Primary Care, 6*(1), 39–45.

Leiser, A.L., & Aghajanian, C. (2006). Evaluation and management of gestational trophoblastic disease. *Community Oncology, 3*(3), 152–156.

Lurain, J.R. (2002). Treatment of gestational trophoblastic tumors. *Current Treatment Options in Oncology, 2*(3), 113–124.

Lurain, J.R., Singh, D.K., & Schink, J.C. (2006). Role of surgery in the management of high-risk gestational trophoblastic neoplasia. *Journal of Reproductive Medicine, 51*(10), 773–776.

Machtinger, R., Gotlieb, W.H., Korach, J., Fridman, E., Apter, S., Goldenberg, M., et al. (2005). Placental site trophoblastic tumor: Outcome of five cases including fertility preserving management. *Gynecologic Oncology, 96*(1), 56–61.

Morrow, P., Nakamura, R., Schlaerth, J., Gaddis, O., Jr., & Eddy, G. (1985). The influence of oral contraceptives on the postmolar human chorionic gonadotropin regression curve. *American Journal of Obstetrics and Gynecology, 151*(7), 906–114.

Mosher, R., Goldstein, D.P., Berkowitz, R., Bernstein, M., & Genest, D.R. (1998). Complete hydatidiform mole: Comparison of clinicopathologic features, current and past. *Journal of Reproductive Medicine, 43*(1), 21–27.

Newlands, E.S. (2003). The management of recurrent and drug resistant gestational trophoblastic neoplasia (GTN). *Best Practice and Research: Clinical Obstetrics and Gynecology, 17*(6), 905–923.

Newlands, E.S., Hancock, B.W., Cole, L.A., & Berkowitz, R.S. (2003). Future prospects. In B.W. Hancock, E.S. Newlands, R.S. Berkowitz, & L.A. Cole (Eds.), *Gestational trophoblastic disease* (2nd ed., pp. 380–394). Orange, CT: International Society for the Study of Trophoblastic Diseases. Retrieved June 20, 2007, from http://www.isstd.org/gtd.html

Ngan, H., Odicino, F., Maisonneuve, P., Creasman, W.T., Beller, U., Quinn, M.A., et al. (2006). Gestational trophoblastic neoplasia: FIGO 6th annual report on the results of treatment in gynecological cancer. *International Journal of Gynecology and Obstetrics, 95*(Suppl. 1), S193–S203.

Palmer, J.R. (1994). Advances in the epidemiology of gestational trophoblastic disease. *Journal of Reproductive Medicine, 39*(3), 155–162.

Paradinas, F.J., Sebire, N.J., & Rees, H.C. (2003). Pathology. In B.W. Hancock, E.S. Newlands, R.S. Berkowitz, & L.A. Cole (Eds.), *Gestational trophoblastic disease* (2nd ed., pp. 77–128). Orange, CT: International Society for the Study of Trophoblastic Diseases. Retrieved June 20, 2007, from http://www.isstd.org/gtd.html

Parul, A.N., Kriplani, A., & Vijayaraghavan, M. (2002). Placental site trophoblastic tumour. *Journal of Postgraduate Medicine, 48*(3), 211–212.

Pisal, N., Tidy, J., & Hancock, B. (2004). Gestational trophoblastic disease: Is intensive follow-up essential in all women? *British Journal of Obstetrics and Gynecology, 111*(12), 1449–1451.

Royal College of Obstetricians and Gynaecologists (2004). *The management of gestational trophoblastic neoplasia. Guideline No. 38.* Retrieved June 9, 2007, from http://www.guidelines.gov/summary/summary.aspx?view_id=1&doc_id=7678

Smith, H.O. (2003). Gestational trophoblastic disease epidemiology and trends. *Clinical Obstetrics and Gynecology, 46*(3), 541–556.

Smith, H.O., & Kim, S.J. (2003). Epidemiology. In B.W. Hancock, E.S. Newlands, R.S. Berkowitz, & L.A. Cole (Eds.), *Gestational trophoblastic disease* (2nd ed., pp. 39–76). Orange, CT: International Society for the Study of Trophoblastic Diseases. Retrieved June 20, 2007, from http://www.isstd.org/gtd.html

Smith, H.O., Qualls, C.R., Prairie, B.A., Padilla, L.A., Rayburn, W.R., & Key, R.K. (2003). Trends in gestational choriocarcinoma: A 27-year perspective. *Obstetrics and Gynecology, 102*(5, Pt. 1), 978–986.

Soper, J.T. (2006). Gestational trophoblastic disease. *Obstetrics and Gynecology, 108*(1), 176–187.

Soper, J.T., Mutch, D.G., & Schink, J.C. (2004). Diagnosis and treatment of gestational trophoblastic disease (ACOG Practice Bulletin No. 53). *Gynecologic Oncology, 93*(3), 575–585.

Soto-Wright, V., Bernstein, M., Goldstein, D.P., & Berkowitz, R.S. (1995). The changing clinical presentation of complete molar pregnancy. *Obstetrics and Gynecology, 86*(5), 775–779.

Steigrad, S.J. (2003). Epidemiology of gestational trophoblastic diseases. *Best Practice and Research Clinical Obstetrics and Gynecology 17*(6), 837–847.

Thaker, H.M., Berlin, A., Tycko, B., Goldstein, D.P., Berkowita, R.S., Castrillon, D.H., et al. (2004). Immunohistochemistry for the imprinted gene product IPL/PHLDA2 for facilitating the differential diagnosis of complete hydatidiform mole. *Journal of Reproductive Medicine, 49*(8), 630–636.

Tham, B.W., Everard, J.E., Tidy, J.A., Drew, D., & Hancock, B.W. (2003). Gestational trophoblastic disease in the Asian population of northern England and north Wales. *British Journal of Obstetrics and Gynecology, 119*(6), 555–559.

Tidy, J. (2003). The role of surgery in the management of gestational trophoblastic disease. In B.W. Hancock, E.S. Newlands, R.S. Berkowitz, & L.A. Cole (Eds.), *Gestational trophoblastic disease* (pp. 348–358). Retrieved August 20, 2007, from http://www.isstd.org/gtd/index.html

Tidy, J.A., Gillispie, A.M., Bright, N., Radstone, C.R., Coleman, R.E., & Hancock, B.W. (2000). Gestational trophoblastic disease: A study of mode of evacuation and subsequent need for treatment with chemotherapy. *Gynecologic Oncology, 78*(3, Pt. 1), 309–312.

Wells, M. (2007). The pathology of gestational trophoblastic disease: Recent advances. *Pathology, 39*(1), 88–96.

Wenzel, L.B. (2003). Psychosocial consequences of gestational trophoblastic disease. In B.W. Hancock, E.S. Newlands, R.S. Berkowitz, & L.A. Cole (Eds.), *Gestational trophoblastic disease* (2nd ed., pp. 359–366). Orange, CT: International Society for the Study of Trophoblastic Diseases. Retrieved June 20, 2007, from http://www.isstd.org/gtd.html

Wenzel, L., Berkowitz, R.S., Newlands, E., Hancock, B., Goldstein, D.P., Seckl, M.J., et al. (2002). Quality of life after gestational trophoblastic disease. *Journal of Reproductive Medicine, 47*(5), 387–394.

Zivaljevic, M., Tesic, M., Vujkov, T., Rajovic, J., & Popovic, M. (2002). Gestational trophoblastic disease. *Archive of Oncology, 10*(2), 71–75.

CHAPTER 11

Vulvar and Vaginal Cancers

Blanca Vasquez-Clarfield, MA, RN, and Jane Duffy-Weiser, MS, RN, ANP-BS

Vulvar Cancer

Introduction

Vulvar cancer is a rare disease accounting for only 5%–8% of all gynecologic cancers (Stehman & Look, 2006). According to the American Cancer Society (ACS, 2008b), approximately 3,460 women in the U.S. will be diagnosed with vulvar cancer, and 870 women will die of the disease. It is primarily a disease of older women, although the prevalence is increasing in younger women (Tyring, 2003). Self-image is compromised when a woman is diagnosed with vulvar cancer. Women often experience painful intercourse and are confronted with issues of intimacy (Spinelli, 2000). However, if it is detected early, vulvar cancer has a high cure rate, and the treatment options may be less invasive, preserving sexual function. Unfortunately, the prognosis for late-stage disease is poor (Tyring).

Both women and their physicians contribute to the delayed diagnosis of vulvar cancer. Approximately 40% are diagnosed at a late stage because women often delay seeking medical attention for early symptoms as a result of embarrassment or denial (Tyring, 2003). The symptoms of vulvar cancer can be caused by other benign conditions. Thus, women may fail to recognize the serious nature of their symptoms and attempt to self-medicate with over-the-counter treatments (Moore, Koh, McGuire, & Wilkinson, 2005; Tyring). Providers, unfamiliar with this rare disease, may not recognize the condition and may prescribe topical therapies without proper vulvar examination or tissue biopsy confirmation (Moore et al., 2005). The key to a cure is early medical attention, examination, biopsy, and referral to a gynecologic oncologist who specializes in treatment of this rare cancer (Moore et al., 2005).

Squamous cell carcinoma (SCC) accounts for 95% of vulvar carcinomas (Moore et al., 2005). Recent evidence suggests that SCC of the vulva may develop as two separate diseases (van der Avoort et al., 2006). The first type is vulvar intraepithelial neoplasia (VIN) caused by human papillomavirus (HPV) infections and is increasingly prevalent among young women (van der Avoort et al.). The second type, seen more frequently in older women, is vulvar non-neoplastic epithelial disorder (VNNED) and occurs because of chronic inflammation known as lichen sclerosis (Jones, Rowan, & Stewart, 2005; Smith & Haefner, 2004). Seventy percent of tumors will involve the labia majora and labia minora; 15%–20% will involve the clitoris, and a small percentage will exhibit extensive local spread involving the vagina, urethra, anus, and in some cases the pubic bone (Eifel, Berek, & Markman, 2005). Definitive diagnosis is based on histology after biopsy of the suspicious lesion. Once diagnosed, vulvar cancer is staged using a combination of two classification systems, the International Federation of Gynecology and Obstetrics (FIGO) System of Staging and the American Joint Committee on Cancer TNM (tumor, node, metastasis) system (Moore et al., 2005). Treatment is surgical resection, with the goal of complete removal of the tumor using conservative surgery to decrease psychosexual complications (Tyring, 2003).

Etiology and Epidemiology

Vulvar cancer usually develops slowly over a period of years. Abnormal cells can grow on the surface of the vulvar skin for a long time as a precancerous condition, VIN, or dysplasia (Jones, Rowan, et al., 2005; Moore et al., 2005). If VIN is diagnosed and treated early, an invasive vulvar malignancy may be avoided (Jones, Rowan, et al., 2005). No specific medical comorbidities have been identified as independently causing vulvar cancer (Tyring, 2003), but 25% of women have comorbid conditions such as hypertension, diabetes, and obesity at the time of diagnosis (Hacker, 2000).

The first type of SCC of the vulva is associated with HPV infection leading to VIN and is known as Bowen disease. This premalignant lesion predisposes a woman to invasive vulvar cancer (Joura, Losch, Haider-Angeler, Breitenecker, & Leodolter, 2000). The incidence of Bowen disease has increased over the past decade, becoming more common in women 20–35 years old (Joura et al.). Studies suggest that risk factors for this type of vulvar cancer are similar to cervical cancer, including the number of lifetime sexual partners, a history of sexually transmitted diseases such as gonorrhea and venereal warts, cigarette smoking, and a history of abnormal cervical Pap smears (Stehman & Look, 2006). VIN in young women presents as a cauliflower-like lesion, and if untreated, up to 80% may develop invasive disease (Moore et. al., 2005).

The second type of SCC involves VNED and is usually seen in women ages 55–85 (Joura et al., 2000). These cancers are not linked to HPV infections or VIN but are associated with lichen sclerosis, a chronic itchy vulvar skin disorder (Jones, Sadler, et al., 2005). This type may have no evidence of preinvasive disease, only invasive cancer (Stehman & Look, 2006). See Table 11-1 for differences in types of vulvar SCC. Although different in etiology, treatment for each type is similar. However, in the future, prevention strategies and appropriate treatment for older and younger women with SCC may change (Tyring, 2003). Therapies such as photodynamic therapy and topical immunotherapy may be used in the future but require further studies (Tyring).

Because other histologic types of vulvar cancers are much rarer than SCC, less is known about how these cancers develop (Govindan & Arquette, 2002). Rare types of vulvar cancer are listed in Table 11-2.

Table 11-1. Two Different Manifestations of Vulvar Squamous Cell Carcinoma

Characteristic	HPV Related	Non–HPV Related
Age	Younger (35–65 years old)	Older (55–85 years old)
Human papillomavirus DNA	Frequent (more than 60%)	Seldom (less than 15%)
Preexisting lesion	Vulvar intraepithelial neoplasia	Vulvar inflammation, lichen sclerosus
History of condyloma	Strong association	Rare association
History of sexually transmitted diseases	Strong association	Rare association
Cigarette smoking	High incidence	Low incidence

Note. From "Carcinoma of the Vulva: Epidemiology and Pathogenesis," by C.P. Crum, 1992, *Obstetrics and Gynecology, 79*(3), p. 449. Copyright 1992 by American College of Obstetricians and Gynecologists. Adapted with permission.

Clinical Presentation

Early symptoms of invasive vulvar cancer may appear similar to those of symptomatic VIN (Stehman & Look, 2006). The most frequently reported symptoms of vulvar cancer include chronic pruritis lasting longer than one month and a lump or mass (Stehman & Look). Less common presenting symptoms include vulvar bleeding not related to menstruation, discharge, dysuria, and pain, as well as a change in size, color, or texture of a vulvar birthmark or mole (Stehman & Look).

Table 11-2. Histologic Types of Vulvar Cancer

Disease	Description
Squamous cell carcinoma	Two types; see Table 11-1
Bartholin gland carcinoma	Usually HPV-associated squamous cell carcinoma or adenocarcinoma; lymph node metastases are common.
Verrucous carcinoma	Also known as the giant wart or Buschke/Lowenstein condyloma A type of invasive squamous cell vulvar cancer with good prognosis; appears as cauliflower-like growths similar to genital warts
Paget disease	A sweat gland carcinoma arising from the basal layer of the vulva Erythematous, crusting, weeping, oozing lesion recurs locally because of residual disease, but it does not metastasize. Good prognosis if no invasive disease is present because it does not metastasize Low mortality rate
Melanoma	3%–10% of vulvar cancers The appearance of a darkly pigmented growth or a change in a mole that has been present for years may indicate melanoma. The most important sign of melanoma is a change in size, shape, or color of a mole.
Basal cell	Very rare; only 2%–4% of vulvar cancers Correlates with sun exposure and older age Appears as an ulcer
Sarcoma	Very rare; only 1%–2% of vulvar cancers Aggressive in vulva; most die of the disease May recur locally or metastasize, usually to lymph nodes

Note. Based on information from AshrafGanjooie, 2004; Naziri & Omranipour, 2006; Sugiyama et al., 2007.

As the cancer advances, a distinct tumor is more likely to form displaying bumps with a wart-like feature (Tyring, 2003). It is very uncommon for a patient to present with a large fungating mass (Hacker, 2000).

Diagnosis

The definitive histologic diagnosis is made by biopsy of the suspicious vulvar lesion (Moore et al., 2005). A complete medical history is needed to assess for risk factors, symptoms, health habits, past illnesses, and treatments. The physical examination includes a thorough visual examination of the vulva, bimanual pelvic exam, and a clinical assessment of groin lymph nodes to assess for evidence of metastasis. Although no standard protocol defines when to perform a biopsy, it is recommended that biopsy be performed when the patient experiences any changes in a vulvar lesion, such as size, color, elevation or surface, or an unusual condyloma or warty appearance that does not respond to therapy or persistent ulceration or itchy area in the vulva (Hacker, 2000). A colposcopic exam may be performed in combination with the biopsy (Furniss, 2000), but it rarely is helpful in diagnosis (Govindan & Arquette, 2002). Depending on the biopsy results, several other diagnostic tests may be performed to determine the extent of the disease (see Table 11-3).

Table 11-3. Diagnostic Imaging and Exams

Diagnostic Test	Rationale
Cystoscopy	Some advanced cases of vulvar cancer can spread to the bladder, so any suspicious areas noted by this exam are removed for biopsy.
Proctoscopy	Some advanced cases of vulvar cancer can spread to the rectum. A biopsy is performed on any suspicious areas.
Examination of the pelvis under anesthesia	This permits a more thorough manual and visual examination that can better evaluate the extent of cancer spread to internal organs of the pelvis.

Imaging Tests to Assist in Diagnosis Include
- Chest x-ray
- Computed tomography
- Magnetic resonance imaging

Note. Based on information from Chang, 2002; Eifel et al., 2005; Moore et al., 2005.

Staging Vulvar of Carcinoma

The stage of SCC of the vulva is described using the FIGO System of Staging combined with the American Joint Committee on Cancer TNM system. The TNM system classifies the diseases in stages 0 through IV depending on the extent of the tumor (T), whether the cancer has spread to lymph nodes (N), and whether it has spread to distant sites (M) (Stehman & Look 2006). (See Appendix for FIGO stages.)

Prognosis

The prognosis for women with invasive vulvar cancer is good when appropriate and timely treatment is provided. The overall five-year survival is 70% (Hacker, 2000). The stage, tumor size, and number of positive groin nodes are the most important factors affecting prognosis and treatment (Hacker).

Overall, the incidence of lymph node metastasis is about 30%. The risk of nodal metastasis increases as the stage of disease, size of the lesion, and depth of invasion increase (Hacker, 2000).

Treatment

Surgery is the treatment of choice for vulvar cancer. For decades, the surgery has been consistent with a radical approach. From the early 1900s until the 1980s, the standard approach was to perform an *en bloc* (removal of all structures together) radical vulvectomy and removal of inguinal femoral lymph nodes. This procedure was known as the Bassett-Way operation and used a curvilinear incision made from one anterior iliac spine to the other and then down to the bilateral groin nodes (Stehman & Look, 2006). This radical procedure was associated with significant physical and psychological complications (Eifel et al., 2005). Wound breakdown, infection, chronic lymphedema, and sexual dysfunction were common results (Landrum, Skaggs, Gould, Walker, & McMeekin, 2008). In 1981, Hacker and colleagues developed a technique where separate incisions are made, one to excise the vulvar lesion and the other to excise the inguinal lymph nodes (Stehman & Look, 2006). The five-year survival rates for both the radical and less radical approach were about 60%–70% (Eifel et al.). This initiated a trend for less radical surgery for early-stage disease (Eifel et al.). Today, the trend continues with the inclusion of chemoradiation followed by surgery for locally advanced disease to reduce tumor size and avoid radical, and possibly exenterative, procedures (Moore et al., 1998).

A rich network of lymphatics drains the vulva. Invasive vulvar lesions can spread to regional lymph nodes, which are the inguinal and femoral nodes. Metastatic spread to regional lymph nodes can then lead to metastasis to distant nodes or pelvic nodes (Eifel et al., 2005). Therefore, addressing nodal involvement, or the risk of nodal involvement, is paramount. Benedet, Bender, Jones, Ngan, and Pecorelli (2000) noted that appropriate groin dissection is the single most important factor in reducing mortality in early vulvar cancer.

Sentinel lymph node mapping, as is performed in early-stage breast cancer, is being studied in the surgical treatment of early-stage vulvar cancer to evaluate who best benefits from inguinal lymphadenectomy (Van der Zee et al., 2007).

Stages I and II Disease

In stage I disease, where lesions are confined to the vulva and are less than 2 cm in diameter, a radical wide local excision alone is recommended. Because the incidence of groin node involvement at this stage is so low, it is considered safe to omit the inguinofemoral lymphadenectomy (de Hullu, Oonk, & Van der Zee, 2004). The radical wide local excision procedure extends down to the fascia of the urogenital diaphragm, which is composed of the sphincter muscle of the urethra and the deep transverse muscle of the perineum, with an effort to obtain 2 cm of normal tissue in all directions (Eifel et al., 2005). Obtaining adequate surgical margins is a significant prognostic factor in reducing local recurrence. Heaps, Fu, Montz, Hacker, and Berek (1990) showed a recurrence rate of 48% if surgical margins were less than 8 mm compared to 0% recurrence if the margins were greater than 8 mm.

Aside from the size of a vulvar lesion, other factors need to be taken into consideration regarding risk of regional metastasis. These include depth of invasion, tumor thickness, and the presence of lymphovascular space invasion (LVSI) (Eifel et al., 2005). Depth of invasion of greater than 1 mm puts the regional lymph nodes at risk (Stehman & Look, 2006), and up to 75% of women with LVSI have positive inguinal nodes (Eifel et al., 2005). With these risk factors, in early-stage disease, treatment would include radical wide local excision and inguinal node dissection. Eifel et al. (2005, p. 1332) recommended that "all patients with greater than 1 mm of invasion have bilateral radical inguinal node dissection." Stehman and Look (2006, pp. 723–724) recommended "radical wide local incision with a 1 cm surgical margin to address the primary lesion and ipsilateral groin dissection through a separate incision," as well as "bilateral groin dissection if there is a positive ipsilateral node or in the setting of a midline lesion."

Stages III and IV Disease

Advanced-stage disease usually involves critical structures such as the vagina, urethra, and anus. Procedures such as *en bloc* radical vulvectomy along with exenterative surgery and bilateral groin dissection often are needed to obtain acceptable surgical margins and reduce the risk of recurrence.

Over the past decade, locally advanced disease has been treated with neoadjuvant chemoradiation followed by resection for any residual disease. The results of a phase II Gynecologic Oncology Group (GOG) study showed favorable results treating stage III and IVA tumors with twice-daily radiation to the primary tumor and to the regional groin nodes for five weeks (Moore et al., 1998). Cisplatin and 5-flurouracil (5-FU) were administered during the first and last week. This resulted in improved rates of successful tumor resection and local control. In another study, Gerszten, Selvaraj, Kelley, and Paul (2005) treated women with earlier stage disease, stages II and III. They used a dosing schedule modified to that of the GOG study and found they were able to decrease the extent of surgery for advanced disease.

Radiation Therapy

Radiation therapy (RT) was once thought to have a very limited role in the treatment of vulvar cancers. In the early part of the 20th century, radical surgery was the mainstay despite the associated morbidity and physical disfigurement. In the 1970s, RT started to be used in the adjuvant and definitive settings (Barnes & Thomas, 2006). Today, RT has an integral role in the treatment of vulvar cancer.

The indications for using adjuvant radiation in a postoperative setting include (Bradley & Petereit, 2006)

- Positive surgical margins
- When the surgical margin is less than 8 mm
- When there are two or more positive inguinal lymph nodes
- A grossly positive lymph node
- Capsular nodal extension.

In a landmark study by Homesley, Bundy, Sedlis, and Adcock (1986), adjuvant RT was found to be superior over surgery in preventing regional and distant recurrence when inguinal nodes were found to be positive at the time of surgery. Patients with positive nodes were randomized to receive 4,500–5,000 cGy to the bilateral groins and midline of the pelvis versus surgical resection of the pelvic nodes in the study by Homesley and colleagues. The trial was stopped early as the two-year survival advantage was 68% for the RT group and 54% for the group that underwent pelvic lymph node resection. The recommended adjuvant RT doses used today are 4,500–5,000 cGy daily over 5–5.5 weeks (Bradley & Pretereit, 2006).

Preoperative or neoadjuvant RT is used in combination with chemotherapies to reduce the need for more radical surgeries in stage III and IV disease. The concurrent use of chemotherapy with RT was first studied in the 1970s with vulvar cancer and other disease sites and found to have a synergistic effect, improving the response rates with the addition of RT (Barnes & Thomas, 2006). Today, these combined modalities are part of standard treatment for cervical, head and neck, vulvar, and anal cancers (Barnes & Thomas).

Palliative RT can be used in cases of vulvar cancer with extensive, advanced local disease, and metastatic spread, when radical surgery is not an option. Advanced local disease can cause ulceration, bleeding, necrosis, pain, and foul-smelling discharge (Barnes & Thomas, 2006). Low-dose regimens over a short time period are effective in reducing symptoms and improving the woman's quality of life. The recommended total RT dose is 2,500 cGy given over 10 fractions (Barnes & Thomas).

Chemotherapy

No standard single-modality chemotherapy regimens are available to treat vulvar cancers, particularly in the neoadjuvant setting. However, in a review of data regarding neoadjuvant trials, good outcomes were found in one trial using 5-FU and cisplatin prior to radical vulvectomy with bilateral inguinal-femoral lymphadenectomy (Gadducci, Cionini, Romanini, Fanucchi, & Genazzani, 2006). Another trial in the same review noted poor results in stage IV patients treated with combination cisplatin, bleomycin, and methotrexate (Gadducci et al.). Cisplatin and 5-FU have been used alone or in combination with radiation therapy with good results.

Recurrent Disease

The rate of recurrence of vulvar cancer after primary treatment with or without RT is about 24% (Salom & Penalver, 2002). Attributable factors of multifocal tumors and advanced age of the patient limits the range of surgical interventions (Weikel, Schmidt, Steiner, Knapstein, & Koelbl, 2006). Recurrence usually is detected during the first two years after primary treatment (Salom & Penalver, 2002). The usual sites of recurrence include vulva (57%), groin (22%), and pelvis or other distant sites (14%–22%) (Salom & Penalver).

Recurrent disease that is limited to the vulva can be successfully treated with the intent to cure. A localized, lateral lesion can be treated with wide radical local excision and inguinal lymphadenectomy with cure rates up to 70% (Salom & Penalver, 2002). RT should be offered to those who have had no prior radiation and who have inadequate or positive surgical margins and positive lymph nodes. For lesions that recur on the vulva but involve midline structures such as the urethra, vagina, and rectum, exenterative procedures (e.g., anterior, posterior, or both) may be offered if prior definitive doses of RT already have been delivered (Salom & Penalver). See Chapter 12 for detailed information about exenterative procedures.

Unfortunately, recurrences in the groin and in distant areas such as the pelvic lymph nodes have a very poor prognosis and often result in death. Stehman and Look (2006) reported that in a GOG series, 91% of patients with groin recurrences died, and the median time of survival after groin recurrence was only 9.4 months. These tumors often originally had high-risk features and a higher stage of disease at the time of diagnosis. Most women already have had maximum doses of RT, thus limiting further treatment. Re-excision in previously radiated fields has resulted in significant morbidity and usually is avoided (Salom & Penalver, 2002). Systemic chemotherapies can be administered to palliate symptoms but will do little to extend survival (Stehman & Look).

Vaginal Cancer

Introduction

Primary vaginal cancers are rare, accounting for only 1%–2% of all gynecologic malignancies (National Cancer Institute [NCI], 2008). Most malignant vaginal lesions result from metastasis from another type of cancer. For example, cancers of the vulva, cervix, and uterus can metastasize to the vagina by direct invasion (Cardenes, Roth, McGuire, & Look, 2005). The majority (70%–80%) of women who develop primary invasive vaginal cancer are postmenopausal and older than 60 years of age (Eifel, 2005). Studies suggest that 10%–50% of women diagnosed with vaginal cancer had previously undergone hysterectomy for cervical carcinoma (Cardenes et al., 2005; Creasman, 2005). It has been suggested that with the cervix absent, the vagina is at risk for developing vaginal intraepithelial neoplasia (VAIN), a preinvasive dysplastic condition that can lead to invasive vaginal disease. It is believed that the risk develops because of a *field effect* (Cardenes et al.; Creasman) among the vulva, vagina, and cervix because each of these structures is lined with squamous epithelium. Field effect also is called *field defect* and *field cancerization* and explains "the development of multiple primary tumors within the same organ and locally recurrent cancer" (Giovannucci & Ogino, 2005, p. 1317). VAIN can develop many years later in women who previously have been treated for cervical or vulvar cancers. Rarely, an abnormal cervical Pap smear result will reveal no cervical lesions, and further evaluation finds the primary lesions to be within the vagina.

Because of the rarity of VAIN and invasive vaginal cancer, research regarding management is limited to retrospective reviews. Thus, treatment options vary and depend on factors such as women's age, general medical condition, and stage of disease at diagnosis.

Treatments may include local excision or radical surgery, RT, or a combination of both. However, the usual treatment of this rare cancer is RT (Grigsby, 2002). Chemotherapy does not have a curative role in the treatment of advanced vaginal cancer, and no standard regimens are available (NCI, 2008). However, the use of chemotherapy as a radiosensitizer has shown a benefit in the treatment of cervical cancer in randomized trials; thus, investigators have suggested that women with vaginal cancer who have high-risk features for recurrent disease would likely benefit from concurrent chemotherapy and radiation (Dalrymple et al., 2004; Frank, Jhingran, Levenback, & Eifel, 2005).

Squamous cell carcinomas and adenocarcinomas account for 85% and 15% respectively of the histologic types seen in vaginal cancer. A small percentage includes very rare types such as melanomas and sarcomas (Creasman, 2005).

Women with this rare type of gynecologic malignancy should be referred to and treated by a gynecologic oncologist and a radiation oncologist, preferably at a comprehensive cancer center where providers have the most experience.

Anatomy and Natural History

The vagina is a tubular structure that averages 7.5 cm in length. It extends from the vulva to the uterine cervix and lies posterior to the bladder and anterior to the rectum. The vaginal mucosa is lined with squamous epithelium. Beneath the mucosa is a double muscularis layer that is highly vascular and innervated and has a complex system of lymphatic drainage (Cardenes et al., 2005). The lymphatics of the upper two-thirds of the vagina drain to the pelvic, obturator, hypogastric, and external iliac nodes. The lower third of the vagina drains to the inguinal and femoral nodes (Benedet et al., 2000; Creasman, 2005).

The distribution of lymphatic drainage leaves the pelvic and bilateral groin nodes at risk for metastatic disease. Beyond stage I disease, there is significant risk for metastatic nodal involvement (Creasman, 2005). Additionally, the location of the lesion within the vagina, the upper two-thirds versus the lower third, will affect treatment decisions and outcome. Fifty-seven to 85% of primary lesions occur in the upper third of the vagina, usually in the posterior wall. Approximately 31% of lesions develop in the lower third of the vagina. Lesions in the middle third are uncommon (Creasman).

Incidence and Risk Factors

ACS (2008c) estimated 2,210 new cases of vaginal cancer with 760 deaths in 2008. Vaginal cancer is one of the rarest of human cancers and accounts for only 0.1%–0.2% of all human cancers (Creasman, Phillips, & Menck, 1998). The majority of women diagnosed with vaginal cancer are 60–70 years old. According to the National Cancer Data Base (NCDB), squamous cell type (85%) is more common in older women, and adenocarcinoma (15%) occurs more commonly in women age 20 years or less (Creasman, 1998; NCI, 2008).

Thirty percent of women with primary vaginal cancer have a history of an in situ or invasive cervical cancer treated at least five years earlier (Aho, Vesterinen, Meyer, Purola, & Paavonen, 1991). Fifty to 66% of women diagnosed with VAIN have a prior history of a cervical or vulvar cancer (Creasman, 2005). Thus, a prior history of a lower genital tract cancer is a risk factor for developing a vaginal primary.

The exact cause of primary vaginal cancer is not known. However, because the predominant cell type is squamous, it is assumed that one of the risk factors may be HPV, similar to that of cervical cancer (Benedet et al., 2000).

Clinical Presentation

Most women with preinvasive or small volume disease are asymptomatic. However, the most common symptom is irregular bleeding or vaginal discharge. Tjalma et al. (2001) reported that 62% of the women presented with vaginal discharge, 16% had no symptoms but positive cytology, 13% had a tumor mass, 4% had pain, and 2% had dysuria. Some reports identify urinary symptoms more commonly because of the proximity of the anterior vaginal wall to the neck of the bladder (Creasman, 2005).

Diagnosis

Because secondary malignancies of the vagina are much more common than primary vaginal cancers, the diagnosis of vaginal cancer will depend on the involvement of disease to either the cervix or vulva. As per FIGO guidelines, if disease is present on the cervix, the diagnosis will be a cervical primary, and if disease is on the vulva, it will be considered a vulvar primary cancer (Benedet et al., 2000; Cardenes et al., 2005). In addition, a primary vaginal cancer should not be considered if the patient has a history of invasive cervical cancer within the past five years (Cardenes et al.). This emphasizes the importance of careful tissue sampling and histologic verification when making this diagnosis.

In most cases, the diagnosis starts with an abnormal Pap smear in women who are having routine vaginal cytologic examinations after prior hysterectomy. The area most commonly involved is the upper vagina. ACS recommends that routine vaginal surveillance cytology for women who have had a hysterectomy be limited to those who had a history of cervical intraepithelial neoplasia or invasive cervical cancer. The reasoning for this is that the incidence of developing VAIN after a hysterectomy for a benign condition is very low (Benedet et al., 2000; Cardenes et al., 2005; Creasman, 2005). However, the ACS guidelines remain controversial (Creasman et al., 1998).

The diagnosis requires a comprehensive history, physical, and complete pelvic examination. The pelvic examination should include a speculum examination, digital palpation including bimanual and rectovaginal examination, cytologic evaluation, and biopsy if possible (Cardenes et al., 2005). If the cervix is present, it should be biopsied to rule out a cervical primary. In women who have had prior hysterectomy, acetic acid can be applied to the entire vaginal vault to evaluate for areas appropriate for colposcopic sampling (Cardenes et al). Postmenopausal women who commonly have vaginal atrophy may benefit from the use of local estrogen cream used once or twice a week for a month to prepare the lining of the vaginal epithelium for optimal visualization prior to further evaluation (Cardenes et al.). Acetic acid can be used to identify areas of the vagina that should be biopsied, as the suspicious areas will appear as white epithelium after the acetic acid is applied (Cardenes et al.).

Suspicious lesions are raised, white, well-defined areas visualized through the colposcope, and some may be gross lesions directly visualized by the examiner. Most lesions involve the upper vagina, but some "skip lesions" can be present at another area of the vagina (Creasman, 2005). Examination under anesthesia can be considered for thorough evaluation and sampling, especially if the woman is having symptomatic pain (Cardenes et al., 2005).

Other routine diagnostic tests are a complete blood count and serum biochemical analysis including liver function tests. Chest radiograph and abdominal and pelvic computed tomography (CT) may be used to evaluate for extent of disease and pelvic, inguinal, and femoral nodal involvement. However, CT and magnetic resonance imaging are not used for the staging of vaginal cancer according to the FIGO guidelines (Chang, 2002).

Staging and Survival Rates

Primary vaginal cancer, like cervical cancer, is clinically staged. Staging is defined by FIGO and the American Joint Committee on Cancer's TNM classification (see Appendix).

According to the NCDB study (Creasman et al., 1998), most women have invasive disease at the time of diagnosis and staging. Only 25% are staged with carcinoma in situ or VAIN, and these women were younger than those with invasive disease. Survival rates correlate with the stage of disease at the time of diagnosis. NCDB reported five-year survival rates as follows (Creasman et al.).

- Stage 0—96%
- Stage I—73%
- Stage II—58%
- Stages III and IV—36%

Histology

The most common histologic type seen in primary vaginal cancer is SCC. The precursor to invasive vaginal cancer is VAIN. These are atypical cells of the squamous epithelium, which lines the vagina. VAIN is graded I–III depending on the degree of nuclear atypia, crowding, and the proportion of epithelium involved (Cardenes et al., 2005). VAIN I involves the lower one-third to one-half of the epithelium; VAIN II involves one-half to two-thirds thickness of the epithelium; VAIN III involves more than three-quarters the thickness of the epithelium; and carcinoma in situ (CIS) involves the full thickness of the epithelium (Cardenes et al.). The progression of high-grade VAIN to invasive cancer is in the range of 10%–20% (Graham, Wright, Cadwallader, Reed, & Symonds, 2007). Aho, Vesterinen, Meyer, Purola, and Paavonen (1991) followed the course of 23 patients who were untreated over 3–15 years and found a spontaneous regression rate of 78%.

Several authors (Benedet et al., 2000; Cardenes et al., 2005; Creasman et al., 1998) have reported on the various histologic types of vaginal cancer and corresponding patient characteristics. Table 11-4 identifies histologic types with reported characteristics.

Treatment

Because of the rarity of vaginal cancer, no gold-standard treatment is available. Treatment for all stages of vaginal cancer can be individualized based on factors such as medical condition of the patient, extent of disease location of tumor within the vagina, clinical stage, operator experience, referral center experience, and patient choice (Graham et al., 2007; Indermaur, Martino, Florica, Roberts, & Hoffman, 2005; Tjalma et al., 2001). Treatment recommendations and choices for patients differ for preinvasive and invasive disease. A multitude of treatment modalities are available that can be used for preinvasive disease. The goals of treatment for VAIN are to eradicate the lesions, prevent the development of invasive disease, prevent severe toxicity, and preserve the function of the vagina (Benedet et al., 2000; Indermaur et al.; Tjalma et al., 2001). The goals of treatment for invasive disease are to eradicate the disease, prevent local spread, avoid radical change in body image, and preserve anatomy and function of the vagina and nearby anatomy and organs such as the bladder and rectum (Grigsby, 2002).

Preinvasive Disease

VAIN is considered a very uncommon clinical entity, and the treatment of it remains controversial. Although multiple approaches are available to treat VAIN, the provider should consider the number of lesions, location of lesions, previous radiation therapy, and previous treatment for VAIN (Indermaur et al., 2005).

The number of lesions is important, as the distribution of vaginal dysplasia or in situ lesions often is multifocal. This type of distribution may preclude focal interventions such as cryotherapy or local excision (Graham et al., 2007). Treatments that can cover the entire length of the vagina are better suited for diffuse lesions and include carbon dioxide laser vaporization, topical 5-fluorouracil, and intracavitary brachytherapy (Dodge, Eltabbakh, Mount, Walker, & Morgan, 2001; Graham et al., 2007; Indermaur et al., 2005).

Approximately 50%–90% of the lesions will occur in the upper vagina (Cardenes et al., 2005; Creasman, 2005; Graham et al., 2007; Indermaur et al., 2005). Lesions in the upper vagina can be treated surgically by performing an upper vaginectomy. Although no one treatment option for VAIN has proved superior, a surgical approach allows for detailed

Table 11-4. Histologic Types of Vaginal Cancer and Patient and Tumor Characteristics

Cell type	Percent of Primary Vaginal Cancer	Risk Factor(s)	Average Age	Most Likely Location
Squamous	80%–90%	CIN, HPV	60–70	Upper, posterior vagina
Clear cell adenocarcinoma	Rare	In utero exposure to DES, vaginal adenosis	19	Upper third vagina
Melanoma	2.8%–5%	Almost all cases occur in white women.	66	Lower third and anterior vaginal wall
Sarcomas	3%	Prior pelvic RT	Diverse	Deep within vaginal wall

CIN—cervical intraepithelial neoplasia; DES—diethylstilbestrol; HPV—human papillomavirus

Note. Based on information from Benedet et al., 2000; Cardenes et al., 2005.

tissue diagnosis and in some cases can reveal occult invasive disease. Indermauer et al. found a 12% prevalence of occult invasive cancer in their retrospective review of 105 patients who had undergone upper vaginectomy. Hoffman et al. (1992) reported a 28% prevalence of occult invasive cancer in a similar retrospective review.

A woman's history of pelvic radiation will affect treatment decisions. If the woman has undergone whole pelvic radiation for cervical cancer, further radiation to the vaginal area may have limited benefit. Prior treatment for VAIN may necessitate a change to a different approach that previously has not been used. Table 11-5 lists various treatment options for VAIN.

Invasive Disease and Surgical Approaches

Surgical approaches for invasive disease mostly have been replaced with RT. Because of the proximity of the vagina to the bladder and the rectum, surgical techniques tend to be radical with some requiring urinary and fecal diversion to obtain clear margins (Tewari et al., 2001). In addition, most women who are diagnosed with vaginal cancer are older adults and may have increased risks of morbidities associated with a radical surgical procedure. However, for early-stage disease (stages I and II), the literature supports surgical approaches, and improved five-year survival rates are reported (Tjalma et al., 2001).

In a retrospective study, Tjalma et al. (2001) compared the survival rates of women who underwent surgery, varying from local excision to exenteration with or without adjuvant radiotherapy versus women who received only brachytherapy and/or external beam RT (EBRT) to the whole pelvis. These findings were compared to all other publications within the past 20 years. Tjalma et al. concluded that the overall five-year survival for women with stages I and II disease who received surgery followed by selective radiotherapy showed modest improvement versus women who received radiotherapy alone ($p = 0.003$). The five-year survival rates were 92% for surgery alone, 71% for surgery plus RT, and 44% for radiation alone. NCDB reported similar five-year survival rates for women who received surgery with or without RT versus women who received RT alone (Creasman et al., 1998). Therefore, although RT is more commonly used to treat vaginal cancer, surgery with curative intent has a role for use in early-stage disease and improved five-year survival rates. Table 11-6 lists the types of surgical approaches that can be used based on FIGO stage of disease for invasive vaginal cancer.

Pelvic exenteration can be performed with a curative intent in a few very select cases. The disease must be central and nonmetastatic (Cardenes et al., 2005). Patients should have a good performance status and be carefully screened for emotional and physical deficits because it is a radical surgery resulting in major alterations of body image (see Chapter 12).

Invasive Disease and Radiation Therapy

RT for the treatment of vaginal cancer was first described in 1929 at the Barnard Free Skin and Cancer Clinic in Boston, where only 2 of 18 patients survived more than five years (Tewari et al., 2001). Today the outcomes have improved along with the science of radiobiology and newer methods of treatment. The different types of RT used in the treatment of vaginal cancer include brachytherapy and EBRT.

Brachytherapy is internal radiation as opposed to external beam radiation (Bradley & Petereit, 2006). Intracavitary brachytherapy utilizes a vaginal cylinder in which the radiation source is placed (Frank et al., 2005). Interstitial brachytherapy utilizes radiation loaded needles placed directly into the tumor (Frank et al.). Depending on the type of brachytherapy used, the treatments can be delivered in either the inpatient or outpatient setting (Kushner et al., 2003).

Historically, low-dose brachytherapy has been used, but high-dose treatment is being used more frequently because the dose amount can be delivered over a shorter period of time and safely in the outpatient setting (Bradley & Petereit, 2006).

EBRT utilizes high-energy linear accelerators to generate electron beams like an x-ray, only in much higher doses (Frank

Table 11-5. Treatment Options for Vaginal Intraepithelial Neoplasia

Treatment	Number of Lesions	Location of Lesions	Rate of Recurrence
Local excision	Single, well defined	Upper or lower one-third of vagina	Low
Upper vaginectomy	–	Upper third of vagina	Cure rate 88% (Dodge et al., 2001; Indermaur et al., 2005)
Loop excision	Multiple abnormal cervical cells	Vaginal apex	Low (Fanning et al., 2000; Indermaur et al., 2005)
Laser CO_2 vaporization	Multiple focal lesions	Lower third of vagina	25–50% (von Gruenigen et al., 2007)
Topical 5-fluorouracil	Multiple	Cervix	59% (Dodge et al., 2001)
Medium dose intracavitary radiation	–	Upper vagina	16% (Graham et al., 2007)

et al., 2005). Both EBRT and brachytherapy are important treatment modalities for vaginal cancer.

Controversy exists regarding the use of RT for stage 1 disease. Bradley and Petereit (2006) recommend brachytherapy alone as the reported local control rates (80%–100%) are the same (78%–100%) for women who underwent external pelvic radiation. Tewari et al. (2001) recommend EBRT and brachytherapy for early-stage disease only if the tumor is poorly differentiated or for patients with greater tumor infiltration thus, posing a greater risk for lymph node metastasis.

Women with stages II and III disease appear to have improved pelvic tumor control with a combination of EBRT and brachytherapy as opposed to EBRT alone (Bradley & Petereit, 2006; Frank et al., 2005; Perez, Grigsby, Garipagaoglu, Mutch, & Lockett, 1999). However, brachytherapy should be individualized to the characteristics of the tumor (Bradley & Petereit; Frank et al.; Perez et al.). Tewari et al. (2001) recommended interstitial brachytherapy, which employs a template and needles that implant directly into the tumor for tumors greater than 0.5 cm in thickness or if tumors are located in the distal portion or at the apex of the vagina to more optimally expose the radiation source to the tumor. Tewari et al. use the following two algorithms to stress the point of achieving local control.

- Local failure→pelvic failure→distant failure→death from disease
- Local control→pelvic control→distant control→survival

Stage IV disease usually is treated with EBRT alone with a palliative intent. The incidence of distant metastasis with stage IV disease is 47% with five-year survival rates of 36%–46% (Cardenes et al., 2005; Creasman, 2005; Creasman et al.,1998).

Radiotherapy and surgical treatment options by stage are presented in Table 11-7.

Table 11-6. Surgical Treatment Options for Invasive Vaginal Cancer by Stage of Disease

FIGO Stage	Surgical Treatment
I	Partial or total vaginectomy Radical hysterectomy/vaginectomy, + pelvic node, +/– para-aortic node dissection; inguinal node dissection for lower third of vaginal lesions
II / III	Partial or total vaginectomy + parametrectomy + paracolpectomy + pelvic node, +/– para-aortic node dissection Radical hysterectomy/vaginectomy, + parametrectomy + pelvic/inguinal node, +/– para-aortic node dissection
IV	Exenterative surgery, usually total, with formation of urinary and bowel bypasses

Note. From "The Role of Surgery in Invasive Squamous Carcinoma of the Vagina," by W.A.A. Tjalma, J.M. Monaghan, A. de Barros Lopes, R. Naik, A.J. Nordin, and J.J. Weyler, 2001, *Gynecologic Oncology, 81*(3), p. 363. Copyright 2001 by Elsevier. Reprinted with permission.

Chemotherapy

Chemotherapy as a radiosensitizer has been studied extensively in locally advanced cervical cancer and advanced vulvar cancer (Cardenes et al., 2005; Eifel et al., 2005). In this setting, the cisplatin given with radiation has shown superior results when compared to patients who received radiotherapy alone (Eifel et al., 2004). Concurrent chemotherapy and RT has become the mainstay of treatment for locally advanced cervical cancer (see Chapter 5) and advanced vulvar cancer. Because of the rarity of vaginal cancer, prospective trials have not been conducted; given the similarities in histology and natural history of the other

Table 11-7. Surgical and Radiation Treatment Options by Stage of Disease

Stage	Radiation	Surgery
I (lesion < 0.5 cm)	Intracavitary, 6,000–7,000 cGy over 5–7 days. External beam for lesions of the lower third of the vagina delivered to the pelvic and/or inguinal lymph nodes (LNs) at total dose of 4,500–5,000 cGy.	Wide local excision or total vaginectomy with reconstruction. (Adjuvant radiation if margins are close or positive.)
I (lesion > 0.5cm)	Combination interstitial and intracavitary, 7,500 cGy to primary tumor. External beam for poorly differentiated or infiltrating lesions with high probability of LN metastasis. Elective external beam delivered to pelvic and/or inguinal LNs at dose of 4,500 cGy for lesions in lower third of vagina	Radical vaginectomy and pelvic lymphadenectomy for lesions in the upper one third of vagina. Inguinal lymphadenectomy for lesions in the lower third of vagina. Construction of neovagina if feasible. (Adjuvant radiation if margins close or positive.)
II	Combination brachytherapy and external beam for a total dose of 7,000–8,000 cGy to primary tumor. Elective external beam for lesions in lower third of vagina delivered to pelvic and/or inguinal LNs at dose of 4,500–5,000 cGy.	Radical vaginectomy or pelvic exenteration with or without radiation therapy.
III	External beam radiation including pelvic nodes over 5–6 weeks followed by interstitial and/or intracavitary implant for a total dose 7,500–8,500 and a doses of 5,500–6,000 cGy to the lateral pelvic walls.	Surgery rare but may be combined with radiation.
IVA	Combination of external beam and interstitial and intracavitary radiation.	Surgery rare but may be combined with radiation.
IVB	Radiation for palliation of symptoms with or without chemotherapy.	

Note. From "Vaginal Cancer Treatment (PDQ®)" [Health professional version], by National Cancer Institute, 2008. Retrieved May 26, 2009, from http://www.cancer.gov/cancertopics/pdq/treatment/vaginal/HealthProfessional

lower genital tract cancers, oncologists may endorse the use of concurrent chemoradiation to achieve better local control in vaginal cancer (Dalrymple et al., 2004; Tewari et al., 2001).

Recurrent Disease

The majority of women who develop recurrent disease will recur locally within the vagina and regionally within the pelvis. The median time to recurrence is 6–12 months (Cardenes et al., 2005). Not surprisingly, the highest recurrence rates are for women who were originally diagnosed with locally advanced disease (stages III and IV). About 50%–70% of these women will have persistent or recurrent disease in the pelvis despite prior initial treatment with whole pelvic radiation and brachytherapy (Cardenes et al.). The local regional failure rate for stage I patients is 10%–20% and is 30%–40% for stage II (Cardenes et al.). As illustrated with a previous algorithm, pelvic failure leads to distant failure that leads to death. This is the pattern of spread with recurrent disease, and generally, the prognosis is very poor.

Some women however, may have a small local recurrence and no evidence of metastatic disease; these women have a potential for cure. If the woman has not received prior EBRT, treatment with whole pelvic RT is an option. On the other hand, if she has received prior EBRT and has only a central recurrence with no other metastasis, she would be a candidate for exenterative surgery.

Response rates to chemotherapy are low especially when treating central recurrences in a previously radiated field. In addition, toxicities such as pancytopenia can be more pronounced because the pelvic bone marrow, in which blood cells originate, has been previously exposed to high-dose radiation. Chemotherapy is used to treat disease recurrence as salvage therapy and for palliation of symptoms. For some chemosensitive women, acceptable palliative response is seen, particularly when lesions occur in distant areas that have not been exposed to prior treatment. Some of the agents used include cisplatin, 5-FU, and mitomycin C, as well as combinations such as methotrexate, vinblastine, doxorubicin, and cisplatin (Cardenes et al., 2005).

Summary

Vaginal and vulvar cancers primarily affect postmenopausal women. Both have good cure rates if detected early. However, there are obstacles to early detection and diagnosis. Forty percent of women with vulvar cancer are diagnosed at a late stage because of delay in seeking medical attention. Additionally, providers may prescribe inappropriate topical therapies without proper exam and biopsy to confirm the diagnosis. Primary vaginal cancer is exceedingly rare and usually occurs in women who have previously undergone hysterectomy for cervical cancer. The diagnosis of primary vaginal cancer is difficult, as most vaginal malignancies are secondary. Additionally, patients with small-volume disease are usually asymptomatic. Most vaginal cancers are invasive at the time of diagnosis. It is important for postmenopausal women to continue to receive routine gynecologic exams for screening. Although no specific screenings are recommended for vaginal or vulvar cancer, ACS has recommendations for cervical cancer screening. Educating women in the 60–70 year age group about these recommendations may encourage them to continue gynecologic care. The current ACS (2008a) *Guidelines for Early Detection of Cancer* recommends for women age 30–70 to receive Pap smear screening every two to three years providing they have had a history of prior normal Pap smears. Women age 70 and older who have had three normal Pap smears in a row and no abnormal pap smears in the past 10 years can elect to discontinue screening. Women age 70 and older with a history of cervical cancer should continue screening as long as they are in good health. The ACS recommends that routine vaginal surveillance cytology be limited to women who have had a hysterectomy secondary to cervical cancer and not for women who have had hysterectomy for benign reasons; however, that guideline is not universally accepted.

Although vaginal and vulvar cancers are rare, they remain important female diseases to prevent as each can have a significant impact on a woman's self-image and sexuality. Thankfully, advances in conservative surgical management and radiation oncology have improved survival and reduced radical changes in body image.

References

Aho, M., Vesterinen, E., Meyer, B., Purola, E., & Paavonen, J. (1991). Natural history of vaginal intraepithelial neoplasia. *Cancer, 68*(1), 195–197.

American Cancer Society. (2008a). *American Cancer Society guidelines for the early detection of cancer.* Retrieved May 26, 2009, from http://www.cancer.org/docroot/ped/content/ped_2_3x_acs_cancer_detection_guidelines_36.asp

American Cancer Society. (2008b). *Cancer facts and figures, 2008.* Retrieved May 6, 2008, from http://www.cancer.org/downloads/STT/2008CAFFfinalsecured.pdf

American Cancer Society. (2008c). *What are the key statistics about vaginal cancer?* Retrieved April 28, 2008, from http://www.cancer.org/docroot/CRI/content/CRI_2_4_1X_What_are_the_key_statistics_for_vaginal_cancer_55.asp

AshrafGanjooie, T. (2004). Case report of liposarcoma. *Journal of Obstetrics and Gynecology, 30*(2) 80–83.

Barnes, E.A., & Thomas, G. (2006). Integrating radiation into the management of vulvar cancer. *Seminars in Radiation Oncology, 16*(3), 168–176.

Benedet, J.L., Bender, H., Jones, H., 3rd., Ngan, H.Y., & Pecorelli, S. (2000). FIGO staging classifications and clinical practice guidelines in the management of gynecologic cancers. *International Journal of Gynecology and Obstetrics, 70*(2), 209–262.

Bradley, K.A., & Petereit, D.G. (2006). Radiation therapy for gynecologic malignancies. *Hematology/Oncology Clinics of North America, 20*(20), 347–361.

Cardenes, H.R., Roth, L.M., McGuire, W.P., & Look, K.Y. (2005). Vagina. In W.J. Hoskins, R.C. Young, M. Markman, C.A. Perez, R. Barakat, & M. Randall (Eds.), *Principles and practice of gynecologic oncology* (pp. 707–742). Philadelphia: Lippincott Williams & Wilkins.

Chang, S.D. (2002). Imaging of the vagina and vulva. *Radiologic Clinics of North America. 40*(3), 637–658.

Creasman, W.T. (2005). Vaginal cancers. *Current Opinion in Obstetrics and Gynecology, 17*(1), 71–76.

Creasman, W.T., Phillips, J.L., & Menck, H.R. (1998). The National Cancer data base report on cancer of the vagina. *Cancer, 83*(5), 1033–1040.

Dalrymple, J.L., Russell, A.H., Lee, S.W., Scudder, A., Leiserowitz, G.S., Kinney, W.K., et al. (2004). Chemoradiation for primary invasive squamous carcinoma of the vagina. *International Journal of Gynecological Cancer, 14*(1), 110–117.

de Hullu, J.A., Oonk, M.H.M., & Van der Zee, A. (2004). Modern management of vulvar cancer. *Current Opinion in Obstetrics and Gynecology, 16*(1), 65–72.

Dodge, J.A., Iltabbakh, G.H., Mount, S.L., Walker, R.P., & Morgan, A. (2001). Clinical features and risk of recurrence among patients with vaginal intraepithelial neoplasia. *Gynecologic Oncology, 83*(2), 363–369.

Eifel, P.J., Berek, J.S., & Markman, M.A. (2005). Cancer of the cervix, vagina, and vulva. In V.T. DeVita, S. Hellman, & S.A. Rosenberg (Eds.), *Cancer: Principles and practice of oncology* (5th ed., pp. 1295–1341). Philadelphia: Lippincott Williams & Wilkins.

Eifel, P.J., Winter, K., Morris, M., Levenback, C., Grisby, P.W., Copper, J., et al. (2004). Pelvic irradiation with concurrent chemotherapy versus pelvic and para-aortic irradiation for high-risk cervical cancer: An update of Radiation Therapy Oncology Group trail (RTOG) 90-01. *Journal of Clinical Oncology, 22*(5), 872–880.

Fanning, J., Manahan, K.J, & McLean, S.A. (2000). Loop electrosurgical excision procedure for partial upper vaginectomy. *American Journal of Obstetrics and Gynecology, 181*(6), 1382–1385.

Frank, S.J., Jhingran, A., Levenback, C., & Eifel, P.J. (2005). Definitive radiation therapy for squamous cell carcinoma of the vagina. *International Journal of Radiation Oncology, Biology, Physics, 62*(1), 138–147.

Furniss, K. (2000). Tomatoes, Pap smears, and tea? Adopting behaviors that may prevent reproductive cancers and improve health. *Journal of Obstetrics, Gynecology, and Neonatal Nursing, 29*(6), 641–652.

Gadducci, A., Cionini, L., Romanini, A., Fanucchi, A., & Genazzani, A.R. (2006). Old and new perspectives in the management of high-risk, locally advanced or recurrent, and metastatic vulvar cancer. *Critical Reviews in Oncology/Hematology, 60*(3), 227–241.

Gerszten, K., Selvaraj, R.N., Kelley, J., & Faul, C. (2005). Preoperative chemoradiation for locally advanced carcinoma of the vulva. *Gynecologic Oncology, 99*(3), 640–644.

Giovannucci, E., & Ogino, S. (2005). DNA methylation, field effects, and colorectal cancer. *Journal of the National Cancer Institute, 97*(18), 1317–1319.

Govindan, R., & Arquette, M.A. (Eds.). (2002). *Washington manual of oncology*. Philadelphia: Lippincott Williams & Wilkins.

Graham, K., Wright, K., Cadwallader, B., Reed, N.S., & Symonds, R.P. (2007). 20-year retrospective review of medium dose rate brachytherapy in VAIN3. *Gynecologic Oncology, 106*(1), 105–111.

Grigsby, P.W. (2002). Vaginal cancer. *Current Treatment Options in Oncology, 3*(2), 125–130.

Hacker, N.F. (2000). Vulvar cancer. In J.S. Berek & N.F. Hacker (Eds.), *Practical Gynecologic Oncology* (4th ed., pp. 543–583). Philadelphia: Lippincott Williams & Wilkins.

Heaps, J.M., Fu, Y.S., Montz, F.J., Hacker, N.F., & Berek, J.S. (1990). Surgical variables predictive of local recurrence in squamous cell carcinoma of the vulva. *Gynecologic Oncology, 38*(3), 309–314.

Hoffman, M.S., DeCesare, S.L., Roberts, W.S., Fiorca, J.V., Finan, M.A., & Cavanagh, D. (1992). Upper vaginectomy for in situ and occult, superficially invasive carcinoma of the vagina. *American Journal of Obstetrics and Gynecology, 166*(1, Pt. 1), 30–33.

Homesley, H.D., Bundy, B.N., Sedlis, A., & Adcock, L. (1986). Radiation therapy versus pelvic node resection for carcinoma of the vulva with positive groin nodes. *Obstetrics and Gynecology, 68*(6), 733–740.

Indermaur, M.D., Martino, M.A., Fiorica, J.V., Roberts, W.S., & Hoffman, M.S. (2005). Upper vaginectomy for the treatment of vaginal intraepithelial neoplasia. *American Journal of Obstetrics and Gynecology, 193*(2), 577–581.

Jones, R.W., Rowan, D.M., & Stewart, A.W. (2005). Vulvar intraepithelial neoplasia: Aspects of the natural history and outcome in 405 women. *Obstetrics and Gynecology, 106*(6), 1319–1326.

Jones, R.W., Sadler, L., Grant, S., Whineray, J., Exeter, M., & Rowan, D. (2005). Clinically identifying women with vulvar lichen sclerosus at increased risk of squamous cell carcinoma. *Obstetrical and Gynecological Survey, 60*(2), 98–99.

Joura, E.A., Losch, A., Haider-Angeler, M.G., Breitenecker, G., & Leodolter S. (2000). Trends in vulvar neoplasia. Increasing incidence of vulvar intraepithelial and squamous cell carcinoma of the vulva in young women. *Journal of Reproductive Medicine. 45*(8), 613–615.

Kushner, D.M., Fleming, P.A., Kennedy, A.W., Wilkinson, D.A., Lee, E., & Saffle, P.A. (2003). High dose rate (192)lr afterloading brachytherapy for cancer of the vagina. *British Journal of Radiology, 76*(910), 719–725.

Landrum, L.M., Skaggs, V., Gould, N., Walker, J.L., & McMeekin, S.D. (2008). Comparison of outcome measures in patients with advanced squamous cell carcinoma of the vulva treated with surgery or primary chemoradiation. *Gynecologic Oncology, 108*(3), 584–590.

Moore, D.H., Koh, W., McGuire, W.P., & Wilkinson, E.J. (2005). Vulva. In W.J. Hoskins, C.A. Perez, R.C. Young, R.R. Barakat, M. Markman, & M.E. Randall (Eds.), *Principles and practice of gynecologic oncology* (4th ed., pp. 665–706). Philadelphia: Lippincott Williams & Wilkins.

Moore, D.H., Thomas, G.M., Montana, G.S., Saxer, A., Gallup, D.G., & Olt, G. (1998). Preoperative chemoradiation for advanced vulvar cancer: A phase II study of the Gynecologic Oncology Group. *International Journal of Radiation Oncology, Biology, Physics, 42*(1), 79–85.

National Cancer Institute. (2008, May 22). *Vaginal cancer treatment (PDQ®)*. Retrieved May 24, 2009, from http://www.cancer.gov/cancertopics/pdq/treatment/vaginal/HealthProfessional

Naziri, Z., & Omranipour, R. (2006). Unusual location of vulvar basal cell carcinoma. *Journal of Lower Genital Track, 10*(4), 242–244.

Perez, C.A., Grigsby, P.W., Garipagaoglu, M., Mutch, D.G., & Lockett, M.A. (1999). Factors affecting long-term outcome of irradiation in carcinoma of the vagina. *International Journal of Radiation Oncology Biology Physics, 44*(1), 37–45.

Salom, E.M., & Penalver, M. (2002). Recurrent vulvar cancer. *Current Treatment Options in Oncology, 3*(1), 143–153.

Smith, Y.R., & Haefner, H.K. (2004). Vulvar lichen sclerosus pathophysiology and treatment. *American Journal of Dermatology, 5*(2),105–125.

Spinelli, A. (2000). Preinvasive diseases of the cervix, vulva, and vagina. In G.J. Moore-Higgs, L.A. Almadrones, B. Colvin-Huff, L.M. Gossfeld, & J. Huang Erickson (Eds.), *Women and cancer* (pp. 50–81). Sudbury, MA: Jones and Bartlett.

Stehman, F.B., & Look, K.Y. (2006). Carcinoma of the vulva. *Obstetrics and Gynecology, 107*(3), 719–733.

Sugiyama, V. E., Chan, J. K., Shin, J.Y., Berek, J.S., Osann, K., Kapp, D.S. (2007). Vulvar melanoma: A multivariable analysis of 644 patients. *Obstetrics and Gynecology 110*(2, Pt. 1), 296–301.

Tewari, K.S., Cappuccini, F., Puthawala, A.A., Kuo, J.V., Burger, R.A., Monk, B.J., et al. (2001). Primary invasive carcinoma of the vagina treatment with interstitial brachytherapy. *Cancer, 91*(4), 758–770.

Tjalma, W.A.A., Monaghan, J.M., de Barros Lopes, A., Naik, R., Nordin, A.J., & Weyler, J.J. (2001). The role of surgery in invasive squamous carcinoma of the vagina. *Gynecologic Oncology, 81*(3), 360–365.

Tyring, S. (2003). Vulvar squamous cell carcinoma: Guidelines for early diagnosis and treatment. *American Journal of Obstetrics and Gynecology, 189*(Suppl. 3), S17–S23.

van der Avoort, I.A., Shirango, H., Hoevenaars, B.M., Grefte, J.M., de Hullu, J.A., de Wilde, P.C., et al. (2006). Vulvar squamous cell carcinoma is a multifactorial disease following two separate and independent pathways. *International Journal of Gynecological Pathology, 25*(1), 22–29.

Van der Zee, A.G.J., Oonk, M.H., de Hullu, J.A., Ansink, A.C., Vergote, I., Verheijen, R.H., et al. (2008). Sentinel node dissection is safe in the treatment of early stage vulvar cancer. *Journal of Clinical Oncology, 26*(6), 884–889.

Weikel, W., Schmidt, M., Steiner, E., Knapstein, P.G., & Koeble, H. (2006). Surgical therapy of recurrent vulvar cancer. *American Journal of Obstetrics and Gynecology, 195*(5), 1293–1302.

CHAPTER 12

Pelvic Exenteration and Reconstruction

Altagracia (Grace) I. Mota, RN, MSN, OCN®, and Nasrin Vaziri-Kermani, RN, CPSN

Introduction

Cancers arising in the pelvis often are treated with multimodality therapies, including surgical resection and radiation. When these cancers recur, many may be locally advanced but limited to the pelvis. Prior treatment with high doses of radiation makes limited surgical resection difficult and may result in multiple complications. In some instances, the only opportunity for cure may lie with a complete resection (Juretzka, Husain, & Teng, 2006).

Brunschwig (1948) first introduced pelvic exenteration surgery for cervical cancer. Goldberg et al. (2006) reported that initially pelvic exenteration was utilized for the palliative management of advanced and recurrent cancer, but it has evolved into a curative intervention for advanced and recurrent gynecologic cancers confined to the central pelvis. Currently, potential candidates include women with cervical cancer, endometrial cancer, ovarian cancer, and other rarer pelvic neoplasms (Lambrou, Pearson, & Averette, 2005). This procedure evolved from a purely exenterative one to one that includes a reconstructive phase. This phase, according to Goldberg et al., has assumed even greater importance in recent years with refinements in urinary diversion, colon-sparing surgery, preservation of the anal sphincter, and vaginal and pelvic floor reconstruction. Disaia and Creasman (1997) stated that extensive experience with pelvic reconstruction has accumulated, and the surgical techniques and patient selection have steadily improved; therefore, this procedure has attained an important role in the treatment of gynecologic malignancy. Although pelvic exenterative surgery was initially severely criticized, it is now accepted as a respectable procedure that offers life to selected patients when no other possibility of cure exists. The criticism of this exenterative procedure has lessened because mortality and morbidity have steadily improved, and a gratifying five-year survival rate has been achieved (Disaia & Creasman, 1997). As explained by Juretzka et al. (2006, p. 3), "Since Brunschwig's time, improvements in critical care, antibiotics, hyperalimentation, thromboembolism prophylaxis, accompanied by similar advances in surgical technique, including the use of stapling devices, separate urinary conduits, and pelvic reconstruction have improved the morbidity and mortality rates associated with this procedure. Currently, operative mortality rates are 3%–5%, the major perioperative complication rate is 30%–44%, and the overall five-year survival rate in patients who successfully undergo the procedure is 20%–50%." Appropriate patient selection is vital. Metastasis outside the pelvis, found preoperatively or discovered at laparotomy, is an absolute contraindication to pelvic exenteration. In addition to metastasis, the triad of unilateral leg edema, sciatic pain, and ureteral obstruction is classic of unresectable disease in the pelvis (Disaia & Creasman, 1997; Lambrou et al., 2005) (see Figure 12-1).

A thorough clinical assessment must be performed to avoid denying a potentially curable patient a chance of

Figure 12-1. Indications and Contraindications for Pelvic Exenteration

Indications
- Local advanced cervical cancer
- Cancer of vulva invading the rectum
- Centrally recurrent cervical, vaginal, or endometrial cancer after radiation therapy
- Ovarian cancer
- Need for more radiation therapy

Contraindications
- Simpler options available
- Distant metastasis
- Serious cardiopulmonary disease
- Pelvic bone invasion
- Tumor invasion of major vessels
- Intraperitoneal disease
- Ipsilateral leg edema, sciatic pain

Note. Based on information from Disaia & Creasman, 1997; Lambrou et al., 2005; Larrison & Cloutier, 2004.

survival and to prevent inappropriate surgery on an unsuitable patient. Preoperatively, the patient's medical or comorbid conditions are evaluated to ensure a candidate can withstand the rigors of a lengthy surgery, anesthesia, and the extended rehabilitation time required. Diagnostic evaluations include but are not limited to chest x-ray, computed tomography of abdomen and pelvis, magnetic resonance imaging to evaluate liver and kidney function, and a bone scan to rule out bone metastasis. A psychological consult as part of a preoperative evaluation is standard management or at least highly advisable. This surgery may result in an ileal conduit and/or colostomy and vaginal and vulval disfigurement. The patient must be emotionally and psychologically able to cope with these changes and have a good network of support.

Exenterative Surgery

The normal pelvic structure (Figure 12-2) is altered during this exenterative surgery. Total pelvic exenteration combines several major procedures: radical hysterectomy with dissection of lymph nodes and bilateral salpingo-oophorectomy, total cystectomy, and abdominal perineal resection of the rectum. A colostomy and urinary conduit are created, and vaginal reconstruction may or may not be performed (Figure 12-3). In selected cases the procedure may be limited to anterior exenteration with removal of the bladder and preservation of the rectosigmoid (Figure 12-4) or posterior exenteration with removal of the rectosigmoid and preservation of the bladder (Figure 12-5) (Disaia & Creasman, 1997).

Figure 12-2. Normal Pelvis

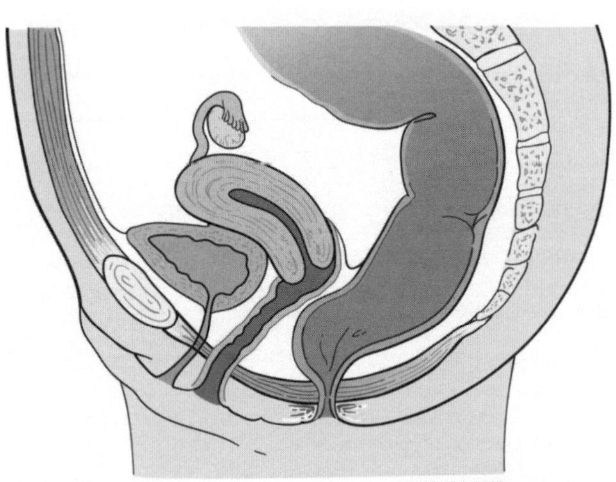

Note. Illustration courtesy of Memorial Sloan-Kettering Cancer Center. Used with permission.

The choice of anterior or posterior exenteration versus total pelvic exenteration is made based on well-defined criteria. Surgeons rely on well-defined criteria to determine whether a procedure will be an anterior, posterior, or total pelvic exenteration. Estape and Angioli (1999) emphasized that although an exenteration is the last available option for salvage therapy, the surgeon should strive to achieve negative margins, even if that means extremely radical surgery. The location of the tumor determines the type of exenteration that will be performed. Tumors confined to the vesicovaginal space require an anterior exenteration, and tumors in the rectovaginal space require a posterior exenteration. A total pelvic exenteration should be done if the tumor is found to extend superiorly or laterally to the vesico- and rectovaginal spaces (Estape & Angioli). These cancers should be treated and surgeries performed by a gynecologic oncologist who has been trained in this surgical technique and the postoperative management of these patients (Gynecologic Cancer Foundation, 2008). Lambrou et al. (2005) described a pelvic exenteration, aside from radical hysterectomy, as perhaps the most defining surgical procedure for practicing gynecologic oncologists. The surgical skill and anatomic knowledge required to complete this procedure safely and successfully are a tribute to the teachings of the predecessors of the subspecialty of gynecologic oncology (Lambrou et al.).

Vaginal and Pelvic Reconstruction

These extensive surgical resections often leave the patient with a large physical defect in the pelvic, perineal, and vaginal region. These defects require pelvic reconstruction or complex closure at the time of the exenteration or at a later date. Primary closure is not possible because of the size of the surgical defects, as well as potential poor healing caused by preoperative, intraoperative, or postoperative radiotherapy. Specialized reconstructive procedures can be performed to correct the pelvic surgical defect (Cordeiro, Pusic, & Disa, 2002). The goals of reconstruction are

- To eliminate the pelvic dead space
- To prevent herniation of abdominal contents by restoring the pelvic floor
- To promote rapid wound healing, which in turn will allow for an early start of adjuvant therapy
- To reconstruct the vagina if surgically possible or desired by patient.

According to Cordeiro et al. (2002), the vagina is a distensible cylindrical pouch, with the opening as the introitus. The anterior vaginal wall is in close proximity to the urethra and bladder, the lateral wall of the vagina is adjacent to pelvic musculature and pelvic side walls, and the posterior of the vagina is in close relation to the rectum. Depending on the structures resected and type of vaginal defect, the requirement of the reconstruction will differ (Cordeiro et

Figure 12-3. Total Exenteration

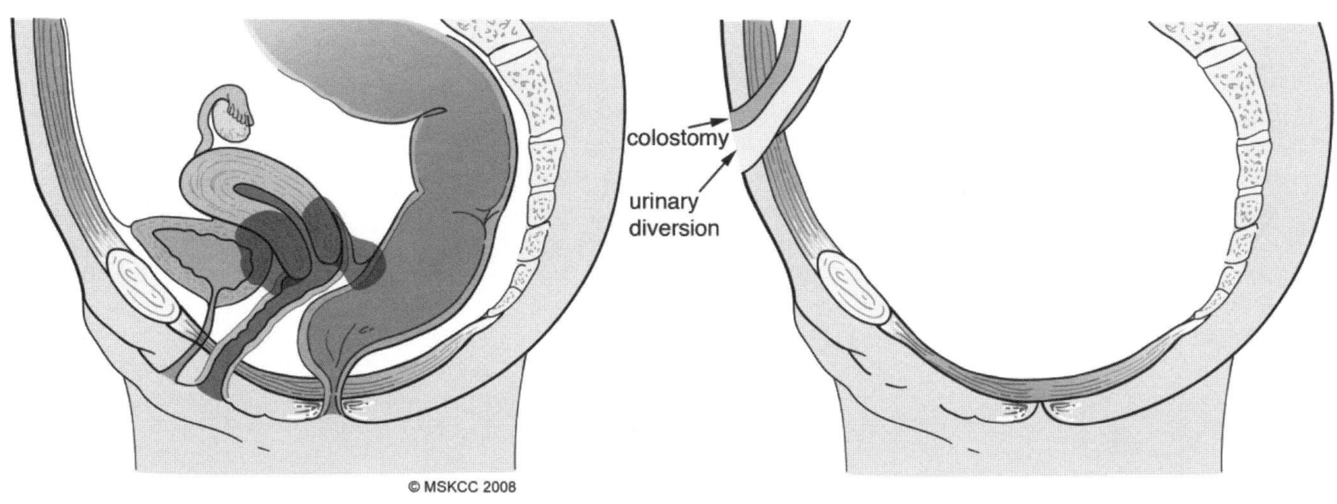

Note. Illustration courtesy of Memorial Sloan-Kettering Cancer Center. Used with permission.

Figure 12-4. Anterior Exenteration

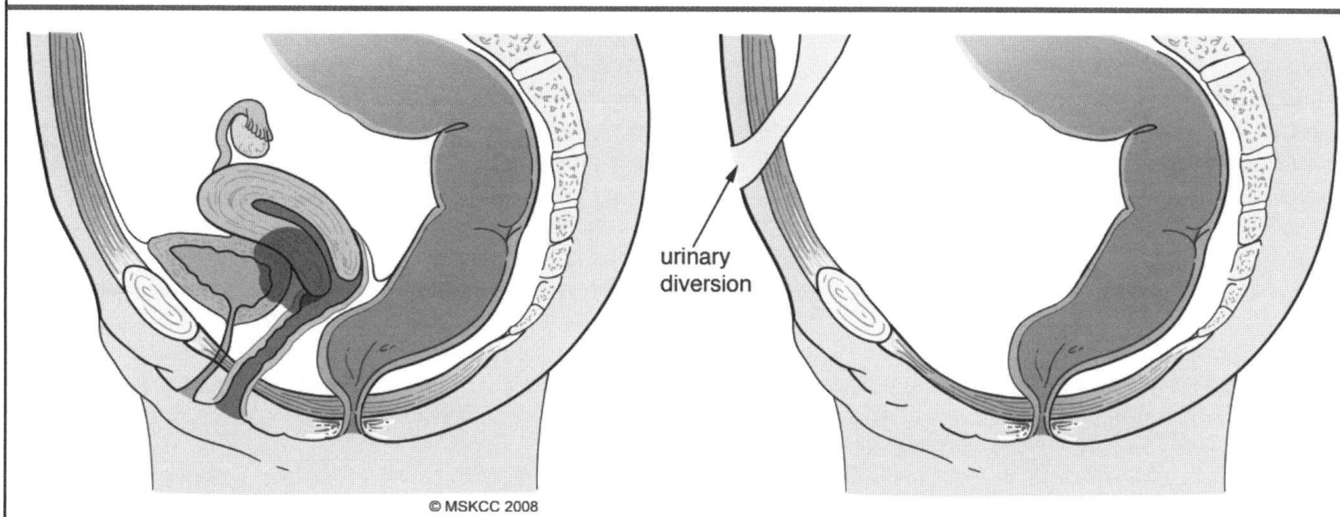

Note. Illustration courtesy of Memorial Sloan-Kettering Cancer Center. Used with permission.

al.). Successful reconstruction of vaginal defects results from careful evaluation of the specific defect. These vaginal defects may be classified based on their anatomic location (Figure 12-6).

The two basic types of defects are partial (type I) and circumferential defects (type II). These can be further subclassified into type IA, IB, IIA and IIB (Pusic & Mehrara, 2006). IA (partial) is characterized by the anterior or lateral wall involvement, as seen in urinary tract or primary vaginal malignancies. IB (partial) is characterized by posterior vaginal wall involvement, which usually results from extension of colorectal carcinomas (most common defects). IIA (circumferential) involves two-thirds of the vagina, resulting primarily from uterine and cervical disease. IIB (circumferential) is typified by total involvement of the vagina (Pusic & Mehrara).

To assist with decision making, a reconstructive algorithm (Figure 12-6) was developed based on defect type (Pusic & Mehrara, 2006). Three pedicle flaps can be used to successfully reconstruct the majority of defects: the modified Singapore flap (or pudendal thigh), the rectus abdominis myocutaneous (RAM) flap, and the gracilis flap.

Figure 12-5. Posterior Exenteration

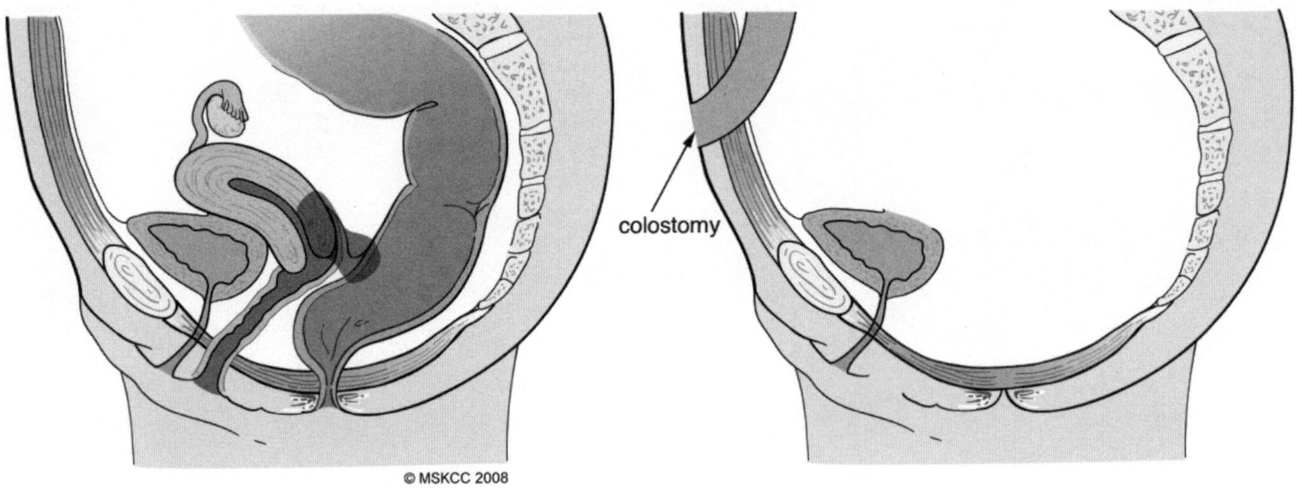

Note. Illustration courtesy of Memorial Sloan-Kettering Cancer Center. Used with permission.

Modified Singapore Flap (Pudendal Thigh Flap)

As Cordeiro et al. (2002, p. 1062) explained, "Type IA defects involve the anterior and lateral walls of the vagina and tend to be limited by the close proximity of the pelvic and side walls and pubic symphysis. These are small to moderate surface area/small volume defects." Bilateral modified Singapore flaps (Figure 12-7) can be used to reconstruct half the circumference or more of the vaginal cylinder. The flap is quite reliable even in the post-irradiated setting and involves primary closure of bilateral groin donor sites (Cordeiro et al.).

In an attempt to decrease the rate of wound complications after an abdominoperineal resection, surgeons have developed the technique of myocutaneous flap coverage of the perineum. Myocutaneous flap reconstruction achieves perineal closure with well-vascularized, nonirradiated tissue and fills the pelvic dead space with bulky, healthy tissue, thus improving wound healing and decreasing infection rates (Chessin et al., 2005).

Rectus Abdominis Myocutaneous Flap

Type IB defects involve the posterior vaginal wall requiring greater soft tissue bulk to close dead space created by resection of the rectum. Pusic and Mehrara (2006) stated that the RAM flap is ideal in this situation.

The advantages of the RAM flap include a wide arc of rotation based on the consistent inferior epigastric artery pedicle, large tissue bulk, consistent viability, minimal donor site morbidity, and the relative ease and speed with which the flap can be raised (see Figure 12-8). The RAM flap can be used to reconstruct the vagina and to decrease the periurethral fibrosis and contraction associated with anorectal resection (Chessin et al., 2005).

Gracilis Flap

Type IIB defects are circumferential defects involving the entire vagina and frequently the introitus. Given the need for a large skin island, bilateral gracilis flaps are an excellent reconstructive choice. The subcutaneous tissue and muscle of the two conjoined flaps will also provide a large volume of soft tissue that completely fills the pelvis. Here, the flaps are rotated, tunneled into the perineum, sutured together, and inset to form the vaginal pouch (see Figure 12-9) (Cordeiro et al., 2002). The location of the gracilis pedicle can sometimes limit the rotation of the flap (see Figure 12-9, a and b). The gracilis is a minor leg adductor, and transposition will not result in functional disability (Vermaas et al., 2005).

Complications of Pelvic Exenteration and Reconstruction

Teran-Porcayo, Zeichner-Gancz, Gomez del Castillo, Beltrán Ortega, and Solorza-Luna (2006) reported that pelvic exenteration continues to be a morbid procedure in spite of advances in perioperative care, surgical techniques, and better patient selection. Their study reported a complication rate as high as of 52.5%, which they said compares to reports published by other institutions. The dilemma faced by gynecologic oncologists is the unpredictable healing capacity of irradiated tissue and the balance of the increased risk of complications versus the potential gain in patient comfort with complex reconstructive techniques (Hockel & Dornhofer, 2006). The usual postoperative complications include infection, blood loss, and respiratory problems. After an exenteration (see Figure 12-10), additional

Figure 12-6. Classification of Acquired Vaginal Defect and Reconstruction Algorithm for Acquired Vaginal Defects

Shaded area of cones delineate area of vaginal defect.

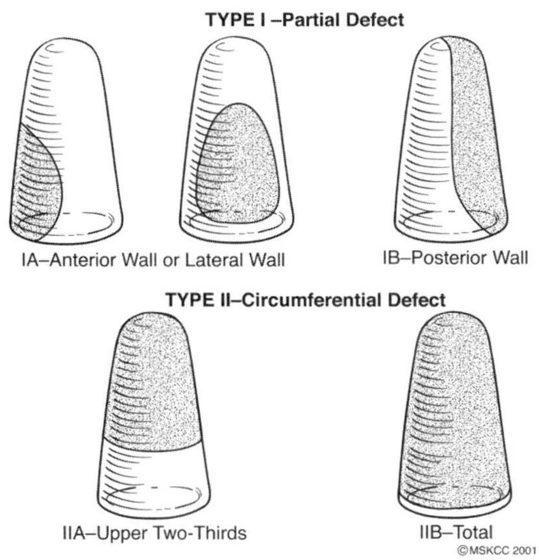

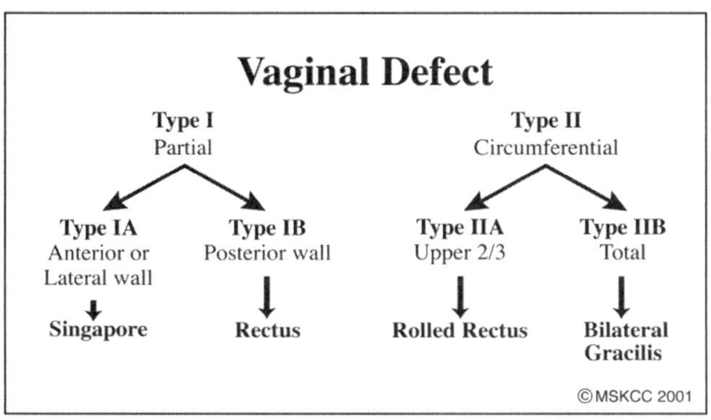

Note. Illustration courtesy of Memorial Sloan-Kettering Cancer Center. Used with permission.

complications are possible, including wound breakdown, fistulas, deep vein thrombosis (DVT), intestinal obstructions, anastomotic breakdown or leak, ureteral stricture, pyelonephritis, flap failure, and flap necrosis (Larrison & Cloutier, 2004).

Psychosocial Impact of Pelvic Exenteration

Patients' psychosocial issues must be given importance in the rehabilitative process of pelvic exenteration. Patients and families are overwhelmed by the emotional impact of the cancer diagnosis or news of recurrence. The list of patients' real and exaggerated as well as current and potential concerns is lengthy (Hampton, 1986).The radical nature of pelvic exenteration places these women at high risk for body-image disturbances, as well as self-esteem and abandonment issues. Lamont, De Petrillo, and Sargent (1978) reported that the patient's reaction to cancer may result in anxiety because of the patient's association with pain and mutilation. The patient often feels damaged or crippled by her physical loss and often suffers guilt, shame, and self-disgust in anticipation that her partner will also see her this way. Carter et al. (2004) reported that the literature supports the view that consequences of this radical surgery affect not only the integrity of the body but the emotional, functional, social, and sexual aspects of the individuals. Patients report feelings of depression, anxieties about sexual desirability, fear, and embarrassment (Carter et al.).

Krebs (2006) reported that sexual and reproductive function is affected by all aspects of cancer, which result in changes in body appearance, fertility, and ability to have sexual intercourse. Krebs supports early assessment and intervention and identified models such as the PLISSIT, ALARM, and BETTER methods of sexual assessment to aid the nurse and multidisciplinary team. Patient and family education is needed, and it is essential to include information on the impact of the disease and therapy on sexual and reproductive functioning. Alternative sexual options need to be discussed, in addition to side effect management, including lubrication, dilators, and management of hot flashes. Supportive services information should also be available.

Carter et al. (2004) reported on results of 6 of 11 women retrospectively identified and interviewed with a history of gynecologic cancer and pelvic exenteration. Seven themes emerged from the interviews.

- Concerns about recovery (length of time needed to recover, feelings of depression/despair, and loss of independence)
- Complications (feelings of unpreparedness for complications, such as the need for physical therapy, abscesses, and infections)
- Ostomies (concerns regarding appearances, postoperative support)
- Social support (reported as a critical need, relating to fatigue/emotional support, transportation)
- Sexuality (Three patients opted not to have vaginal reconstruction because they did not feel it was necessary and because of the longer surgical time. Three had reconstruction; one was unable to use neovagina successfully; two were unwilling to attempt to use neovagina; and only one patient out of the six reported any sexual interest or activity.)
- Disclosure (not wanting to reveal bodily changes with others, fear of rejection, embarrassment)
- Fear of recurrence (no treatment options, issues of death and dying)

Nurses and the multidisciplinary team must address early preoperative and postoperative assessments and rec-

Figure 12-7. The Modified Singapore Flap (Pudendal Flap)

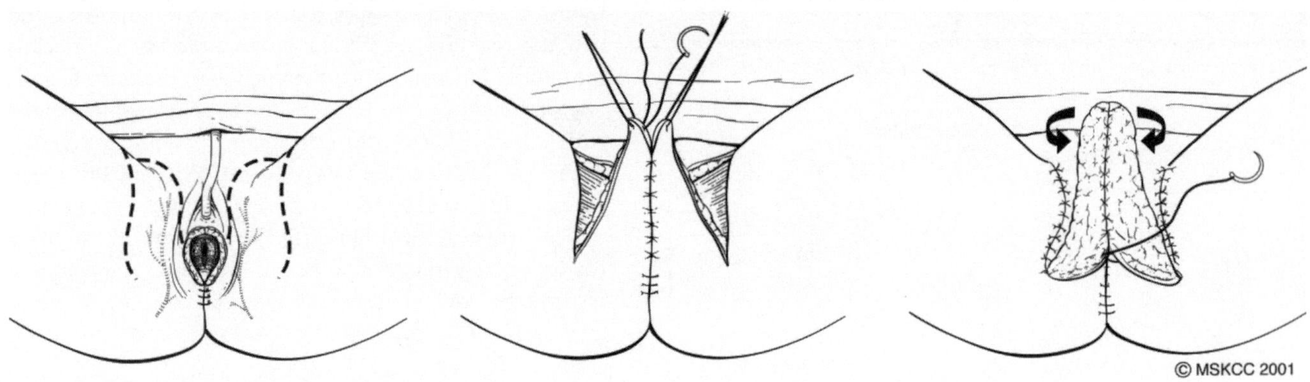

Use of bilateral Singapore flaps for reconstruction of a vaginal defect. The flaps are sewn together in the midline. Here, you see primary closure of donor sites within the bilateral groin creases.

Note. Illustration courtesy of Memorial Sloan-Kettering Cancer Center. Used with permission.

Figure 12-8. Rectus Abdominal Flap

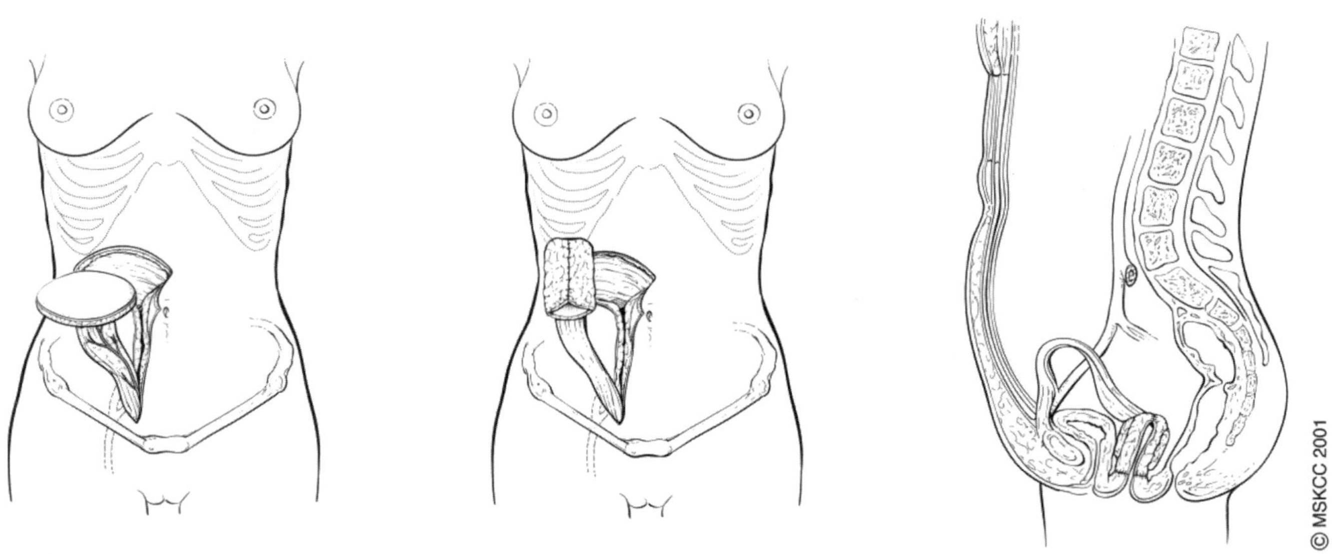

Rectus abdominis myocutaneous (RAM) flap is elevated, the RAM flap is designed into a new vagina (skin in the inside), and RAM flap is rotated down to fill the perineal defect.

Note. Illustration courtesy of Memorial Sloan-Kettering Cancer Center. Used with permission.

ognize potential problems. Care relating to these psychosocial needs must be implemented immediately. Patients undergoing these complicated procedures require extensive preoperative and postoperative education and support. Oncology nurses play an essential role in helping patients and families to cope with the diagnosis, understand implications of surgery, and identify needs upon discharge home.

Nursing Care

Preoperative

The nursing care of patients undergoing pelvic exenteration is a tremendous challenge that places heavy demands on all healthcare providers. Because of its extensive nature,

Figure 12-9. Vaginal Reconstruction With Gracilis Flap

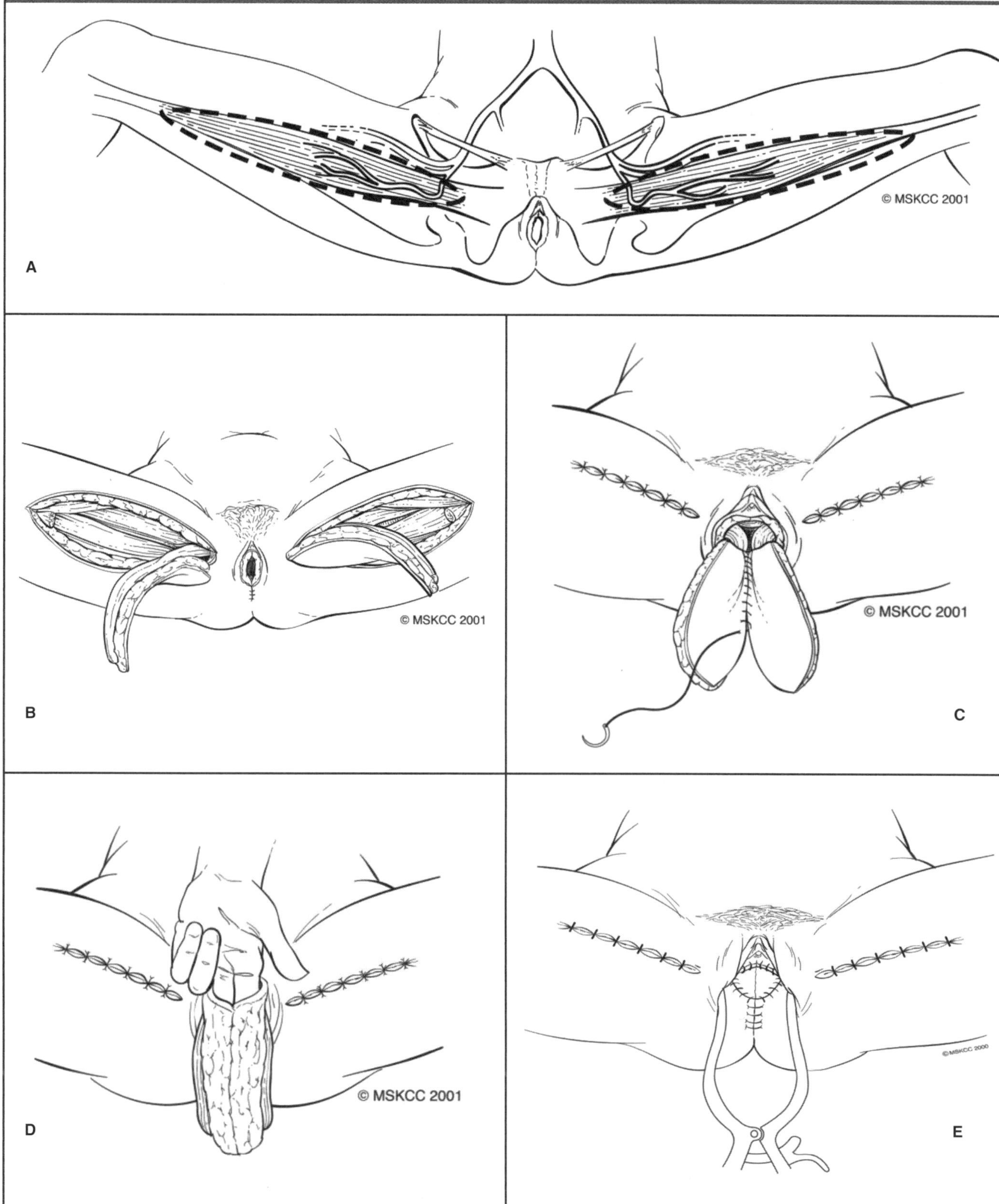

Note. Illustration courtesy of Memorial Sloan-Kettering Cancer Center. Used with permission.

Figure 12-10. Complications of Pelvic Exenteration With Pelvic and Vaginal Reconstruction

General Complications
- Fluid imbalances
- Deep vein thrombosis
- Stoma complications (e.g., retraction, necrosis)
- Ileus/bowel obstruction
- Prolapse of small intestine
- Sepsis
- Fistulas (gastrointestinal or genitourinary)
- Urinary tract infections
- Delayed healing at surgical, donor, or reconstructed sites
- Anastomotic leaks

Donor Site Complications
- Infected Gore-Tex® (W.L. Gore and Associates, Inc.) patch
- Incision line separation
- Tension on incision line
- Abdominal hernia if rectus is used
- Bleeding or seroma
- Functional loss (early postoperative)

Reconstructed Site Complications
- Fat necrosis
- Partial or total flap loss
- Size issues (flap too bulky)
- Vaginal stenosis
- Shortening of the vagina
- Vulvar pain
- Vaginal discharge
- Loss of coital function

Note. Based on information from Goldberg et al., 2006; Lambrou et al., 2005; Salom & Penalver, 2003.

the procedure itself is almost incomprehensible to patients and their significant others during the preoperative period (Ruth-Sahd & Zulkosky, 1999). Holistic nursing care requires respect and dedication from a multidisciplinary healthcare team that recognizes that extensive preoperative counseling and teaching are often the keys to successful recovery (see Figure 12-11).

A psychosocial and self-care assessment is of the utmost importance prior to surgery. This assessment can be achieved through a collaborative interdisciplinary approach from physicians, nurses, psychiatry, social work, case management, patient, and family. This includes ability of patient to manage self-care needs at home, need for visiting nurse services, long-term needs, education from enterostomal nurse regarding the challenges of managing bowel and urinary diversions, and psychological issues such as body image and relationship issues (including sexuality) (Carter et al., 2004; Corney, Everett, Howells, & Crowther, 1992; Krebs, 2006; Larrison & Cloutier, 2004).

Early preoperative and family education is also very important in facilitating the patient and family understanding of this extensive procedure. Preoperative education should

Figure 12-11. Preoperative Recommended Consults

- Gynecologic surgeon
- Genitourinary surgeon
- Colorectal surgeon
- Plastic and reconstructive surgeon
- Cardiac and pulmonary consults
- Nursing
- Social work
- Oncologists
- Psychiatry
- Enterostomy therapist
- Radiologist
- Rehabilitation consult
- Case management

Note. Based on information from Carter et al., 2004; Corney et al., 1992, Gurganus & Morris, 1991; Krebs, 2006; Larrison & Cloutier, 2004.

be thorough and understood by the patient and significant others. Education should entail review of extent of procedure to be performed, reconstructive options, and temporary and permanent changes to body structure and function (see Figures 12-12 and 12-13), including reproductive and sexual function. Other topics to discuss are dietary restrictions and bowel prep regimens, potential intesive-care unit admission, postoperative pulmonary toileting, pain management, and need for physical therapy (Larrison & Cloutier, 2004).

Postoperative

Postoperative nursing care consists of management of potential disorders relating to multiple systems. Potential cardiac complications relate to fluid and electrolyte imbalances and DVTs. Nurses should expect generalized edema postoperatively, including lower extremity edema. Patients are at high risk for DVTs caused by prolonged surgery (8–14 hours) and immobility. Nursing assessment and action plan should include monitoring patients closely for fluid imbalances via central venous pressure readings, strict intake and output, and daily weights. Early ambulation, anticoagulant therapy, and compression devices are essential for DVT prevention (Larrison & Cloutier, 2004).

Patients' respiratory status must be closely monitored as they are at high risk for respiratory complications, such as atelectasis, fluid overload, pulmonary embolus, pneumonia, and hypoxemia. Nurses need to encourage aggressive pulmonary toileting and pulse oximetry monitoring. Prophylactic antibiotics may also be administered (Larrison & Cloutier, 2004).

Gastrointestinal complications may be related to postoperative ileus and bowel obstruction or complications from bowel resection with posterior or total exenteration. These complications can be anastomotic leaks, fistula formations, and ostomy complications. Patients will have a nasogastric

Figure 12-12. Immediately Postoperative: Abdominal Dressing, Colostomy, Urinary Diversion, Multiple Wound Drains at Incision and Donor Reconstruction Sites

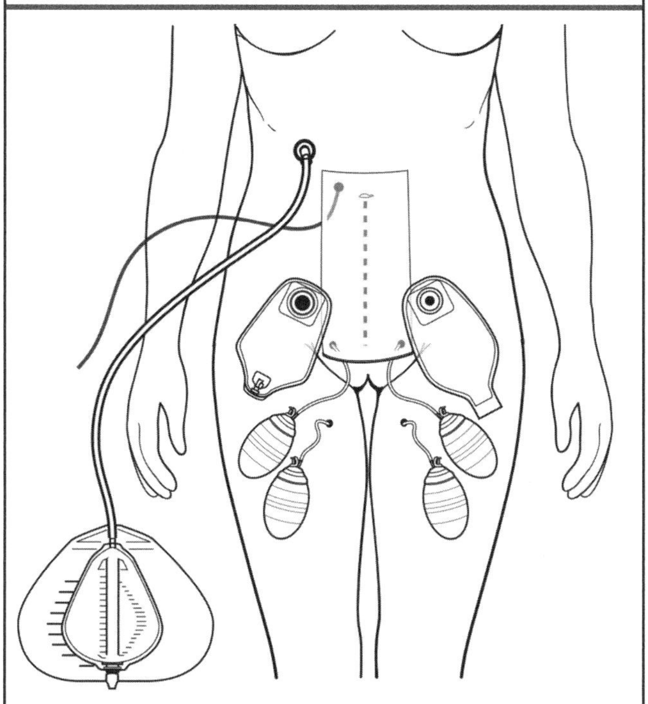

Note. Illustration courtesy of Memorial Sloan-Kettering Cancer Center. Used with permission.

Figure 12-13. Later in the Postoperative Phase: Colostomy and Urinary Diversion

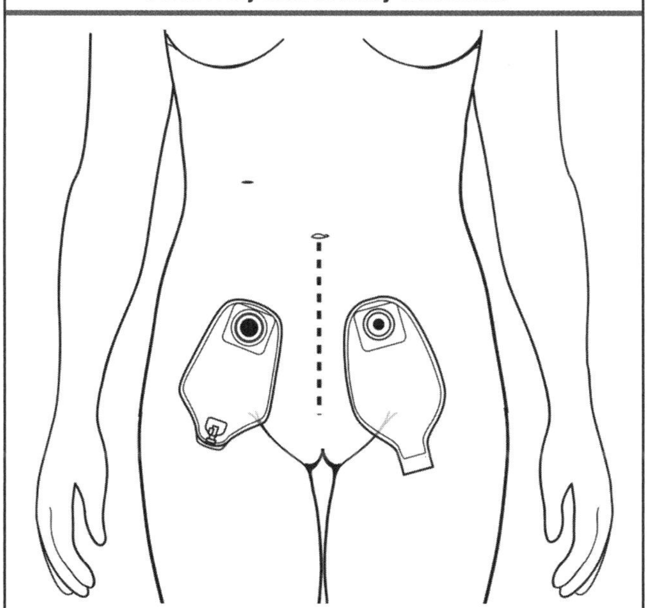

Note. Illustration courtesy of Memorial Sloan-Kettering Cancer Center. Used with permission.

tube in place and possible extended NPO (nothing by mouth) status. (Nurses should refer to their specific institution's protocol.) Nurses must monitor for return of bowel function or signs and symptoms of ileus such as distention, absent or tympanic bowel sounds or symptoms of obstruction such as distention, high-pitched bowel sounds, and cramping pain. Anastomotic leaks may present as abdominal pain, firmness, and localized tenderness. The patient may experience fecal drainage from the vagina or surgical incision indicating presence of fistula.

Nurses must monitor colostomy stoma for healing and viability. Stomal complications may include stenosis, mucocutaneous separation, retraction, prolapse, and necrosis. The stoma should be beefy red; any signs of graying or "dusky" color is a sign that stoma is not surviving. In addition, the stoma should lie above cutaneous level and be patent for easy passage of stool (Larrison & Cloutier, 2004).

In anterior or total exenteration, the presence of continent (neobladder formed from bowel) or incontinent (ileal conduit) urinary diversions requires nursing assessment of urinary functional status and potential complications, which can include low urine output immediately following surgery that may indicate third spacing or urinary obstruction. Nursing interventions also include stoma management and education. An enterostomal/wound ostomy care nurse (if available) may be consulted preoperatively for education and stomal site marking and postoperatively for continued education on skin, appliance, and ostomy care (see Figure 12-14) (Carter et al., 2004; Larrison & Cloutier, 2004).

With all pelvic and vaginal reconstructive methods, the care of the flap is very important. Nurses must routinely assess the flap for signs and symptoms of bleeding, such as new swelling or increased size or if it feels hard to the touch. Flap color should be assessed frequently; it should be pink with capillary refill of five to six seconds. Flap should blanch with gentle pressure; mottling and/or cyanosis may indicate a hematoma. When repositioning, direct pressure on the flap should be avoided, and it is recommended that patients do not sit or lie on flap for the first three postoperative weeks. The sutures are usually removed 21 days after surgery if the patient has had prior radiation therapy or on day 15 if no prior radiation.

Summary

Pelvic exenteration offers a select group of women a chance for cure or palliation. Availability of new reconstructive surgical procedures and advancement in colon and urinary diversion techniques has made it possible to offer new hope and better quality of life to patients with the diagnosis of pelvic malignancies. As part of a multidisciplinary team, nurses play a vital role in helping this patient population to meet the numerous physical, psychological, and educational challenges of pelvic exenteration and reconstruction.

Figure 12-14. Teaching Ostomy Care

Ileal Conduit
- Pouch emptying
- Pouch removal and disposal
- Peristomal skin care
- Pouch preparation
- Pouch application
- Night drainage bag
- Procurement of pouches and supplies
- Dietary issues

Continent Urostomy
- Care of red rubber catheter in stoma
- Care of Malecot catheter draining bladder
- Care of urinary stents
- Local care and pouching
- Self-catheterization

Colostomy
- Pouch emptying
- Pouch removal and disposal
- Peristomal skin care
- Pouch preparation
- Pouch application
- Procurement of pouches and supplies
- Dietary Issues
- Odor control
- Irrigation

Note. Based on information from Gurganus & Morris, 1991; Larrison & Cloutier, 2004.

References

Brunschwig, A. (1948). Complete excision of the pelvic viscera for abdominal carcinoma: A one-stage abdominoperineal operation with end colostomy and bilateral ureteral implantation in the colon above the colostomy. *Cancer, 1*(2), 177–183.

Carter, J., Chi, D., Abu-Rustum, N., Brown, C.L., McCreath, W., & Barakat, R. (2003). Brief report: Total pelvic exenteration—A retrospective clinical needs assessment. *Psycho-Oncology, 13*(2), 125–131.

Chessin, D.B., Hartley, J., Cohen, A.M., Mazumdar, M., Cordeiro, P., Disa, J., et al. (2005). Rectus flap reconstruction decreases perineal wound complications after pelvic chemoradiation and surgery: A cohort study. *Annals of Surgical Oncology, 12*(2), 104–110.

Cordeiro, P.G., Pusic, A.L., & Disa J.A. (2002). A classification system and reconstructive algorithm for acquired vaginal defects. *Plastic and Reconstructive Surgery, 11*(4), 1058–1065.

Corney, R., Everett H., Howells, A., & Crowther, M. (1992). The care of patients undergoing surgery for gynecological cancer: The need for information, emotional support and counseling. *Journal of Advanced Nursing, 17*(6), 667–671.

Disaia, P.J., & Creasman, W.T. (1997). Invasive cervical cancer. In P.J. Disaia & W.T. Creasman (Eds.), *Clinical gynecologic oncology* (5th ed., pp. 93–106). St. Louis, MO: Mosby.

Estape, R., & Angioli R. (1999). Surgical management of advanced and recurrent cervical cancer. *Seminars in Surgical Oncology, 16*(3), 236–241.

Goldberg, G.L., Sukumvanic, P., Einstein, M.H., Smith, H.O., Anderson, P.S., & Fields, A.L. (2006). Total pelvic exenteration: The Albert Einstein College of Medicine/Montefiore Medical Center experience (1987 to 2003). *Gynecologic Oncology, 101*(2), 261–268.

Gurganus, E.S., & Morris, E.J. (1991). Pelvic exenteration: The challenge of rehabilitation in a patient with multiple psychological problems. *Journal of Enterostomal Therapy, 18*(2), 52–55.

Gynecologic Cancer Foundation. (2008). *State of the state of gynecologic cancers*. Retrieved May 6, 2008, from http://www.thegcf.org/sos_2007final081507.pdf.

Hampton, B.G. (1986). Nursing management of a patient following pelvic exenteration. *Seminars in Oncology Nursing, 2*(4), 281–286.

Hockel, M., & Dornhofer, N. (2006). Pelvic exenteration for gynaecological tumours: Achievement and unanswered questions. *Lancet Oncology 7*(10), 837–847.

Juretzka, M., Husain, A., & Teng, N. (2006). *Pelvic exenteration*. Retrieved on May 22, 2008, from http://www.emedicine.com/med/topic3332.htm.

Krebs, L.U. (2006).What should I say? Talking with patients about sexuality issues. *Clinical Journal of Oncology Nursing 10*(3), 313–315.

Lambrou, N.C., Pearson, J.M., & Averette, H.E. (2005). Pelvic exenteration of gynecologic malignancy: Indications, and technical and reconstructive considerations. *Surgical Oncology Clinics of North America, 14*(2), 289–300.

Lamont, J.A., De Petrillo, A.D., & Sargeant, E.J. (1978). Psychosexual rehabilitation and exenterative surgery. *Gynecologic Oncology, 6*(3), 236–242.

Larrison, E.H., & Coultier, L. (2004). Pelvic exenteration: Patient care and education. *Journal of Gynecologic Oncology Nursing 14*(2), 11–16.

Pusic, A., & Mehrara, B. (2006). Vaginal reconstruction: An algorithm approach to defect classification and flap reconstruction. *Journal of Surgical Oncology, 94*(6), 515–521.

Ruth-Sahd, L.A., & Zulkosky, K.D. (1999). Cervical cancer: Caring for patients undergoing total pelvic exenteration. *Critical Care Nurse 19*(1), 46–57.

Salom, E.M., & Penalver, M.A. (2003). Pelvic exenteration and reconstruction. *Cancer Journal, 9*(5), 415–420.

Teran-Porcayo, M.A., Zeichner-Gancz. I., Gomez del Castillo, R.A.C., Beltran Ortega, A., & Solorza-Luna, G. (2005). Pelvic exenteration for recurrent or persistent cervical cancer. *Medical Oncology, 23*(2), 219–223.

Vermaas, M., Ferenschild, F.T., Hofer, S.O., Verhoef, C., Eggermont, A.M., & de Wilt, J.H. (2005). Primary and secondary reconstruction after surgery of the irradiated pelvis using a Gracilis flap transposition. *European Journal of Surgical Oncology, 31*(9), 1000–1005.

CHAPTER 13

Acute Symptom Management

Catherine Hydzik, RN, MS, AOCN®, and Kathleen A. O'Connor, RN, BSN

Introduction

Women diagnosed with a gynecologic malignancy may be treated with one or all of the following standard interventions: surgery, chemotherapy, and radiation therapy (RT). New approaches are being researched in clinical trials sponsored by the Gynecologic Oncology Group, as well as other cooperative groups and organizations worldwide. The treatment plan is always dependent on the woman's diagnosis, stage, grade, medical history, and performance status. This chapter summarizes the potential acute effects related to the three standard treatment modalities administered to women with gynecologic cancers and the nursing management of each in care plan format.

The management of gynecologic cancers can be extremely complex, with the nursing management requiring comprehensive nursing assessment, patient and caregiver education, and interventions that are tailored to meet each individual's specific needs during the trajectory of treatment. At diagnosis, the focus of nursing care must include education regarding the disease, the immediate treatment plan, and coping strategies. Information is needed about preparation for surgery, chemotherapy, and/or RT, and the potential side effects of each. The management of potential side effects should be discussed, and written information and instructions should be given to the patient.

Because patient anxiety is high, especially at diagnosis and the initiation of a new treatment, nurses can be pivotal in providing information and education that facilitates their ability to cope and lessen anxiety. Fatigue and anxiety may be experienced by all patients regardless of the modality of treatment. Table 13-1 provides the general care plan for these ubiquitous side effects.

Surgery

The most common potential problems in postoperative patients treated for a gynecologic malignancy are (National Comprehensive Care Network [NCCN], 2009a; Smith, Lee, & Skootsky, 2005)

- Alteration in body image
- Alteration in sexuality patterns
- Possible high risk for infection
- Possible high risk for bleeding
- Possible high risk for pain
- Possible high risk for constipation
- Alteration in urinary output
- Risk for possible pulmonary embolism
- Lymphedema.

These side effects and the associated nursing management are outlined in Table 13-2.

Chemotherapy

Common agents used for the treatment of gynecologic cancers and their potential toxicities are listed in Table 13-3. These therapies are often provided in the outpatient setting. The major side effects include the following (Chu & DeVita, 2008; NCCN, 2009d, 2009e, 2009f; Polovich et al., 2009).

- Myelosuppression
- Fatigue
- Mucositis
- Constipation
- Diarrhea
- Nausea and vomiting
- Alopecia
- Alteration in electrolytes
- Potential for hypersensitivity reactions
- Cardiac toxicity
- Fluid retention

The incidence and severity of any of these side effects is largely dependent on the patient's characteristics such as diagnosis, stage, performance status, comorbidities, and individual treatment regimen (e.g., agent, dosage, schedule). The acute side effects related to chemotherapy usually occur during treatment or within a few weeks. Therefore, patient and caregiver education should first address the specific agent(s) and then the agent's potential acute side effects that may occur before the next treatment and their management. It is important that the patient knows when to call the provider to report or discuss the side effect (e.g., fever) and possible medical intervention. A follow-up phone call from the nurse, especially after the first treatment or change in treatment, may relieve anxiety and reinforce teaching. Table 13-4 summarizes the nursing management of acute side effects of chemotherapy frequently used in gynecologic treatment. Nausea and vomiting is one of the most common side effects but can be effectively managed with specific antiemetic regimens (Eilers, 2004; Epstein & Schubert, 2003; Friese, 2004; Joanna Briggs Institute for Evidence Based Nursing and Midwifery, 1998; Köstler, Hejna, Wenzel, & Zelinski, 2001; McGuire, 2003; Miller & Kearney, 2001; Multinational Association of Supportive Care in Cancer, 2006; NCCN, 2009b; National Institute of Dental and Craniofacial Research, 2008a, 2008b; Plevova, 1999; Polovich et al., 2009; Rhodes & McDaniel, 2004; Rubenstein et al., 2004; Stricker & Sullivan, 2003; Sonis et al., 2004; Tipton et al., 2007; Worthington, Clarkson, & Eden, 2007).

Table 13-1. General Symptom Management

Nursing Diagnosis/ Problem	Intervention and Rationale	Patient Education and Instruction
Anxiety related to diagnoses, treatment, or prognosis	• Assess the patient's level of understanding of the disease, treatment, and prognosis. • Provide the patient with opportunities to verbalize concerns and questions. • Provide the patient with understanding of what to expect. • Assess patient's ability to cope and effective past coping strategies. • Assess support systems. • Assess for signs and symptoms of anxiety. • Administer medications to decrease anxiety as ordered. • Monitor changes in level of anxiety. • Provide a calm, reassuring environment.	Instruct patient regarding • What to expect • Signs and symptoms of anxiety • What increases their anxiety • Strategies to minimize anxiety, including relaxation exercises, meditation, distraction • Ways to decrease environmental stimuli • When to notify a healthcare professional.
Fatigue	• Assess for fatigue. • Assess ability to perform activities of daily living. • Assess for contributing factors: pain, emotional distress, sleep disturbances, anemia, nutritional status, and comorbidities. • Screen for potential etiologic factors. • Monitor blood counts (computed blood count, hemoglobin, and hematocrit). • Treat with erythropoiesis-stimulating agents such as darbepoetin alfa or epoetin alfa as ordered. • Transfuse as ordered. • Develop an exercise program appropriate to the patient's condition. • Encourage rest as needed. • Consider physical therapy, nutrition, or psychosocial referral.	Explain the facts about blood and blood cells. Instruct the patient regarding • Signs and symptoms of fatigue • Practicing energy conservation, including setting priorities, planning and pacing activities, delegating, scheduling activity at peak energy time, napping, structured routine, and distraction • Self-administration technique for erythropoiesis-stimulating agents if appropriate • Importance of adequate intake of iron • When to notify a healthcare professional.
Alteration in bowel: constipation	• Assess patient's normal pattern. • Assess fluid and fiber intake. • Review medications used for constipation. • Consider nutrition referral. • Assess for signs and symptoms of obstruction and/or impaction (i.e., nausea/vomiting, abdominal distention, decreased bowel sounds, no passage of flatus, abdominal pain, presence of impacted stool in rectum). • If obstruction/impaction is suspected, consult with physician or nurse practitioner regarding an abdominal x-ray and management. • Implement regimen and reassess.	Explain to patient about bowel function. Establish a pattern of toileting. Teach the signs and symptoms of constipation. Encourage diet/hydration and physical activity. • Drink 2 L/day. • Encourage high fiber foods. • Exercise as tolerated. Instruct patient regarding • Use of bowel regimen and laxatives • Stool softeners • Stimulant laxatives • Saline laxatives • Bulk-forming laxatives • Medications requiring a prescription • When to notify the healthcare professional.

(Continued on next page)

Table 13-1. General Symptom Management *(Continued)*

Nursing Diagnosis/ Problem	Intervention and Rationale	Patient Education and Instruction
Alteration in bowel: diarrhea	• Assess patient's elimination pattern. • Assess frequency and amount of diarrhea. • Assess if patient is receiving concurrent chemotherapy. • Assess orthostatic blood pressure. • Assess skin and mucosal skin turgor. • Administer antidiarrheal medications as ordered. • Monitor intake and output. • Assess for signs and symptoms of dehydration. • Administer IV hydration as ordered. • Monitor weight and chemistries. • Assess patient's nutritional status. • Send stool cultures as ordered.	Instruct patient regarding • Oral intake • Eating a low residue diet • Avoiding foods that are highly sweet, highly seasoned or greasy, extreme temperature changes, and lactose-containing products and caffeine • Small, frequent meals • Keeping a food diary to monitor response • Administering antidiarrheal medications • Caring for perianal skin (i.e., sitz baths) • Administering anti-inflammatory agents such as creams or foams as ordered • Administering antispasmodic medications as needed/ordered • Gently cleansing the perianal region (after each bowel movement) with warm water, patting dry and use barrier cream • When to notify the healthcare professional.

Note. Based on information from Beck & Erickson, 2004; Brandt et al., 2005; Campbell et al., 2001; Folden et al., 2002; Hinrichs et al., 2001; Hsieh, 2005; Locke et al., 2000; Marlett et al., 2002; Muller-Lissner et al., 2005; National Cancer Institute, 2006; National Comprehensive Cancer Network, 2009c; Polovich et al., 2009; Stern & Ippoliti, 2003; Towers et al., 1994; Tramonte et al., 1997.

Table 13-2. Nursing Care for the Patient Undergoing Gynecologic Surgery

Nursing Diagnosis/ Problem	Intervention and Rationale	Patient Education and Instruction
Knowledge deficit regarding surgery	Assess patient's knowledge regarding disease and treatment options. Explain • Type of surgery/outcome • Preparation for operation • Medication and smoking history • Advance directives • Postoperative course • Side effects and potential complications • Symptom management strategies • When/where to call.	Instruct the patient regarding • A diagram or model of the female genital tract to explain the procedure • Literature on prep routine and advance directives • Deep breathing exercises • Strategies to prevent infection and manage pain • When to notify the healthcare professional.
Alteration of body image	• Acknowledge that the woman may see her body differently. • Encourage the patient to express feelings of loss, violation, and grief to begin emotional healing. • Enlist the help of the patient's partner to reassure her that she is still loved and desirable.	Instruct the patient regarding • Relearning that the body can be a source of pleasure • Use of nonsexual activities such as manicures and pedicures to reintroduce touch in a nonthreatening manner • Sensate focus exercises that can be performed with the patient's partner to reestablish intimacy.
Potential alteration in sexuality patterns	• Address the issue of sexuality with the patient and encourage communication. • Identify specific problems early and plan strategies to manage problem. • Assess understanding of sexuality and physiology. • Obtain sexual history.	Instruct the patient regarding • Vaginal dilation techniques • Use of vaginal lubricants (Water- or silicone-based lubricants that are free of dyes and perfumes are preferred.) • Strategies to manage menopause

(Continued on next page)

Table 13-2. Nursing Care for the Patient Undergoing Gynecologic Surgery *(Continued)*

Nursing Diagnosis/ Problem	Intervention and Rationale	Patient Education and Instruction
	• Explain the sexual side effects of surgery, including – Hormonal changes – Vaginal dryness – Painful intercourse – Changes in desire, arousal, and orgasm.	• Support and resources for the patient and partner, including sex therapy and literature such as the American Cancer Society booklet *Sexuality and Cancer: For the Woman Who Has Cancer and Her Partner.*
High risk for infection related to surgical procedure	• Monitor blood counts (complete blood count with differential). • Monitor for signs and symptoms of infection. • Assess skin and wound site for drainage. • Monitor vital signs • Administer antibiotics and antipyretic as ordered • Obtain blood culture and sensitivity as ordered	Explain the facts about blood and blood cells. Instruct the patient regarding • The signs and symptoms of infection • Signs of healing • Wound care • When to notify the healthcare professional.
High risk for bleeding related to surgical procedure	• Monitor blood counts (computed blood count, hemoglobin, and hematocrit). • Monitor for signs and symptoms of bleeding, including site, duration, amount, and color. • Monitor vital signs. • Institute safety precautions. • Institute thrombocytopenic precautions for a platelet count of 50,000/mm^3. • Avoid aspirin-containing agents and agents that interfere with platelet function. • Administer blood and blood products as ordered.	Explain the facts about blood and blood cells. Instruct the patient • About the signs and symptoms of bleeding • To check the surgical incision site for bleeding or drainage • On strategies to alleviate or stop the bleeding (e.g., applying pressure to the site). • About bleeding precautions if appropriate • To avoid heavy lifting • About abstinence from sexual intercourse • About when to notify the healthcare professional.
Pain	• Assess for pain. – Location – Quality – Severity using the 0 to 10 scale – Onset/duration – Association with an activity (e.g., eating) • Administer pain medications as ordered. • Use nonpharmacologic strategies. • Evaluate effectiveness of pain management plan. • Monitor for analgesic side effects and treat as needed. • If pain is not controlled well, refer to a specialist.	Explain to patient the importance of reporting pain and adhering to the pain management plan. Instruct the patient regarding • Medication • Potential side effects of medications and strategies to manage these side effects • Use of relaxation exercises/distraction techniques • When to notify the healthcare professional.
Urinary alteration	• Assess the patient's normal pattern. • Assess for bladder distention. • Monitor intake and output. • Assess for residual urine as needed.	Instruct patient to report changes in normal urination pattern.
Risk for pulmonary embolism	• Assess for risk, especially in patients with a prior history of a pulmonary embolism. • Monitor vital signs. • Assess for leg pain and signs of thrombophlebitis. • Apply antiembolic compression or devices to both lower extremities. • Assess color. • Perform active range-of-motion exercises to prevent embolism. • Ambulate as soon as possible. • Administer anticoagulants as ordered. • Auscultate breath sounds. • Assess for shortness of breath.	Instruct patient regarding • Potential risk of pulmonary embolism • Importance of wearing the antiembolic compression stockings or devices • Rationale for performing range-of-motion exercises • When to notify the healthcare professional.
Lymphedema	See Chapter 14.	–

Note. Based on information from Katz, 2007; National Comprehensive Cancer Network, 2009a; Smith et al., 2005.

Table 13-3. Chemotherapy Agents Used to Treat Gynecologic Cancers

Classification	Agent	Side Effects
Alkylating agent	Carboplatin	Myelosuppression, nausea and vomiting, hypersensitivity reactions; less renal toxicity than cisplatin
	Cisplatin	Myelosuppression, nausea and vomiting, hypomagnesemia, hypersensitivity reactions, nephrotoxicity, neurotoxicity, ototoxicity
	Cyclophosphamide	Myelosuppression, nausea and vomiting, alopecia, hemorrhagic cystitis, secondary malignancy, testicular/ovarian failure
	Ifosfamide	Myelosuppression, nausea and vomiting, alopecia, hemorrhagic cystitis, neurotoxicity
Antibiotic agent	Bleomycin	Hypersensitivity reactions; pulmonary, renal, and hepatic toxicity; photosensitivity; fever and chills
	Doxorubicin	Myelosuppression, nausea and vomiting, mucositis, alopecia, cardiac toxicity, radiation recall, red urine, photosensitivity
	Epirubicin	Myelosuppression, nausea and vomiting, mucositis, diarrhea, alopecia, radiation recall, red urine, cardiac toxicity
	Liposomal doxorubicin	Myelosuppression, nausea and vomiting, mucositis, alopecia, hand-foot syndrome, cardiac toxicity, red urine, photosensitivity
	Mitomycin	Myelosuppression, nausea and vomiting, mucositis, anorexia, alopecia, pulmonary and renal toxicity, fatigue
Antimetabolite agent	5-fluorouracil	Myelosuppression, nausea and vomiting, mucositis, diarrhea, anorexia, alopecia, darkening of veins, photosensitivity
	Gemcitabine	Myelosuppression, nausea and vomiting, mucositis, rash, flu-like symptoms
	Methotrexate	Myelosuppression, nausea and vomiting, mucositis, renal toxicity, photosensitivity, hepatic toxicity, neurotoxicity
Aromatase inhibitor	Letrozole	Myelosuppression, hot flashes, bone pain, headache, chest pain, arthralgia, dyspnea, fatigue
Epipodophyllotoxin group	Etoposide	Myelosuppression, nausea and vomiting, mucositis (at high doses), anorexia (at high doses), hypersensitivity reactions, alopecia, hypotension, secondary malignancies
Experimental agent	Bevacizumab	Diarrhea, hypertension, hemorrhage, proteinuria, congestive heart failure, leucopenia, thromboembolism, hyponatremia
Plant alkaloid	Irinotecan	Myelosuppression, diarrhea, alopecia
	Vinorelbine	Myelosuppression, nausea and vomiting, constipation, alopecia, neurotoxicity
Selective estrogen receptor modulator	Tamoxifen	Nausea and vomiting, hypercalcemia, menstrual irregularity, vaginal discharge/bleeding, hot flashes
Taxane	Docetaxel	Myelosuppression, nausea and vomiting, mucositis, hypersensitivity reactions, alopecia, fluid retention, skin and nail changes, neurotoxicity
	Paclitaxel	Myelosuppression, mucositis, diarrhea, hypersensitivity reactions, alopecia
Topoisomerase-I inhibitor	Topotecan	Myelosuppression, mucositis, diarrhea, alopecia, headache

Note. Based on information from Chu & DeVita, 2008; National Comprehensive Cancer Network, 2009d, 2009e, 2009f; Polovich et al., 2009.

Table 13-4. Nursing Care for the Patient Receiving Chemotherapy

Nursing Diagnosis/ Problem	Intervention and Rationale	Patient Education and Instruction
Knowledge deficit regarding treatment	• Assess patient's knowledge regarding disease and treatment options. • Assess patient's concerns and fears.	Explain and instruct regarding chemotherapy agents. • Routes of administration (IV & IP) • Treatment schedule • Side effects • Symptom management strategies • When to notify the healthcare professional
High risk for infection related to neutropenia	• Monitor blood counts (complete blood count with differential) • Monitor for signs and symptoms of infection • Monitor vital signs • Administer colony-stimulating factors (filgrastim, sargramostim, and pegfilgrastim) as ordered. • Institute neutropenic precautions for an absolute neutrophil count < 1,000 mm^3. • Administer antibiotics as ordered. • If patient is febrile and neutropenic, the patient must be assessed and cultured. • Chemotherapy treatment may be held/dose modified. • Administer the influenza and pneumococcal vaccine as ordered.	Explain the facts about blood and blood cells. Instruct the patient • To wash hands with soap and water and dry especially if visibly soiled (if hands not visibly soiled, use alcohol-based hand rub or soap and water) • To dry hands properly so they do not remain colonized with microorganisms • About the signs and symptoms of infection • About neutropenic precautions • About self-administration technique for colony-stimulating factors if appropriate • To report temperature of > 100.5°F • When to notify the healthcare professional.
High risk for bleeding related to thrombocytopenia	• Monitor blood counts (complete blood count and platelet count). • Monitor for signs and symptoms of bleeding. • Monitor vital signs. • Institute safety precautions. • Institute thrombocytopenic precautions for a platelet count of 50,000/mm^3. • Avoid aspirin-containing agents and agents that interfere with platelet function • Chemotherapy treatment may be held/dose modified	Explain the facts about blood and blood cells. Instruct the patient • About the signs and symptoms of bleeding and to report these signs and symptoms • About bleeding precautions • About creating a safe environment at home to reduce the risk of injury • When to notify the healthcare professional.
Anemia	• Monitor blood counts (complete blood count, hemoglobin, and hematocrit). • Assess for signs and symptoms of anemia: palpitations/chest pain on exertion, dyspnea, dizziness, fatigue, headache, anorexia, tinnitus, and/or insomnia. • Monitor for signs and symptoms of bleeding. • Monitor orthostatic vital signs. • Assess for contributing factors: pain, emotional distress, sleep disturbances, nutritional status, and comorbidities. • Screen for potential etiologic factors. • Treat with erythropoiesis-stimulating agents such as darbepoetin alfa or epoetin alfa as ordered. • Transfuse as ordered. • Develop an exercise program appropriate to the patient's condition. • Institute energy conservation practices. • Consider physical therapy, nutrition, or psychosocial referral as appropriate.	Explain the facts about blood and blood cells. Instruct the patient regarding • The signs and symptoms of anemia: pallor, fatigue, shortness of breath, tachycardia, headache, dizziness, irritability, and/or palpitations • Possible causes • The signs and symptoms of fatigue • Energy-conservation practices, including setting priorities, planning and pacing activities, delegating, scheduling activity at peak energy time, napping, structuring routine, and distraction • About self-administration technique for erythropoiesis-stimulating agents if appropriate • About the importance of adequate intake of iron • When to notify the healthcare professional.

(Continued on next page)

Table 13-4. Nursing Care for the Patient Receiving Chemotherapy *(Continued)*

Nursing Diagnosis/ Problem	Intervention and Rationale	Patient Education and Instruction
Mucositis	• Assess the patient's risk for mucositis. • Assess current oral hygiene and dental care status. • Inspect all surfaces of the oral cavity. • Assess ability to swallow solids, soft foods, and liquids. • Assess nutritional status. • If appropriate, refer for a nutritional consult and encourage dietary supplements. • Maintain adequate hydration and nutrition. • Perform oral care. • Brush all tooth surfaces after each meal and at bedtime. • Floss teeth with unwaxed dental floss once daily. If not flossing regularly prior to treatment, do not initiate flossing now. • Rinse mouth every four to six hours or more often for comfort • Any of the following solutions may be used. – One quart water mixed with one teaspoon salt and one teaspoon baking soda or one quart normal saline with one teaspoon baking soda – One quart water mixed with one teaspoon salt – One quart water mixed with one teaspoon baking soda – Water – Alcohol-free unsweetened mouthwash (e.g., Biotene® [GlaxoSmithKline]); commercial mouthwashes with alcohol should not be used. – Each day, unused solution should be discarded and a new solution should be mixed. • Apply moisturizer to lips four to six times a day. Use water-based moisturizer to protect lips. • For signs of thrush or infection, consult with physician or nurse practitioner regarding initiation of antibiotics. • For mouth dryness, instruct patient to take frequent sips of water or other liquids throughout the day. • Assess for pain and medicate per orders. • Obtain dental consult as needed. • For patients receiving IV bolus of 5-fluorouracil use cryotherapy (the use of ice chips five minutes prior to administration of the IV medication and continuing for 30 minutes after treatment).	Explain risk factors for mucositis. Instruct the patient regarding • The signs and symptoms of mucositis • How to perform an oral assessment • Oral hygiene and care • Removal and cleaning of dental appliances each time mouth is cleaned. Keep dental appliances out at night and if the mucous membranes become irritated, wear them during the day only when eating or out in public. • Avoiding substances that may irritate the mucous membranes during treatment: Chemical irritants (e.g., tobacco, alcohol, commercial mouthwash that contains alcohol, spices); physical irritants (e.g., loose or ill-fitting dentures, hard, dry or coarse foods); thermal irritants (e.g., very hot foods or liquids) • The importance of adequate nutrition intake • Cryotherapy if appropriate • When to notify the healthcare professional.
Nausea and vomiting	• Assess patient for risk factors. – Emetogenic potential of agent – History of poor control of nausea and vomiting – Female gender – Younger age – History of motion or morning sickness – Low chronic alcohol intake – Anxiety – Renal and hepatic dysfunction • Assess patient's patterns of nausea and vomiting. • Assess for signs and symptoms of fluid volume deficit. • Administer antiemetic(s) as ordered based on agent and patient specific risk factors. • Perform oral care before/after each meal and emesis. • Monitor intake and output.	Instruct patient regarding strategies to minimize or prevent nausea and vomiting. • Small, frequent meals • Rest periods, especially before and after eating • Minimizing stimuli • Avoiding foods that are highly sweet, highly seasoned, or greasy or with strong aromas • Taking antiemetics as prescribed • Nonpharmacologic interventions (e.g., relaxation exercises) • When to notify the healthcare professional

(Continued on next page)

Table 13-4. Nursing Care for the Patient Receiving Chemotherapy *(Continued)*

Nursing Diagnosis/ Problem	Intervention and Rationale	Patient Education and Instruction
	• Encourage oral intake. • Administer IV hydration as ordered. • Encourage small, frequent meals. • Monitor weight. • Refer for nutritional consult as appropriate. • Monitor electrolytes. • Use nonpharmacologic techniques such as relaxation exercises.	
Alopecia	• Inform the patient about expected time frame of hair loss and duration. • Assess the importance of hair loss to the patient and significant other. • Encourage patient to verbalize feelings about alopecia. • Identify strategies to manage hair loss. • Evaluate how patient is coping with hair loss.	Instruct patient regarding • Strategies to minimize alopecia • Considering cutting hair short to prepare for any hair loss • Rinsing hair thoroughly and gently patting it dry • Using a hair net, turban, or scarf to contain falling hair • Using a satin pillowcase • Using a wide-tooth comb or bristle brush on hair; can also "finger-comb" hair by using moistened fingers • Using a shampoo and conditioner with a sunscreen to prevent damage from sun exposure • Informing hairstylist that the patient is receiving chemotherapy • Keeping head covered in the summer to prevent sunburn or using sunscreen on scalp • Avoiding the following products – Hair sprays, coloring, dye, bleach, or permanent waves or straightening agents – Clips, barrettes, and bobby pins – Braids or corn rows – Hair dryers, curlers, or curling irons – Rubber bathing or swimming caps • Resources to obtain a wig.
Anorexia	• Assess nutritional status. • Obtain diet history. • Monitor weight. • Monitor albumin, transferrin, lymphocyte count, and electrolytes. • Referral to nutritional services. • Encourage a high-calorie, high-protein diet. • Administer appetite stimulant as ordered. • Ensure nausea and vomiting is managed.	Instruct patient regarding • Eating small, frequent meals • Rest periods especially before and after eating • Maintaining a high-calorie, high-protein diet • Experimenting with foods • Using gravies • Taking antiemetics or pain medications as prescribed • Oral care • Exercise • Monitoring weight weekly • Not drinking fluids with meals • When to notify the healthcare professional.
Potential for electrolyte alterations	• Monitor electrolytes (magnesium, potassium, calcium). • Assess for signs and symptoms of hypomagnesemia, hypokalemia, and hypocalcemia. • Replace electrolytes as ordered.	Instruct patient about diet and supplements.

(Continued on next page)

Table 13-4. Nursing Care for the Patient Receiving Chemotherapy *(Continued)*

Nursing Diagnosis/ Problem	Intervention and Rationale	Patient Education and Instruction
Potential for hypersensitivity reactions	• Record patient's allergy history. • Ensure emergency equipment and medications are available. • Ensure patient has taken premedications as ordered. • Monitor vital signs. • Observe for signs and symptoms of hypersensitivity reactions: itching, urticaria, flushing, skin reactions, dyspnea, wheezing, chest tightness or back pain, stridor, bronchospasms, angioedema, decreased oxygen saturation, hypotension, and tachycardia. • If you suspect a reaction – Stop the infusion of the drug and ensure patent IV access of normal saline to keep vein open. – Notify physician or nurse practitioner. – Administer oxygen therapy via nonrebreather mask for patent airway or via manual resuscitator (e.g., Ambu bag) for signs of airway obstruction or respiratory failure or arrest. – Initiate frequent vital signs and oxygen saturation every five minutes. – Initiate the appropriate interventions/orders based on signs and symptoms of reaction. • Decision to rechallenge will be based on the agent and severity of reaction. The physician will make this decision.	Instruct patient regarding • The importance of taking premedication • When to notify the healthcare professional.
Potential alterations in cardiac toxicity	• Assess patient's risk factors. • Baseline electrocardiogram and multigated acquisition scan as ordered. • Monitor for cumulative dosages (e.g., doxorubicin dose of greater than 300 mg/m^2) • Monitor for increased fatigue, reports of changes in rhythm and respiratory crackles.	Instruct patient • Regarding potential toxicity • Regarding monitoring tests • When to notify the healthcare professional.
Potential fluid retention related to docetaxel	• Provide patient with prophylactic steroid therapy as ordered. • Monitor patient's weight. • Monitor patient's vital signs. • Assess breath sounds.	Instruct patient regarding • Prophylactic steroid therapy as ordered • When to notify the healthcare professional.

Note. Based on information from Eilers, 2004; Epstein & Schubert, 2003; Friese, 2004; Joanna Briggs Institute for Evidence Based Nursing and Midwifery, 1998; Kostler et al., 2001; McGuire, 2003; Miller & Kearney, 2001, Multinational Association of Supportive Care in Cancer, 2006; National Comprehensive Cancer Network, 2008, 2009b; National Institute of Dental and Craniofacial Research, 2008a, 2008b; Plevova, 1999; Polovich et al., 2009; Rhodes & McDaniel, 2004; Rubenstein et al., 2004; Sonis et al., 2004; Stricker & Sullivan, 2003; Tipton et al., 2007; Worthington et al., 2007.

Table 13-5 lists agents and their emetic potential. (See also NCCN, 2009b for additional information on the usual antiemetic treatment and interventions based on emetic potential classification.) However, individuals may have increased emetic risk based on factors such as (NCCN, 2009b; Polovich et al., 2009)

- Their personal history of poor emetic control
- Younger age
- History of motion or morning sickness
- Chronic alcohol intake
- Anxiety level
- Renal or hepatic dysfunction.

In these patients, a higher-level antiemetic regimen, possibly started earlier, may be needed. In addition to the recommended regimens, patients with anticipatory emesis may be treated with benzodiazepines (alprazolam or lorazepam) (NCCN, 2009b). If a patient reports breakthrough emesis, a preventive around-the-clock rather than an as-needed regimen may be used (NCCN, 2009b). If emesis continues despite the use of antiemetics, the need for IV hydration and electrolyte replacement may be needed. Nonpharmacologic interventions such as acupuncture, acupressure, music therapy, relaxation exercises, guided imagery, and psychoeducational support have shown benefit (NCCN, 2009b; Tipton et al., 2007).

In January 2006, NCI recommended that intraperitoneal chemotherapy be added to the standard IV route for the initial treatment of advanced epithelial ovarian cancer (NCI, 2006). Although the agents used are familiar to gynecologic oncology nurses, the management of intraperitoneal therapy presents challenges related to the route of delivery. Table 13-6 outlines the common side effects unique to this type of treatment.

Table 13-5. Agents Classified Based on Emetic Risk Potential

Agent	Emetic Risk Potential
Bleomycin	Minimal
Vinorelbine	Minimal
Bevacizumab	Minimal
Docetaxel	Low
Etoposide	Low
5-fluorouracil	Low
Gemcitabine	Low
Liposomal doxorubicin	Low
Mitomycin C	Low
Paclitaxel	Low
Carboplatin	Moderate
Cisplatin < 50 mg/m^2	Moderate
Cyclophosphamide $\leq 1,500$ mg/m^2	Moderate
Doxorubicin	Moderate
Epirubicin	Moderate
Ifosfamide	Moderate
Irinotecan	Moderate
Cisplatin ≥ 50 mg/m^2	High
Cyclophosphamide $> 1,500$ mg/m^2	High

Note. Based on information from National Comprehensive Cancer Network, 2009b.

Radiation Therapy

Gynecologic oncology patients may receive several types of RT. Side effects vary by RT type and body location. External beam and low- or high-dose brachytherapy usually are administered in the outpatient setting. The major side effects of external RT to the pelvis include diarrhea, cystitis, alterations in vaginal mucous membranes, and fatigue (Bruner, Haas, & Gosselin-Acomb, 2004).

Patient education focuses on the type of radiation and the management of side effects at home. Table 13-7 summarizes nursing management for patients who receive either external beam RT or brachytherapy to the pelvis. In addition, Table 13-8 gives specific patient-education information related to a knowledge deficit of brachytherapy.

Summary

Nurses have an essential role in the management of side effects related to gynecologic cancer treatments. Successful management improves the quality of care for women with gynecologic cancers despite the type of treatment. Patients can be directed to Internet sites that will provide additional helpful information related to their cancers, the treatment, and possible clinical trials for which they may be eligible. Figure 13-1 lists these resources.

Figure 13-1. Resources for Women With a Gynecologic Cancer

Gynecologic Cancer Foundation: www.thegcf.org
Gynecologic Oncology Group: www.gog.org
National Cancer Institute: www.cancer.gov
Oncology Nursing Society: www.ons.org
Ovarian Cancer National Alliance: www.ovariancancer.org
Society of Gynecologic Nurse Oncologists: www.sgno.org
Society of Gynecologic Oncologists: www.sgo.org

Table 13-6. Unique Nursing Management for Intraperitoneal Chemotherapy

Nursing Diagnosis/ Problem	Intervention and Rationale	Patient Education and Instruction
Abdominal distention/pain	Assess abdomen prior to therapy. Assess for pain using the 0–10 scale. • If pain occurs during infusion, slow the infusion until discomfort stops. • Administer pain medications as needed/ordered.	Instruct patient to • Eat a light meal • Wear comfortable clothes • Post-therapy, to turn side to side every 15 minutes for 1 hour.
Frequent urination	Monitor voiding pattern.	Inform patient of this side effect. Instruct patient to • Void prior to treatment • Call if normal urination pattern does not return within 48 hours.
Dyspnea	Assess pretreatment respiratory status. Provide emotional support.	Instruct patient • To report difficulty breathing • That it is a temporary side effect • Regarding measures to relieve shortness of breath. – Elevate head of bed – Sit upright – Increase ambulation

Note. Based on information from Hydzik, 2007; Marin et al., 2007; Potter & Held-Warmkessel, 2008.

Table 13-7. Nursing Care for the Patient Receiving External Beam Radiation

Nursing Diagnosis/ Problem	Intervention and Rationale	Patient Education and Instruction
Knowledge deficit regarding external beam radiation therapy	• Assess patient's knowledge regarding disease and treatment options.	• Explain what external beam radiation therapy is and how it works. • Explain simulation and treatment planning process. • Explain goal of therapy (e.g., prophylaxis, curative, palliative). • Explain importance of patient compliance with positioning. • Educate patient that he or she is not radioactive. • Educate regarding potential acute and late toxicities.
Cystitis	• Assess patient's bladder function: patterns of urinary elimination (e.g., symptoms of urgency, frequency, dysuria, nocturia, past history of urinary tract infections). • Assess baseline hemoglobin, hematocrit, and coagulation values. • Assess for fever. • Assess urinalysis and urine culture and sensitivity. • Administer antibiotic therapy if indicated and ordered. • Administer antispasmodics if indicated and ordered. • Administer anticholinergic drugs if indicated and ordered.	Instruct patient • That signs and symptoms will subside gradually within 2–8 weeks following completion of radiation • To maintain adequate amount of fluid intake: 1–2 L/day • To avoid foods that irritate the bladder mucosa (e.g., coffee, tea, alcohol) and tobacco products • To monitor urinary output • To report signs and symptoms of bladder irritation, dysuria, urgency with decreased urine volume, and signs of hematuria • When to notify the healthcare professional.

(Continued on next page)

Table 13-7. Nursing Care for the Patient Receiving External Beam Radiation *(Continued)*

Nursing Diagnosis/ Problem	Intervention and Rationale	Patient Education and Instruction
Alteration in vaginal mucous membranes	• Assess for vaginal discharge. • Assess for pruritis. • Assess for dyspareunia. • Assess the potential for estrogen depletion. • Assess the impact on sexual activity and satisfaction.	Instruct patient • About the importance of cleansing vaginal area with warm water and mild soap and patting dry skin with towel • To use sitz baths as needed • To keep skin free from moisture • To avoid the use of creams, lotions, or powder to the treated area • To wear loose-fitting, soft cotton clothing • To apply lidocaine ointments as needed • To apply corticosteroid and/or antibiotic if indicated as ordered • To apply medicated cream after daily dose of radiation • Regarding careful positioning and use of water-soluble lubricants with intercourse • To apply estrogen cream as indicated • Regarding use of vaginal dilators • When to notify the healthcare professional.
Small bowel obstruction	• Only a small percentage will develop this serious complication. • Assess for signs and symptoms of obstruction and/or impaction (e.g., nausea/vomiting, abdominal distention, decreased bowel sounds, no passage of flatus, abdominal pain, presence of impacted stool in rectum). • If obstruction/impaction is suspected, consult with physician or nurse practitioner regarding an abdominal x-ray and management. • Administer IV fluids as ordered. • Administer parenteral nutrition as ordered. • Surgery may be necessary.	Instruct patient regarding • Being nothing-by-mouth status • Importance of oral care • Possible options to manage the obstruction.
Alteration in skin integrity	• Assess for treatment-related risk factors. • Assess for patient-related risk factors. • Assess skin at least weekly or when notified by patient. • Assess for erythema, folliculitis (inflammation of hair follicles, presenting as itchy raised red rash), hyperpigmentation, dry desquamation (dryness and itching), moist desquamation (loss of epidermis, exposed dermis, serous exudate, pain), and discomfort. • Assess for signs or symptoms of infection. • Culture the wound if you suspect the possibility of an infection. • Based on skin assessment, institute skin management plan.	Instruct patient regarding • Importance of adequate nutritional intake • Importance of skin care • Gentle washing of skin with tepid water, using soft washcloth and nondeodorant soap • Avoiding removal of any temporary marks • Wearing loose-fitting, soft cotton clothing • Using only recommended skin-care products • Avoiding scratching skin • Protecting skin from extreme temperatures and sunlight • Not using adhesive tape or bandage in treatment field • Seeking advice from healthcare professional regarding swimming • How to care for all stages of skin reactions • When to notify healthcare professional.

Table 13-8. Nursing Care for the Patient Receiving Brachytherapy

Nursing Diagnosis/ Problem	Intervention and Rationale	Patient Education and Instruction
Knowledge deficit regarding brachytherapy	• Assess patient's knowledge regarding disease and treatment options. • Educate about process of brachytherapy. • Educate patient regarding different techniques in brachytherapy—high dose rate and low dose rate. • Educate regarding potential acute and late toxicities. • Educate regarding risks and benefits of brachytherapy.	• Explain what brachytherapy is and how it works. • Explain treatment planning process. • Explain goal of therapy (e.g., prophylaxis, curative, palliative). • Explain importance of patient compliance with positioning.

Special thanks to George Monemvasitis for his editorial assistance.

References

Beck, S.L., & Erickson, J. (2004). *Measuring oncology nursing-sensitive patient outcomes: Evidence-based summary review—Fatigue*. Pittsburgh, PA: Oncology Nursing Society. Retrieved April 15, 2009, from http://www.ons.org/outcomes/measures/pdf/FatigueSummary.pdf

Brandt, L.J., Prather, C.M., Quigley, E.M., Schiller, L.R., Schoenfeld, P., & Talley, N.J. (2005). Systematic review on the management of chronic constipation in North America. *American Journal of Gastroenterology 100*(Suppl. 1), S5–S22.

Bruner, D.W., Haas, M.L., & Gosselin-Acomb, T.K. (Eds.). (2004). *Manual for radiation oncology nursing practice and education* (3rd ed.). Pittsburgh, PA: Oncology Nursing Society.

Campbell, T., Draper, S., Reid, J., & Robinson, L. (2001). The management of constipation in people with advanced cancer. *International Journal of Palliative Nursing, 7*(3), 110–119.

Chu, E., & DeVita, V.T. (2008) *Physician's cancer chemotherapy drug manual 2008*. Sudbury, MA: Jones and Bartlett.

Eilers, J. (2004). Nursing interventions and supportive care for the prevention and treatment of oral mucositis associated with cancer treatment [Review]. *Oncology Nursing Forum, 31*(Suppl. 4), 13–23.

Epstein, J.B., & Schubert, M.M. (2003). Oropharyngeal mucositis in cancer therapy: Review of pathogenesis, diagnosis, and management. *Oncology, 17*(12), 1767–1779.

Folden, S.L., Backer, J.H., Maynard, F., Stevens, K., Gilbride, J.A., Pires, M., et al. (2002). *Practice guidelines for the management of constipation in adults*. Glenview, IL: Rehabilitation Nursing Foundation. Retrieved April 15, 2009, from http://www.rehabnurse.org/pdf/BowelGuideforWEB.pdf

Friese, C. (2004). *Measuring oncology nursing-sensitive patient outcomes: Evidence-based summary review—Prevention of infection*. Pittsburgh, PA: Oncology Nursing Society. Retrieved April 15, 2009, from http://www.ons.org/outcomes/measures/pdf/PreventionSummary.pdf

Hinrichs, M., Huseboe, J., Tang, J.H., & Titler, M.G. (2001). Research-based protocol: Management of constipation. *Journal of Gerontological Nursing, 27*(2), 17–28.

Hsieh, C. (2005). Treatment of constipation in older adults. *American Family Physician 72*(11), 2277–2284.

Hydzik, C. (2007). Implementation of intraperitoneal chemotherapy for the treatment of ovarian cancer. *Clinical Journal of Oncology Nursing, 11*(2), 221–225.

Joanna Briggs Institute for Evidence Based Nursing and Midwifery. (1998). *Prevention and treatment of oral mucositis in cancer patients. Best practice: Evidence based practice information sheets for health professionals, 2*(3), 1–6. Retrieved April 15, 2009, from http://www.oralcancerfoundation.org/dental/pdf/mucositis.pdf

Katz, A. (2007). *Breaking the silence on cancer and sexuality: A handbook for healthcare providers*. Pittsburgh, PA: Oncology Nursing Society.

Köstler, W.J., Hejna, M., Wenzel, C., & Zielinski, C.C. (2001). Oral mucositis complicating chemotherapy and/or radiotherapy: options for prevention and treatment. *CA: A Cancer Journal for Clinicians, 51*(5), 290–315.

Locke, G.R., III, Pemberton, J.H., & Phillips, S.F. (2000). American Gastroenterological Association medical position statement: Guidelines on constipation. *Gastroenterology 119*(6), 1761–1766.

Marin, K., Oleszewski, K., & Muehlbauer, P. (2007). Intraperitoneal chemotherapy: Implications beyond ovarian cancer. *Clinical Journal of Oncology Nursing, 11*(6), 881–889.

Marlett, J.A., McBurney, M.I., Slavin, J.L., & American Dietetic Association. (2002). Position of the American Dietetic Association: Health implications of dietary fiber. *Journal of the American Dietetic Association, 102*(7), 993–1000.

McGuire, D.B. (2003). Barriers and strategies in implementation of oral care standards for cancer patients. *Supportive Care in Cancer, 11*(7), 435–441.

Miller, M., & Kearney, N. (2001). Oral care for patients with cancer: A review of the literature. *Cancer Nursing, 24*(4), 241–254.

Muller-Lissner, S., Kamm, M., Scarpignato, C., & Wald, A. (2005). Myths and misconceptions about chronic constipation. *American Journal of Gastroenterology, 100*(1), 232–242.

Multinational Association of Supportive Care in Cancer. (2006). *Education*. Retrieved May 14, 2009, from http://www.mascc.org/content/444.html

National Cancer Institute. (2006, January 5). *NCI clinical announcement: Intraperitoneal chemotherapy for ovarian cancer.* Retrieved May 13, 2009, from http://ctep.cancer.gov/highlights/docs/clin_annc_010506.pdf

National Comprehensive Cancer Network. (2008). *NCCN Clinical Practice Guidelines in Oncology™: Prevention and treatment of cancer-related infections* [v.1.2008]. Retrieved April 15, 2009, from http://www.nccn.org/professionals/physician_gls/PDF/infections.pdf

National Comprehensive Cancer Network. (2009a). *NCCN Clinical Practice Guidelines in Oncology™: Adult cancer pain* [v.1.2009]. Retrieved April 15, 2009, from http://www.nccn.org/professionals/physician_gls/PDF/pain.pdf

National Comprehensive Cancer Network. (2009b). *NCCN Clinical Practice Guidelines in Oncology™: Antiemesis* [v.3.2009]. Retrieved April 15, 2009, from http://www.nccn.org/professionals/physician_gls/PDF/antiemesis.pdf

National Comprehensive Cancer Network. (2009c). *NCCN Clinical Practice Guidelines in Oncology™: Cancer-related fatigue* [v.1.2009]. Retrieved April 15, 2009, from http://www.nccn.org/professionals/physician_gls/PDF/fatigue.pdf

National Comprehensive Cancer Network. (2009d). *NCCN Clinical Practice Guidelines in Oncology™: Cervical Cancer* [v.1.2009]. Retrieved April 15, 2009, from http://www.nccn.org/professionals/physician_gls/PDF/cervical.pdf

National Comprehensive Cancer Network. (2009e). *NCCN Clinical Practice Guidelines in Oncology™: Ovarian cancer including fallopian tube cancer and primary peritoneal cancer* [v.1.2009]. Retrieved April 15, 2009, from http://www.nccn.org/professionals/physician_gls/PDF/ovarian.pdf

National Comprehensive Cancer Network. (2009f). *NCCN Clinical Practice Guidelines in Oncology™: Uterine neoplasms* [v.2.2009]. Retrieved April 15, 2009, from http://www.nccn.org/professionals/physician_gls/PDF/uterine.pdf

National Institute of Dental and Craniofacial Research. (2008a). *Oral complications of cancer treatment: What the oncology team can do*. Bethesda, MD: Author. Retrieved April 15, 2008, from http://www.nidcr.nih.gov/NR/rdonlyres/AA8E12E6-9D51-4DC3-9721-0FA59DE9CCB2/0/WhatOncologyTeamCanDo.pdf

National Institute of Dental and Craniofacial Research. (2008b). *Oncology pocket guide to oral health.* Bethesda, MD: Author. Retrieved April 15, 2009, from http://www.nidcr.nih.gov/NR/rdonlyres/FB0A632B-10B0-473A-8F29-65A651562458/0/OncologyPocketGuide.pdf

Plevova, P. (1999). Prevention and treatment of chemotherapy- and radiotherapy-induced oral mucositis: A review. *Oral Oncology, 35*, 453–470.

Polovich, M., Whitford, J.M., & Olsen, M. (Eds.). (2009). *Chemotherapy and biotherapy guidelines and recommendations for practice* (3rd. ed.). Pittsburgh, PA: Oncology Nursing Society.

Potter, K.L., & Held-Warmkessel, J. (2008). Intraperitoneal chemotherapy for women with ovarian cancer: Nursing care and considerations. *Clinical Journal of Oncology Nursing, 12*(2), 265–271.

Rhodes, V. & McDaniel, R. (2004). *Measuring oncology nursing-sensitive patient outcomes: Evidence-based summary review—Nausea and vomiting*. Pittsburgh, PA: Oncology Nursing Society. Retrieved April 15, 2009, from http://www.ons.org/outcomes/measures/pdf/NauseaSummary.pdf

Rubenstein, E.B., Peterson, D.E., Schubert, M., Keefe, D., McGuire, D., Epstein, J., et al. (2004). Clinical practice guidelines for the prevention and treatment of cancer therapy-induced oral and gastrointestinal mucositis. *Cancer, 100*(Suppl. 9), 2026–2046.

Smith, M.I., Lee, R.M., & Skootsky, S.A. (2005) Preoperative evaluation, medical management and critical care. In J.S. Berek & N.F. Hacker (Eds.), *Practical gynecologic oncology* (4th ed., pp. 792–793). Philadelphia: Lippincott Williams & Wilkins.

Sonis, S.T., Elting, L.S., Keefe, D., Peterson, D.E., Schubert, M., Hauer-Jensen, M., et al. (2004). Perspectives on cancer therapy-induced mucosal injury: Pathogenesis, measurement, epidemiology, and consequences for patients. *Cancer, 100*(Suppl. 9), 1995–2025.

Stern, J., & Ippoliti, C. (2003). Management of acute cancer treatment-induced diarrhea. *Seminars in Oncology Nursing, 19*(4, Suppl. 3), 11–16.

Stricker, C.T., & Sullivan, J. (2003). Evidence-based oncology oral care clinical practice guidelines: Development, implementation, and evaluation. *Clinical Journal of Oncology Nursing, 7*(2), 222–227.

Tipton, J.M., McDaniel, R.W., Barbour, L., Johnston, M.P., Kayne, M., LeRoy, P., et al. (2007). Putting evidence into practice: Evidence-based interventions to prevent, manage, and treat chemotherapy-induced nausea and vomiting. *Clinical Journal of Oncology Nursing, 11*(1), 69–78.

Towers, A.L., Burgio, K.L., Locher, J.L., Merkel, I.S., Safaeian, M., & Wald, A. (1994). Constipation in the elderly: Influence of dietary, psychological, and physiological factors. *Journal of the American Geriatric Society, 42*(7), 701–706.

Tramonte, S.M., Brand, M.B., Mulrow, C.D., Amato, M.G., O'Keefe, M.E., & Ramirez, G. (1997). The treatment of chronic constipation in adults: A systematic review. *Journal of General Internal Medicine, 12*(1), 15–24.

Worthington, H.V., Clarkson, J.E., & Eden, T.O.B. (2007). Interventions for preventing oral mucositis for patients with cancer receiving treatment. *Cochrane Database Systematic Reviews 2007,* Issue 4. Art. No. CD000978. DOI: 10.1002/14651858.CD000978.pub3.

CHAPTER 14

Long-Term Symptom Management

Kathleen Appollo, RN, BSN, OCN®, Lois Almadrones-Cassidy, RN, MS, FNP, MPA, and Randy E. Gross, MS, RN, NP, WHNP-BC, ACNS-BC, AOCNP®

Introduction

Improved surgical techniques, new chemotherapy combinations, novel biologic agents, targeted radiation therapy, and multimodality therapy have improved overall survival for women with gynecologic cancers in the last two decades (Jemal et al., 2008). Even ovarian cancer, the most lethal and difficult to achieve a durable response and long-term survival, has shown improvement in five-year overall survival (Armstrong et al., 2006). Although survivorship is celebrated, often the cost is less-than-optimal function because of either short- or long-term treatment morbidity. This chapter focuses on three symptoms that may have profound long-term effects on a woman's physical and/or mental functional abilities. They all have the potential to severely compromise quality of life. These symptoms are chemotherapy-induced peripheral neuropathy, lower extremity lymphedema, and menopause.

Peripheral Neuropathy

Peripheral neuropathy (PN) is defined as "any injury, inflammation, or degeneration of the peripheral nerves" (Almadrones, Armstrong, Gilbert, & Schwartz, 2002, p. 5). These nerves are located outside the central nervous system (brain and spinal cord) and include the sensory, motor, and autonomic nerves. Each type of nerve has a different function (Armstrong, Almadrones, & Gilbert, 2005).

- Sensory nerves sense touch, pain, temperature, position, and vibration.
- Motor nerves control voluntary movement, muscle tone, and coordination.
- Autonomic nerves control intestinal mobility, blood pressure, and involuntary muscles.

The sensory nerves are further subdivided into small and large fibers nerves. How PN symptoms manifest depends on both the type of nerve affected and in the case of sensory nerve damage, the particular type of nerve fiber affected. PN may be caused by trauma, infection, and a host of medical conditions and medications (Hausheer, Schilsky, Bain, Berghorn, & Lieberman, 2006; Hughes, 2002; Poncelet, 1998) (see Figure 14-1).

Chemotherapy-Induced Peripheral Neuropathy

The most active and therefore most frequently used chemotherapeutic agents in gynecologic cancers, regardless of the cancer site, are the taxanes (paclitaxel and docetaxel) and platinum analogs (carboplatin and cisplatin) (Bhoola & Hoskins, 2006; Cadron, Van Gorp, Amant, Leunen, Neven, & Vergote, 2007; McMeekin, Alektiar, Sabbatini, & Zaino, in press). Other less frequently used agents are vinca alkaloids (vincristine), etoposide, and bortezomib. All of these, especially the taxanes and platinum analogs, are neurotoxic and cause sensory and motor PN. Chemotherapy-induced PN (CIPN) is often a dose-limiting toxicity of cisplatin and paclitaxel (Wickham, 2007).

CIPN is caused directly by the administration of a neurotoxic agent, but is enhanced by other factors, including cumulative dose, rapid infusion times, high single dose, and prior or concurrent use of other neurotoxic drugs or agents (e.g., paclitaxel concomitantly with cisplatin for ovarian cancer) (Hausheer et al., 2006; Hilkens & ven den Bent, 1997; Ocean & Vahdat, 2004; Quasthoff & Hartung, 2002; Verstappen, Heimans, Hoekman, & Postma, 2003).

It is not uncommon for CIPN to affect more than one type of peripheral nerve, causing a mixed sensorimotor polyneuropathy. For CIPN to occur, the neurotoxic agent must first be able to cross the blood-nerve barrier. The blood-brain barrier protects the central nervous system from harmful substances by inhibiting diffusion of large molecules, highly charged ions, and many drugs from the bloodstream into the brain and spinal cord. However, the peripheral nervous system is not protected by a similar vascular barrier and is more susceptible to affects of neurotoxic chemotherapeutic agents. Second, the

Figure 14-1. Possible Etiologies of Symmetric Peripheral Neuropathies

Endocrine Diseases
- Diabetes mellitus
- Hypothyroidism

Nutritional Diseases
- Alcoholism
- Vitamin B_{12} deficiency
- Thiamine deficiency
- Vitamin E deficiency
- Folate deficiency
- Postgastrectomy syndrome
- Crohn disease

Connective Tissue Diseases
- Rheumatoid arthritis
- Systemic lupus erythematosus
- Polyarteritis nodosa
- Sjögren syndrome

Infectious Diseases
- AIDS
- Lyme disease

Hereditary Diseases
- Charcot-Marie-Tooth syndrome
- Freidreich's ataxia
- Other sensory neuropathies

Metal Neuropathy
- Chronic arsenic intoxication
- Mercury
- Gold
- Thallium

Medications
- Colchicine
- Isoniazid
- Hydralazine
- Metronidazole
- Lithium
- Alfa interferon
- Dapsone
- Phenytoin
- Cimetadine
- Amiodarone
- Pyridoxine
- Amitriptyline

Toxic Neuropathy
- Acrylamide
- Carbon disulfide
- Dichloorphenoxyacetic acid
- Ethylene oxide
- Carbon monoxide
- Glue sniffing

Other
- Amyloidosis
- Sarcoidosis
- Primary biliary cirrhosis
- Uremia
- Vasculitis
- Ischemic lesions

Note. From "Chemotherapy-Induced Peripheral Neuropathy: A Review and Implications for Oncology Nursing Practice," by R. Wickham, 2007, *Clinical Journal of Oncology Nursing, 11*(3), p. 363. Copyright 2007 by Oncology Nursing Society. Reprinted with permission.

nervous system must be sensitive to the agent (Armstrong et al., 2005; Willis, 2000).

The incidence of severe CIPN is unknown but is estimated at 3%–7% when a single treating agent is used and as high as 38% when multiple neurotoxic agents are used (Cavaletti & Zanna, 2002). CIPN is diagnosed after completion of a comprehensive neurologic assessment that includes (Armstrong et al., 2005; England et al., 2005; Marrs & Newton, 2003)

- The patient's subjective report of symptoms
- A comprehensive clinical history to determine preexisting PN
- Objective neurologic testing, including nerve conduction studies
- A neurologic clinical examination to evaluate sensory and motor nerve function.

Emerging evidence suggests that CIPN is substantially underreported in clinical trials because of limitations in available grading scales and challenges in assessing and diagnosing by reliable and reproducible manner in clinical practice (Hausheer et al., 2006). Instead, the patient's self-report of symptoms and ability to perform activities of daily living (ADL), combined with the clinician's observation of motor (gait and strength) and sensory skills (light touch or pin-prick) form the basis on which the diagnosis of CIPN is made. Measurement by a valid and reliable instrument that is easily administered in the clinical setting and accepted by nurses and clinicians remains elusive but necessary (Almadrones, McGuire, Walzak, Florio, & Tian, 2004; Smith, Beck, & Cohen, 2008).

Symptoms manifested by CIPN depend on the type of nerve or nerve fiber affected. Most symptoms begin within hours, days, or weeks after administration of the neurotoxic agent (Armstrong et al., 2005). The exception is cisplatin CIPN, which may progress in severity for several months after the drug is discontinued, a condition known as *coasting* (Armstrong et al., 2005; Wickham, 2007).

Sensory CIPN usually presents in a symmetrical pattern starting in the most distal parts of the extremities and moving proximally up the extremity (e.g., fingertips to fingers to hands, toes to feet to ankles) in a stocking/glove distribution. As CIPN progresses in severity, symptoms extend up the extremity medially toward the trunk. Symptoms range from absent or diminished sensation (hypoesthesia, paresthesia) to extreme sensitivity or abnormal sensation (dysesthesia, allodynia, neuropathic pain).

Neuropathic pain is usually described as tingling or burning sensations. Sensory loss also may cause diminished vibration and position sense (proprioception, ataxia) and inability to distinguish temperature. Lhermitte sign is a shock-like sensation that goes down the back and into the limbs when the neck is flexed. It is a rare symptom, particularly associated with cisplatin, but indicates nerve damage that extends to the level of the spinal cord (Armstrong et al., 2005; Cerosimo, 1989; Wickham, 2007).

One of the first objective symptoms of CIPN is the loss of deep tendon reflexes. Motor CIPN causes symptoms of arthralgia, myalgia, muscle cramps and weakness, and loss of strength mostly confined to the extremities in a symmetrical pattern (Hausheer et al., 2006; Wickham, 2007). These symptoms may affect the ability to bend or stoop or to lift objects.

Autonomic CIPN usually manifests with cardiovascular symptoms, such as orthostatic hypotension or altered heart rate, gastrointestinal effects such as constipation or ileus, or urinary bladder dysfunction manifested by difficulty initiating or controlling urinary stream or incomplete emptying and overflow incontinence (Quastoff & Hartung, 2002; Wickham, 2007). These symptoms are more likely associated with vinca alkaloids but can also occur with cisplatin.

Currently, no effective cytoprotective agents are available to prevent or reduce the occurrence or severity of CIPN

(Armstrong et al., 2005; Visovsky, Collins, Abbott, Aschenbrenner, & Hart, 2007). Visovsky et al. performed an extensive literature review of pharmacologic and nonpharmacologic interventions specific to the prevention and symptom improvement of CIPN and concluded that the studies failed to meet the scientific rigor necessary for practice recommendations. Published studies on chemoprotectants, including amifostine; calcium and magnesium infusions; tricyclic antidepressants; anticonvulsants; acetyl-L carnitine; glutamine; glutathione; alpha lipoic acid; and human leukemia factor were included in the review. Furthermore, the review failed to reveal any effective nonpharmacologic intervention in the oncology population.

A small clinical trial using alpha-tocopherol (vitamin E) 300 mg given orally every day demonstrated decreased incidence and severity of cisplatin induced peripheral neurotoxicity. However, further study in a larger trial was recommended (Pace et al., 2003).

Visovsky et al. (2007) extrapolated from literature about diabetic PN that recommending assistive devices to prevent injury caused by sensory and motor changes, as well as encouraging physical activity and strength training, provide a small benefit. Infrared light therapy, transcutaneous stimulation, and spinal cord stimulation proved to have a limited benefit for diabetic PN; however, more research is needed before applying these strategies to the oncology population. No evidence was available to support the use of topical capsaicin ointment in the treatment of CIPN.

Neuropathic pain is one of the most debilitating symptoms of CIPN and often has a negative effect on quality of life. The exact pathophysiologic mechanism that causes neuropathic pain is complex, but it occurs when peripheral nerves are damaged at the level of the nerve root or spinal cord. It is described as burning, shooting, sharp-cutting, or lancinating pain (Wickham, 2007). It is often characterized by "wind-up" or escalation of pain, even when the offending agent has been removed (Armstrong et al., 2005). Despite the lack of evidence-based data to support their use in oncology, the mainstay of treatment remains anticonvulsants (gabapentin), tricyclic antidepressants, and opioids (see Table 14-1 for complete list). A new analog, oxcarbazepine, is being studied for neuropathic pain in postherpetic neuralgia and may be useful when pain is refractory to carbamazepine and gabapentin (Criscuolo, Auletta, Lippi, Brogi, & Brogi, 2004).

Two interventions for CIPN can be recommended. The first is to recognize and treat any preexisting conditions to prevent toxic synergy (Armstrong et al., 2005). Whenever possible, a woman with preexisting PN should be treated with a less-neurotoxic regimen to prevent a rapid and more severe onset of CIPN (Chaudry, Rowinsky, Sartorius, Donehower, & Cornblath, 1994). The second intervention is education and support to preserve patient safety (Almadrones & Arcot, 1999; Armstrong et al. 2005; Bennett

Table 14-1. Pharmacologic Interventions for Peripheral Neuropathy Pain

Class and Drug	Usual Starting Dose (mg per day)	Usual Effective Dose (mg)
Alpha-2-adreneric agonist		
Clonidine	–	–
Anticonvulsants		
Carbamazepine	200	600–1,200
Phenytoin	300	Dosed to effectiveness
Valproic acid	10–15 per kg per day in 1–3 doses	750–2,000
Gabapentin	300	300–3,600
Antidepressants: tricyclics		
Amitriptyline	10–15	50–150
Clomipramine	10–15	50–150
Desipramine	10–15	50–150
Doxepin	10–15	50–150
Imipramine	10–15	50–150
Nortriptyline	10–15	50–150
Antidepressants: selective serotonin reuptake inhibitors		
Fluoxetine	10–20	20–40
Paroxetine	20	20–40
Sertraline	50	150–200
Citalopram	20	–
Corticosteroids		
Dexamethasone	Initial: 10	–
Prednisone	Chronic: 1–2	–
Local anesthetics		
Mexiletine	150	900–1,200
Tocainide	400	1,200–1,600
Lidocaine	Brief infusion: 2–5 per kg over 20–30 minutes	Same
	Continuous infusion: 2.5 per kg per hour	
	Transdermal 5% patch	Up to three patches
Opioids		
Morphine	Dose determined by patient tolerance	Dose titrated to analgesia
Hydromorphone		
Oxycodone		
Fentanyl		
Methadone		

Note. From "Chemotherapy-Induced Peripheral Neuropathy," by T. Armstrong, L. Almadrones, and M.R. Gilbert, 2005, *Oncology Nursing Forum, 32*(3), p. 309. Copyright 2005 by Oncology Nursing Society. Reprinted with permission.

& Paice, 2007; Marrs & Newton, 2003). These education interventions include teaching
- The signs and symptoms of CIPN
- Personal safety to avoid falls by using well-lighted areas both inside and outside the home, removing throw rugs and clutter from floors, and using skid-free shower and bathroom mats
- To wear properly fitting, closed-toe shoes that give insole support and to inspect feet daily for injury
- To lower water temperature to avoid burns
- To use protective gloves when washing dishes and thick potholders when handling hot plates and pans and to inspect hands for injury
- Ways to avoid constipation with diet and adequate fluids
- To avoid falls caused by postural hypotension by dangling feet and legs before arising.

Nurses can influence the care of women with CIPN. A thorough neurologic assessment prior to and at each chemotherapy and follow-up visit, education about the signs and symptoms of CIPN, and safety and preventive strategies are nursing interventions that will help to promote a positive outcome for those at risk for CIPN. When CIPN is suspected, early referral to a physical or occupational therapist can help the patient to avoid the frustration of difficulties in accomplishing ADLs and help to create a safe home and workplace. Nursing research is vital to develop assessment instruments for CIPN suitable for easy use by the multidisciplinary team. Prevention and treatment strategies across all oncology disciplines remain deficient, and well-designed clinical trials using adequate sample sizes still are needed.

Lower Extremity Lymphedema

Anatomy and Physiology

The lymphatic system is an interconnected network of organs, lymph vessels, and lymph nodes. One function of this system is to drain and transport waste products of cell metabolism from the interstitial or extracellular spaces into the general circulation. This absorption and transport of extracellular fluid away from the cells helps to maintain body fluid balance (Foldi, 1998). Extracellular fluid is composed of water, fats, proteins, bacteria, and waste products of cell metabolism. When this fluid is absorbed into the lymphatic system, it becomes known as lymph.

Lymph nodes are bean-shaped glands located throughout the lymphatic system. They filter lymph of bacteria, viruses, and cell metabolism waste products and release lymphocytes into the circulation.

The superficial lymphatic capillaries are made up of endothelial cells, which overlap but do not form a continuous connection. Each of these cells is anchored to surrounding tissue by filaments, which pull on the cells in response to changes in tissue pressure. As the cell is pulled by the filament, it moves away from an overlapping cell, creating a space for the fluid to drain into a lymphatic capillary. Pressure changes that affect the filament action occur during muscle contraction, during respiration, during arterial pulsation, or when the skin is stretched (Foldi, 1998).

The lymph flows into progressively larger deep vessels containing intrinsic smooth muscles, which contract to promote lymph flow. One-way valves ensure that lymph moves away from tissues in a slow, steady, low-pressure system. Afferent vessels transport lymph into lymph nodes. Here, the lymph is filtered of cellular waste products, pathogens, and cancer cells; exposed to antibodies; and receives lymphocytes. Efferent vessels carry the filtered lymph out of the node. Lymph drains from the lower limbs into the lumbar and intestinal trunks in the abdomen. These trunks merge to form an upward pathway into the thorax called the *cisterna chyli*. The cisterna chyli ends at the thoracic duct, where lymph empties into the subclavian veins (Casely-Smith, 1997; Mortimer, 1998).

Etiology

Lymphedema occurs when the lymphatic system is unable to transport the interstitial filtrate, causing an accumulation of excess water, plasma proteins, blood cells, and waste products or lymph (Foeldi, Foeldi, & Dubik, 2003; International Society of Lymphology, 2003). Primary lymphedema develops as a consequence of a congenital or hereditary etiology whereby lymphatic tissue or structures are absent or abnormal in formation. Secondary lymphedema develops when the flow is interrupted because of malignancies, surgery, infection, trauma, or postradiation fibrosis (Foeldi et al.).

Incidence

To date, no prospective studies have been conducted that primarily assess the incidence of lower extremity lymphedema; therefore, the true incidence rate is not known. Some retrospective studies that include the consequences of gynecologic surgery suggest that the incidence is in the range of 1%–49%. Surgery for vulvar cancer with inguinal lymph node dissection produces the highest incidence (Abu-Rustum et al., 2003, 2006; Rouzier, Haddad, Dubernard, Dubois, & Paniel, 2003; Ryan et al., 2003a; Werngren-Elgstrom, & Lidman, 1994).

Risk Factors

Increased risk for lymphedema development is associated with the disruption of the flow of lymph. This disruption of flow may occur as a result of (Foeldi et al., 2003)
- Surgery involving lymphadenectomy, which cuts the pathway
- Radiation treatments, which can scar lymphatic tissue
- Advanced or recurrent cancer, which invades and blocks the lymph nodes.

The development of lymphedema may be gender linked, with a higher incidence in women with advancing age (Moffat et al., 2003). Because gynecologic cancers occur frequently with advancing age, an inherent risk is added. Infection can occur more easily in the stagnant, protein-rich lymph fluid, which is a perfect medium for the growth of bacteria. Infections with accompanying inflammation and obesity increase the fluid volume, which may not be handled by the compromised lymph system (Brewer, Hahn, Rohrbach, & Baddour, 2000; Rouzier et al., 2003).

Weight gain may be a risk factor in the development of lymphedema. Increased weight requires a change in the vascular and lymphatic flow to an extremity, and this may strain an already impaired lymphatic circulation (Meek, 1998).

Symptoms

Early symptoms (stage 0) of lymphedema include reports of heaviness, pulling, tightness, tingling, fatigue, or aching in the extremity. These sensations may be present before swelling appears (Armer, Radina, Porock, & Culbertson, 2003). Interview of the patient may reveal that shoes or clothing feel tight.

When swelling occurs, it usually starts distally and spreads upward, as pitting edema. In early lymphedema (stage 1), the swelling may resolve with elevation. Patients may delay reporting this if the edema resolves overnight. As the condition progresses (stage 2), the edema persists and eventually results in fibrosis of connective tissue and hyperkeratosis. Late lymphedema (stage 3) is manifested by a grossly enlarged limb with papillomas or skin breakdown (International Society of Lymphology, 2003). See Figures 14-2 and 14-3.

Diagnosis

Any reports of leg swelling after gynecologic treatment should be investigated. A deep vein thrombosis (DVT) or a recurrence of disease may manifest in extremity swelling;

Figure 14-2. Lymphedema Stages

Stage 0: No objective edema even though lymph transport is impaired; patient may report a heavy sensation.
Stage 1: Pitting edema present; relieved with elevation but may take overnight; most easily treated at this stage.
Stage 2: Edema no longer pitting and does not decrease with elevation; fibrosis of connective tissue and brawny skin may be present.
Stage 3: Elephantiasis; limb grossly enlarged and misshapen; skin breakdown and weeping may be present.

Note. From *What Is Lymphedema?* by National Lymphedema Network, 2005. Retrieved June 1, 2009, from http://www.lymphnet.org/lymphedemaFAQs/overview.htm. Copyright 2005 by National Lymphedema Network. Adapted with permission.

Figure 14-3. Stages of Lower Extremity Lymphedema

Stage 1

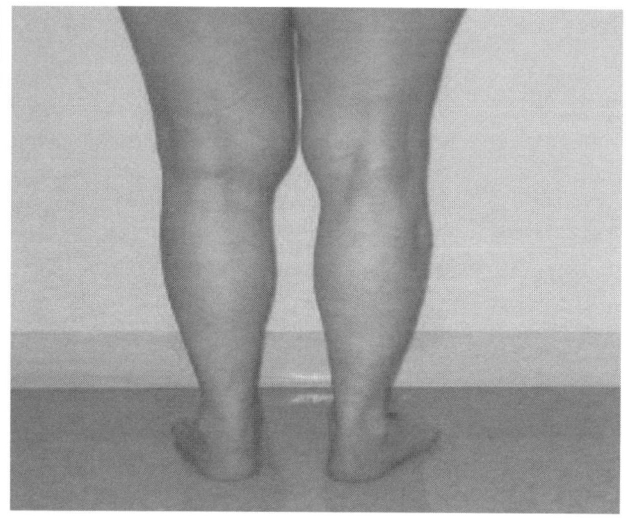

Stage 2

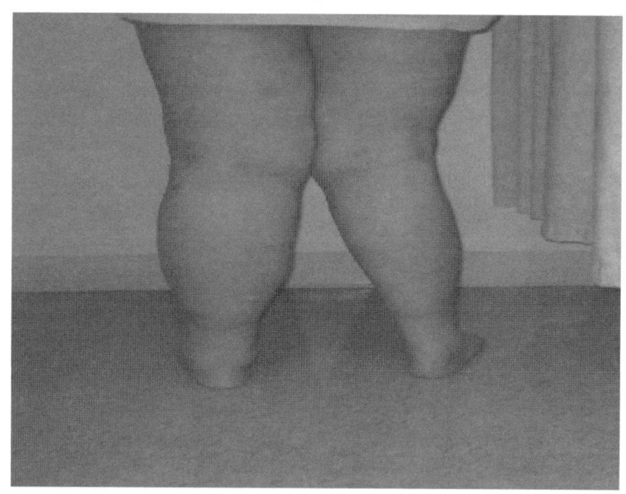

Stage 3

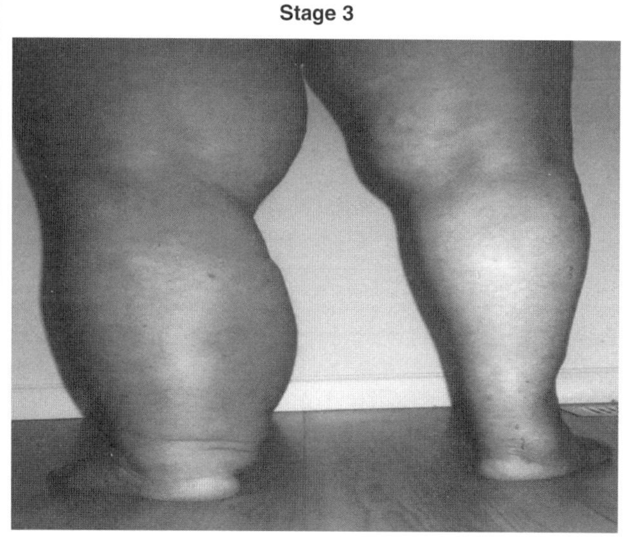

therefore, these causes must be ruled out. If there is no DVT or recurrence, prompt referral to a lymphedema specialist is warranted as early intervention holds the best chance for prevention of long-term sequelae (Armer et al., 2003). Along with pitting edema and evaluation of the skin, a positive Stemmer sign may help to determine lymphedema. A *Stemmer sign* is the inability to pinch the skin on the dorsum of the second toe or the involved extremity between the thumb and forefinger (Gary, 2007).

The most common method and easiest to use in the clinical setting for measuring lymphedema is the tape measure. Measurements are taken at specific points over time and compared to a baseline or to the opposite extremity (Brown, 2004). Water displacement is a method of placing the extremity in a water-filled container with measurement of the amount of fluid which is displaced. This method is cumbersome and difficult to execute in a clinical setting (Lockwood-Rayerman, 2007). A third measurement method is lymphoscintigraphy. This involves intradermal injections of technetium-labeled sulfur colloid into the interdigital web spaces of the dorsal foot (Szuba, Shin, Strauss, & Rockson, 2003). Serial images are taken and the pattern analyzed to assess sluggish or failed arrival of tracer in lymph nodes. Lymphoscintigraphy may be useful in questions of etiology of swelling, but results are subject to inconsistent interpretation and generally are not used for diagnosis (Cheville, 2007).

Treatment

Complex or complete decongestive therapy (CDT) is the current standard of care for lymphedema management (International Society of Lymphology, 2003). This treatment is a two phase system beginning with manual lymphatic drainage (MLD) that involves a gentle massage that starts proximally in the intact nodal areas and proceeds into the congested area. This promotes the drainage of lymph from the intact area by causing a type of siphoning action moving lymph from the congested distal extremity. MLD stimulates smooth muscle contraction in the vessel walls to encourage their inherent pumping, moving lymph into the normally functioning lymphatics (Cheville, 2007; Cheville et al., 2003; Foldi, 1998; Lerner, 1998; Leduc, Leduc, Bourgeois, & Belgrado, 1998). MLD massage is followed by compression in the form of padding and application of short stretch compression bandages. These are applied with gradual pressure changes distally to proximally. Compression is essential during CDT, resulting in improved lymphatic flow, reduction of lymph, enhanced venous return, proper shaping of the limb, sustained volume control, maintenance of skin integrity, and protection of the limb from trauma. Skin care is emphasized because cellulitis is not uncommon (Cheville, 2007; Cheville et al., 2003; International Society of Lymphology, 2003). See Figure 14-4 for an overview of treatment options. The use of pneumatic compression pumps is controversial.

Figure 14-4. Overview of Lymphedema Treatment

Manual Lymphatic Drainage (MLD)
- Start massage at body center and move to the extremities.
- Massage gently and slowly to promote central emptying and allow room for the lymph to flow from the extremity.
- Avoid deep massage or improper sequence, as this may shut down the lymph flow.

Compression Wrapping
- Bandage extremity after MLD to prevent lymph reaccumulation.
- Apply padding to protect the skin.
- Apply short stretch wraps to support without binding.
- Wrap with high pressure distally and decreasing pressure proximally.
- Teach patient to apply, remove, and reapply wrapping as needed.

Exercises
- Promote flexibility by instructing in stretching exercises.
- Encourage deep breathing exercises to increase the flow of lymph.

Skin Care
- Keep limb and skin folds clean.
- Use additive-free lotion after bathing or swimming and prior to and after use of compression garments.
- Observe daily for signs and symptoms of infection.

Compression Hosiery
- Fit individually to cover well without constriction.
- Properly fitted hosiery will help to prevent lymphedema accumulation or reaccumulation after massage.
- Hosiery may provide support during air travel when the atmospheric pressure changes.
- Replace every six months or with weight changes.

Pneumatic Compression Pumps
- Use is controversial.

Note. Based on information from Brewer et al., 2000; Cheville, 2007; Cheville et al., 2003; Foldi, 1998; Lerner, 1998; International Society of Lymphology, 2003; Mortimer, 1998; National Lymphedema Network Medical Advisory Committee, 2008a, 2008b.

It is recommended that lymphedema treatment be done by those who are trained in the proper technique. Certified therapists are often found in physical therapy departments. Patients should be referred to the National Lymphedema Network (NLN) Web site (www.lymphnet.org) for a listing of certified lymphedema specialists.

Risk Reduction Recommendations

Because of the paucity of research in lower extremity lymphedema, guidelines for care and risk reduction are based on upper extremity lymphedema recommendations for post–breast cancer treatment. However, research is lacking that supports many recommendations for prevention of lymphedema (Ridner, 2002).

Guidelines for risk reduction take into consideration that any action or condition that predisposes to or increases swelling may disrupt the fine balance of drainage after surgery (Mortimer, 1998). Mobility is encouraged as muscle contraction will aid in the flow of lymph. Exercises done in a gradual manner will promote flow and decrease the chance of inflammation that may occur as a result of sudden strenuous muscle activity. Deep breathing exercises can be done at any time of the day and in any location and will encourage the flow of lymph through the cisterna chyli. Limb constriction decreases the flow of lymph. Those with a sedentary lifestyle need to be reminded of the importance of frequent change of position and to avoid crossing their legs. The prophylactic use of compression stockings is controversial because it is essential that hose be fitted properly to avoid constriction and replaced periodically to ensure the proper fit and stretch, especially after any weight changes (Cheville, 2007).

As the skin may become fibrotic and easily infected, the use of a mild soap and the application of additive-free lotion will help to keep the skin clean and supple. Special attention to the areas between the toes and in leg creases is essential to ensure an intact skin barrier. The skin should be monitored daily for redness and warmth and the patient encouraged to call for any changes. Antibiotic ointments may be used on open skin for cellulitis prevention. Oral antibiotics may be necessary for treatment.

During air travel, the atmospheric pressure changes, and this may affect the pressure balance in the legs, resulting in swelling (NLM Medical Advisory Committee, 2008a, 2008b). Therefore, patients should be encouraged to request a seat with adequate leg room, to ambulate as often as possible, and to hydrate with nonalcoholic beverages during flights (see Figure 14-5).

Figure 14-5. Patient Education for Risk Reduction of Lower Extremity Lymphedema

Few evidence-based recommendations have been published for the prevention of lower extremity lymphedema. The following education points are meant to be used as guidelines in the prevention of either an increased volume of fluid or decreased flow in the extremity, which are thought to contribute to the development of lymphedema.

Increase Mobility
- Stress the importance of ambulation.
- Change position as often as possible.
- Perform stretching and range of motion exercises when stationary.
- Avoid crossing legs or sitting with legs at 90° angle.
- Elevate extremities whenever sitting for long periods.

Infection Prevention
- Examine extremities daily for swelling, inflammation, redness, or warmth.
- Observe for blisters, rash, change in texture, or weeping of skin.
- Use insect repellent.
- Keep extremities clean using mild soap.
- Pat skin dry; avoid brisk rubbing, especially between toes and skin creases.
- Keep skin soft using an alcohol- and additive-free moisturizer after bathing, swimming, and under compression garments.

Protect From Pressure
- Wear loose-fitting clothing and jewelry, such as toe rings.
- Wear properly fitted closed-toe shoes.
- Avoid extreme temperature changes such as saunas, heating pads, and ice packs.
- Consider the use of an electric razor.
- Use sunscreen.
- Cut nails straight across and use a file; do not cut cuticles.

Exercise
- Maintain hydration.
- Slowly progress exercise to former baseline.
- Stop activity if limb aches or tires, and elevate.

During Air Travel
- Consider the use of personally fitted compression stocking(s).
- Hydrate during flight.
- Ambulate as often as possible during flight.
- Request a seat assignment with adequate leg room.

Note. Based on information from National Lymphedema Network, 2008a, 2008b.

Quality of Life

Lymphedema may have a profound effect on the lives of cancer survivors. Many patients report that they were not notified about this risk prior to surgery (Ryan et al., 2003b). Some are frustrated when care providers have dismissed their concerns as cosmetic or have not addressed this side effect adequately (Musacari, 2004). Changes in wardrobe, employment, and interpersonal interactions often are necessary when swelling occurs. Alteration in body image may result in changes to regular social activities and possibly lead to social isolation (Ryan et al., 2003b).

The healthcare provider must be sensitive to the lifestyle modifications and financial burden that may result and force changes in occupation, wardrobe, and dealings with family and friends. Referrals to support groups or individual therapy sessions may be indicated.

Pain assessment at every physician visit is crucial in helping these patients cope. An over-the-counter medication may suffice, but some may need prescription-strength pain medication.

Fatigue has been noted to be another troublesome symptom affecting the quality of life of patients with lymphedema of the upper extremity (Armer & Porock, 2002). Recommendations to help to decrease fatigue may include pacing activities or decreasing distances to maintain stamina. Pacing activities also may deter swelling that can be associated with strenuous or long-distance exercise. Insomnia caused by leg discomfort may contribute to fatigue and needs to be assessed.

With increased survival after cancer treatment, the long-term sequelae caused by cancer treatment need to be recognized and treated. Healthcare providers must be educated about the risks and early signs of lymphedema development so they may not only assess correctly but also educate patients who are at risk. Continued research is necessary to determine the best interventions to decrease lymphedema caused by cancer treatment and to maximize quality of life.

Menopausal Management

Introduction

Menopause is a transition that normally accompanies midlife for women and signifies the end of child bearing. As women's life expectancies continue to increase into their late 70s, they can be expected to live one-third of their lifetime after this transition. The average age for a healthy woman to enter into menopause is 51 but ranges from 48 to 55 years old and best correlates with the age her mother or older sister entered menopause (Cramer, Xu, & Harlow, 1995). Officially, *menopause* is defined as 12 months after the final menstrual period; this process occurs as part of normal physiologic aging of the hypothalamic, pituitary, and ovarian functions within the body (Alexander & Andrist, 2005). The ovaries produce less estradiol, progesterone, and androgens, thus contributing to the symptoms that many—but not all—women experience. *Perimenopause* is defined as the two to five years prior to total cessation of menstruation (Alexander & Andrist). Many women experience some symptoms of menopause during this time because of the gradual systemic reduction of hormones. Symptoms typically experienced include vasomotor symptoms (hot flashes and night sweats) and irregular menses. Other possible symptoms include (Altman, Granath, Cnattingius, & Falconer, 2007)

- Decreased libido that may lead to decreased sexual function
- Irritability and mood disturbances
- Dyspareunia
- Vaginal dryness
- Itching caused by atrophy
- Nocturia
- Urinary frequency
- Stress and urge incontinence.

These become more prevalent as perimenopause progresses and can persist after the menopause transition. Vasomotor symptoms usually dissipate, but some women report symptoms 10 years into menopause. Moreover, myriad symptoms exist, but not all women experience them. The clinician needs to be sensitive to the individual and consider subjective symptoms as real to the woman and an important component of her quality of life. Other health problems can mimic natural aging and must be incorporated into the treatment plan. Adding to the dimension of the treatment for menopause is managing menopausal symptoms in a woman who is diagnosed with and treated for a gynecologic cancer.

This section focuses on the menopause transition in relation to women who are undergoing treatment and/or have completed treatment for a gynecologic cancer. The HABITS (Hormonal Replacement After Breast Cancer—Is It Safe?) trial demonstrated a fourfold increase in breast cancer events in those who used estrogen therapy or estrogen/progestin therapy (ET/EPT) (Holmberg, Anderson, & HABITS Steering and Monitoring Committees, 2004). A meta-analysis of menopausal hormone therapy after breast cancer performed by Col, Kim, and Chlebowski (2005) also showed an increased risk of recurrence.

These studies confirmed the risks associated with hormonal therapy for menopausal symptoms in women with breast cancer; however, for women with gynecologic cancers, far less evidence-based research exists. In reality, clinical management has been extrapolated from the breast cancer literature because of the paucity of data specific to patients with gynecologic cancer (Antione, Liebens, Carly, & Pastijn, 2007; Bordeleau, Pritchard, Goodwin, & Loprinzi, 2007; Bruno & Feeney, 2006; Graf & Geller, 2003).

Menopause in Patients With Gynecologic Cancer

The current standard treatments for women with gynecologic cancers include surgery, chemotherapy, and radiation, used alone or in combination. Each of these modalities has a potential to exacerbate menopausal symptoms as sequelae or facilitate an earlier than expected menopause (Rees, 2006). The expected morbidities of each modality can be more devastating when the woman experiences symptoms that may impede sexual function, including (Knobf, 2006; Penson, Wenzel, Vernte, & Cella, 2006; Pignata, Ballatori, Favalli, & Scambia, 2001; Tabano, Condosta, & Coons, 2002)

- Loss of ovarian function
- Treatment-related fatigue
- Anemia
- Nausea and vomiting
- Loss of fertility
- Changes in body image
- Alopecia
- Possible altered relationships
- Radiation- or surgery-induced vaginal shortening
- Vaginal dryness
- Atrophy and stenosis
- Urinary and gastrointestinal dysfunction.

All these modalities may have a profound long-term influence on a woman's self-image that may diminish quality of life in a cancer survivor (Auchincloss, 1995; Hamilton, 1999; Houldin, Curtis, & Haylock, 2006; Li, Samioe, & Iosif, 1999a, 1999b).

Hormonal Replacement Therapy

The issue of ET/EPT in cancer survivors remains controversial (Biglia et al., 2006). Standard therapy for a healthy woman without cancer has been ET/EPT, which reduces symptoms by 90%. However, cancer survivors, especially if premenopausal, are apt to have more severe and bothersome symptoms. Because of the controversies, conflicting data, and lack of large-sample randomized clinical trials (RCTs) in gynecologic patients, ET/EPT is generally the last intervention recommended and then only for short-term use to improve quality of life and functioning. However, the risks and benefits need to be discussed with the woman so she can make an informed decision.

The large, longitudinal, randomized Women's Health Initiative Trial suggested EPT increased the risk for breast cancer, but ET did not (Women's Health Initiative Steering Committee, 2004; Writing Group for Women's Health Initiative Investigators, 2002). Additionally, the risks for coronary heart disease, venous thrombotic events, stroke, and dementia were increased in the EPT group, whereas the ET group saw an increase in just stroke and thrombotic events. Limitations of the trial consisted of long-term usage (10 years) at higher doses in an older population of women. Questions remain regarding the safe use of ET/EPT at lower doses and for short-term use.

Because of these concerns and controversies, the majority of clinicians avoid prescribing ET/EPT during active cancer. Clinicians are hesitant to prescribe ET/EPT after treatment because of known concerns and possible long-term risks in the gynecologic cancer population. Although the recurrence risk is the highest during the first two years after diagnosis when menopausal symptoms may be at their most intolerable, clinicians remain hesitant to recommend ET/EPT during this time without concrete scientific evidence of safety gleaned from prospective RCTs. However, in certain subgroups of the gynecologic cancer patients, ET/EPT is definitely contraindicated. Generally, endometrial cancer is considered a hormone-dependent cancer, much like breast cancer, and hormone use is discouraged. The Gynecologic Oncology Group RCT of ET versus no ET for patients with early-stage endometrial cancer demonstrated that the absolute recurrence was very low at 2.1% (Barakat, Bundy, Spirtos, Bell, & Mannel, 2006), suggesting short-term therapy may be safe for women with severe symptoms not responsive to other interventions. However, the study was stopped early because of information regarding the risk of ET/EPT in the Women's Health Initiative Study (Writing Group for Women's Health Initiative Investigators, 2002). The American College of Obstetricians and Gynecologists (2007) recommends an individual approach that covers the woman's personal needs, her medical and family history, her symptoms, and the risk of bone loss. The group further suggest that ET/EPT may be contraindicated in those women with a past history of heart disease, breast cancer, and other diseases, and lifestyle interventions are encouraged. If a woman wants to use ET or EPT for relief of symptoms, it is recommended that she be given the lowest dose for the shortest time. Skouby (2002) suggested that candidates for ET/EPT be chosen based on prognostic indicators, thus permitting women with early-stage disease, minimal invasion, and well-differentiated cancers to use short-term hormones but not beyond two years.

Squamous cell carcinomas of the cervix and ovarian cancers are not hormonally linked; therefore, ET/EPT are not associated with their occurrence (Anderson et al., 2003). However, cervical adenocarcinomas behave more like endometrial cancers, so ET/EPT recommendations are equivocal in this population. The safest and most prudent approach for management of menopausal symptoms is nonhormonal therapy. A variety of interventions can be safely recommended by healthcare providers.

Nurses are at the forefront of patient care, making them key members in the multidisciplinary team that treats and manages women with gynecologic cancer. The nurse's role is to assist the woman from diagnosis through the long-term sequelae of treatments, assessing symptoms and providing education about symptom management. Written information from reliable sources can be great adjuncts to formal and informal teaching. Nurses may assist with management of physical symptoms as well as the psychosocial problems and adjustments that come with a cancer diagnosis, such as libido, sexual problems, and quality-of-life issues. Also, nurses can help women to understand the limited evidence and the unknowns regarding nonhormonal and hormonal interventions, with the goal of resolving any decisional conflict. Zibecchi, Greendale, and Ganz (2003) developed the Comprehensive Menopause Assessment tool to manage the two most common areas of symptom management: vasomotor and urogenital symptoms. This assessment can be incorporated easily into various women's clinical practice cancer care settings. Barton and Loprinzi (2004) provide knowledge and guidance for nurses regarding the management of various menopausal symptoms without the use of hormones.

Nonhormonal Menopausal Management of Vasomotor Symptoms

Vasomotor symptoms—the experience of hot flashes and night sweats—are the most common symptom experienced in menopause. Seventy-five percent of women experience these symptoms at some point during menopause (North American Menopause Society, 2004a). Hot flashes are recurrent, transient episodes of flushing and perspiration along with sensations of warmth or heat arising typically from the feet or torso to the neck and face, sometimes followed by chills; hot flashes that occur with perspiration during sleep are termed night sweats (North American Menopause Society, 2004b).

The risk factors for women experiencing vasomotor symptoms are listed in Figure 14-6. The exact reason for hot flashes is not known. However, as estrogen levels decrease,

Figure 14-6. Risk Factors for Experiencing Vasomotor Symptoms

- Surgical oophorectomy
- Premature ovarian failure
- History of premenstrual syndrome
- Higher body mass index (greater than 27 kg/m^2)
- Younger onset of menopause (before age 51)
- Cigarette smoking (active or history)

luteinizing hormone (LH) is released, which causes changes in nerve pathways, and veins to enlarge for no apparent reason. This leads to the skin flushing to a shade of red, along with an increase in perspiration and changes in blood flow, temperature, and heart rate. The number and length of time of a hot flash varies among woman, with some reporting as few as one day and others having as many as three an hour; some women may not experience any (Alexander & Andrist, 2005). No data exist comparing menopausal symptoms in gynecologic versus breast cancer survivors.

Much has been written about vasomotor and urogenital menopausal symptoms having a negative effect on mood, increasing irritability, and sleep disturbances (Li et al., 2003). However, no direct RCTs explore these direct relationships. Clinical assessment includes the prevalence, frequency, and severity (e.g., mild, moderate, severe) of the vasomotor symptoms and determination of the impact on quality of life and functioning in daily life to guide intervention. Management should focus first on lifestyle modifications, as this may be sufficient to manage mild symptoms. See Figure 14-7 for practical interventions. Although hot flashes' etiology is not truly known, they are associated with small core temperature elevations theorized to be related to the narrowing of the thermoregulatory zone that makes menopausal women more sensitive to temperature changes. Therefore, practical interventions that focus on lowering core temperatures are a first-line option (National Institutes of Health State-of-the-Science Panel, 2005). These suggestions carry no appreciable risk for patients with cancer undergoing treatment or long-term survivors. No RCTs that examine such simple interventions are available, but these recommendations are rooted in observational and anecdotal information. Their practicality makes them very useful for the gynecologic cancer population (Gross, 2006).

Figure 14-7. Practical Interventions for Vasomotor Symptoms

- Wear absorbable fabrics.
- Dress in layers.
- Lower the thermostat.
- Use personal or handheld fans.
- Keep dry linens and sleeping attire close to the bedside.
- Keep well-hydrated (2–3 liters of fluid daily).
- Avoid hot showers or baths two hours before bed.
- Avoid or limit caffeine, alcohol, and spicy foods.

Exercise

Obesity and sedentary lifestyle are related to increased hot flash occurrence in observational studies (Hammar, Berg, & Lindgren, 1990). Therefore, regular physical activity and weight control should be recommended to cancer survivors. Furthermore, daily exercise is associated with a decreased incidence of hot flashes (Wilbur, Miller, McDevitt, Wang, & Miller, 2005). The theory is that endorphins released from regular exercise help to regulate core body temperature, thus minimizing the heightened sensitivity of the thermoregulatory zone. Regular exercise promotes more restorative sleep, strengthens muscles, lessens bone loss, regulates mood, assists in weight maintenance or reduction, and decreases risk for cardiovascular disease (still the leading cause of death for women in United States). Data from the Nurses' Health Study suggests that walking three to five hours weekly significantly reduces a breast cancer survivor's risk from dying from the disease (Holmes, Chen, Feskanich, Kroenke, & Colditz, 2005).

The American Cancer Society's guidelines for exercise for cancer survivors consist of at least 30 minutes daily of moderate physical activity five times per week (Brown et al., 2003). Helpful suggestions to accomplish these goals include using stairs rather than elevators, walking to destinations, reframing activities such as housecleaning as methods of exercise, and making regular plans with friends or family that include some form of regular physical activity. These interventions can be assessed at provider visits and encouraged with positive reinforcement.

Smoking Cessation

Because women who do not smoke have fewer hot flashes than women smokers (Whiteman, Staropoli, Lengenberg, McCarter, Kierulff, & Flaws, 2003), smoking cessation is recommended to help to manage these symptoms. It is a well-accepted fact that smoking cessation significantly reduces the risk for cardiovascular disease, strokes, heart attacks, as well as cancer diagnosis and recurrence (U.S. Department of Health and Human Services [DHHS], 2004b). To date, no studies exist to demonstrate a direct correlation between hot flashes and smoking, but this recommendation should be part of a clinician's approach to management of vasomotor symptoms (Whiteman et al., 2003). Cancer survivors who still smoke may need the help of pharmacotherapy with nicotine replacement and bupropion along with psychosocial and group support (Henningfield, Fant, Buchhalter, & Stitzer, 2005). Referral to a smoking cessation specialist may assist women who have had failed attempts at smoking cessation.

Paced Respirations

Paced respirations are a slow, controlled diaphragmatic breathing that showed efficacy for control of hot flashes in four small prospective RCTs (Freedman, 2005; Freedman & Woodward, 1992; Germaine & Freedman, 1984; Irvin, Donnar, Clark, Zuttmeister, & Freidman, 1996). These studies recommend inhaling deeply and exhaling slowly for a count of 10, done 8–10 times per minute for 15 minutes twice daily. Although RCTs used small sample sizes, results suggest the use of this method to help to manage vasomotor symptoms. All studies consistently demonstrated an approximate 50% reduction in hot flash incidence and severity. In theory, this induces a relaxation response possibly affecting the body's thermoregulatory center similar to that of exercise. It involves no risk, has potential for benefit, and is considered safe for patients undergoing active cancer treatment and cancer survivors (Philip, 2003). Women who practice regular yoga breathing anecdotally report fewer hot flashes, so paced respirations suggest some underlying validity to this intervention. Two pilot studies in healthy women suggest that a structured yoga program improves the women's perceptions of the severity of their menopausal symptoms (Booth-LaForce, Thurston, & Taylor, 2007) and a 34% reduction of vasomotor symptoms (Cohen et al., 2007). These studies need replication in gynecologic cancer populations to evaluate their effectiveness in order to make this an evidence-based intervention. However, paced respirations are relatively safe, lack side effects, and may provide benefit.

Acupuncture

Two small randomized controlled trials were not very suggestive that acupuncture had benefit for vasomotor symptoms (Sandberg, Wijma, Wyon, Nedstrand, & Hammar, 2002; Wyon, Lindgren, Hammar, & Lundeberg, 1994). However, in a direct-comparison RCT of acupuncture versus the gold standard of oral estradiol treatment, both interventions demonstrated significant reduction in hot flash incidence and severity (Wyon, Wijma, Nedstrand, & Hammar, 2004). The estradiol group had a 99% reduction, compared to a 50%–83% reduction in the acupuncture group. In two randomized prospective parallel trials, acupuncture was compared to applied relaxation, ET/EPT, and a placebo. Each intervention arm showed improvement, but no improvement was demonstrated in the placebo arm (Zaborowska et al., 2007). Further investigation is warranted given that this is a viable low-risk option for the management of vasomotor symptoms.

Vitamin E

Since the 1940s, vitamin E supplementation in doses of 50–800 IU has been recommended to reduce hot flash incidence. However, the only randomized placebo-controlled crossover trial showed a clinically small difference between the two groups (one less hot flash daily) although there was a statistically significant reduction in the vitamin E group with a dose of 800 IU (Barton et al., 1998). This benefit was seen after four weeks of use, thus suggesting that it is not the most efficacious intervention. A meta-analysis suggests that more than 400 IU of vitamin E may affect or cause mortality, particularly cardiac-related (Miller et al., 2005). Vitamin E may not be as benign an intervention as once thought, and its use for vasomotor symptom management is now controversial. Until further evidence is available, clinical prudence suggests that vitamin E no longer be recommended, particularly in women at increased risk for cardiovascular disease.

Soy

The use of isoflavones and soy products remains the most popular alternative to ET/EPT in use today (Elkind-Hirsch, 2001). RCTs in the general population have suggested that women who consume soy-derived isoflavones have a lower incidence of hot flashes when compared to placebo controls (Nelson et al., 2006). However, data remain elusive regarding the estrogenicity of isoflavones, thus creating a question as to the potential risk for cancer recurrence in women with hormone-dependent cancers (North American Menopause Society, 2004a). The use of soy products in cancer survivors remains controversial because of scant scientific evidence (Hu, 2004). In clinical practice, the recommendation for use of soy products for cancer survivors should be cautious, with two to four servings weekly from food products, not supplements. Education is needed to understand that such supplements are not U.S. Food and Drug Administration regulated, nor formulated in standardized dosages. Such supplements are best utilized under the auspices of an RCT where informed consent includes standardized dosages, reliable product, and the understanding by the subject of both potential risks and possible benefits.

Black Cohosh

Black cohosh (*Cimicifuga racemosa*) is an herbal preparation known also as Remifemin® (Enzymatic Therapy, Inc.). It is endorsed by German Commission E and has been prescribed for hot flashes for more than 100 years (Blumenthal, Goldberg, & Brinckmann, 2000). Black cohosh is thought to have both estrogen-like action—suppressing LH, binding to estrogen receptors—while also having estrogen agonist properties; however, its true mechanism in the human body is unknown. Three randomized, double-blind, placebo-controlled trials have been done using black cohosh. Two trials showed no advantage over placebo (Jacobsen et al., 2001; Wuttke, Seidlova-Wurttke, & Gorkow, 2003), whereas an older trial suggested that black cohosh was more effective than ET or placebo (Warnecke, 1985). Given that black cohosh's effects on vasomotor symptoms remains contradictory and its mechanisms of action in the body are unknown, caution is necessary for survivors of breast cancer or other hormone-dependent gynecologic cancers. Furthermore, there is suggestion that black cohosh may interfere with cytotoxic drug therapies (Memorial Sloan-Kettering Cancer Center, 2008).

Antidepressants

For problematic vasomotor symptoms, prescription medications may be necessary to improve quality-of-life or function. The body's natural serotonin levels decrease when estrogen levels decrease regardless of the cause. Antidepressants that help to regulate serotonin and norepinephrine in the hypothalmus' thermoregulatory zone have been studied in menopausal women. The most promising is venlafaxine (Effexor®, Wyeth Pharmaceutics, Inc.), a combined serotonin and norepinephrine reuptake inhibitor (SNRI). In a large randomized, double-blind, placebo-controlled trial consisting of women choosing not to take ET/EPT and those with a history of breast cancer, venlafaxine at a dose of 75 mg daily reduced vasomotor symptoms by 60%, compared to a 27% reduction in the placebo group (Loprinzi et al., 2000). The benefit was seen within a one- to two-week period. Recently, a larger trial concurred with the Loprinzi trial (Carpenter et al., 2007). Venlafaxine is not hormonally activating and currently is safe to use in cancer survivors. Typical side effects include nausea, insomnia, and possible sexual dysfunction.

Trials with the selective serotonin reuptake inhibitors (SSRIs) such as paroxetine (Paxil®, GlaxoSmithKline) (Stearns et al., 2000; Stearns, Beebe, Iynengar, & Dube, 2003) and fluoxetine (Prozac®, Eli Lilly) (Loprinzi et al., 2002; Mariani et al., 2005) have shown these to be as efficacious as venlafaxine with a more than 60% reduction in vasomotor symptoms. However, concerns exist with both of these medications because they are potent inhibitors of the cytochrome P450 enzyme. Cytochrome P450 converts tamoxifen, the most widely prescribed anticancer drug, to active metabolites in the body. Given this potential to lower levels of active medication in the body and reduce tamoxifen's potency (Stearns, Johnson, et al., 2003), the benefits of risk recurrence from tamoxifen may be altered (Jin et al., 2005). The use of paroxetine or fluoxetine should not be prescribed in breast cancer survivors taking tamoxifen nor in patients with gynecologic cancer who may be taking a hormone blocker as part of their treatment. No specific RCTs have been conducted with the SSRIs or SNRIs in the gynecologic population, but this does not exclude their usage. In fact, most patients who are moderately to severely symptomatic may benefit. More specific research is needed for this population.

Gabapentin

Gabapentin, a GABA analog that has been used in a variety of neurologic and psychiatric disorders, is effective in controlling hot flashes. Its exact mechanism is unclear, but it may reduce noradrenergic hyperactivity in the central nervous system, thus controlling hot flash episodes. At a dosage of 900 mg daily, hot flashes have been shown to decrease by 45%–54%, significantly better than placebo (Guttoso, Kurlan, McDermott, & Kiebertz, 2003; Pandya et al., 2004, 2005). Although well tolerated and nonhormonal, gabapentin can cause somnolence and dizziness in the short term but resolves within a few days to several weeks. A more long-term side effect and perhaps disturbing to menopausal women is weight gain.

Menopausal Management of Other Symptoms

Urogenital

Many women in menopause experience urogenital complications because the gynecologic organs (vulva, vagina, bladder, urethra, pelvic floor musculature, and endopelvic fascia) have the most estrogen receptors anywhere in the body. Though urogenital symptoms are more insidious than vasomotor symptoms, they can be just as bothersome. Urogenital symptoms include vaginal dryness, dyspareunia, urinary incontinence, and recurrent urinary tract infections (Bruno & Feeney, 2006). Atrophy of the vagina causes dryness, pruritus, burning or soreness, discharge, and dyspareunia. Urinary atrophy causes frequency, nocturia, urgency, dysuria, and incontinence (stress, urge, or mixed) (Zebecchi, Greendale, & Ganz, 2003).

Much of the sexual dysfunction a woman experiences during and after cancer treatments may be attributed to these symptoms (Wenzel et al., 2005). Loss of libido is not related directly to estrogen but to the loss of ovarian production of testosterone that physiologically facilitates a woman's sexual drives. Some women who have had TAH/BSO report sufficient libido, whereas others have significant problems with arousal, function, and orgasm. If urogenital symptoms improve, then sexual satisfaction may improve, as vaginal dryness (the most common urogenital complaint) has the most impact on desire, arousal, and orgasm (Tabano, Condosta, & Coons, 2002).

The first recommended intervention is hydrophilic moisturizers (e.g., Lubrin®, Pharmaderm; Replens®, Lil' Drug Store Products, Inc.) used vaginally every three days. Water-based lubricants such as K-Y® (McNeill-PPC) or Astroglide® (Biofilm, Inc.) can be used as needed, prior to intercourse, masturbation, or with vaginal dilators. A vitamin E capsule can be adjunctively used as a vaginal suppository alternating with the hydrophilic moisturizer to increase relief (Auchincloss, 1995). All of these interventions are available over the counter in most local pharmacies.

Pharmacologic prescriptive interventions include topical estrogens. Prescription estrogen cream three times weekly for two to three months may be used for severe symptoms and then changed to permanent low-dose vaginal estrogen. These medications (Vagifem®, Novo Nordisk, Inc.; Estring®, Pfizer, Inc.) have the advantage of the local estrogen effect with minute systemic effect and can be recommended safely for women with breast or hormone-dependent gynecologic cancer (Knobf, 2006). Education should include encouraging regular stimulation to increase blood flow (whether self-stimulated or with a partner), longer foreplay to facilitate desire and arousal, change in positions to compensate for a shortened vagina (e.g., the woman may want to sit on top of her partner for insertion of his penis). Regular exercise to decrease fatigue and control normal body weight can improve self-image and a woman's emotional well-being that contributes to sexual health (Holmes et al., 2005; Wilbur et al., 2005).

Recommendations for managing urinary incontinence, whether stress, urge, or mixed, should include Kegel exercises. A *Kegel exercise* is a contraction of the muscle that controls urinary flow; for example, stop the urine flow midstream and hold for three to five seconds. These should be done 3 sets of 10, 3 times daily, and can be done anytime or anywhere. These easy exercises over time can increase pelvic floor tone, improve urinary and vaginal blood flow, and enhance sexual pleasure (Penson et al., 2006). After hysterectomy women are more than twice as likely to have stress incontinence (Altman, Granath, Cnattingius, & Falconer, 2007). A 10-year follow-up study showed that 66% of the women had more positive results if initially successful with their Kegel exercises (Cammu, Vany Nylen, & Amy, 2000). If symptoms persist or are more complicated, other urologic treatments may be recommended that include bladder retraining, fluid/diet management, medical devices such as pessaries, anticholinergic medications, or possibly surgery (National Institutes of Health, 2005). Referral to a urogenital specialist may be required for difficult physiologic management issues.

Other referrals for persistent sexual dysfunction may include a sexual counselor or psychologist. The woman's partner should be included in sessions to fully understand the problems and be involved in the resolution. Relationship and sexual problems may be aggravated by the additional stressors and sequelae of a gynecologic cancer.

Osteoporosis

Decreased bone mass and increased bone fragility can happen as a result of failure to achieve optimal peak bone mass by approximately age 35. Bone densitometry, or the more specific term, dual-energy x-ray absorptiometry, commonly referred to as a DEXA scan, is the gold standard for measurement of bone mineral density (Riley & Jan de Beur, 2008). The DEXA scan generates a T score, which reflects how much the bone mineral density (BMD) is above or below normal. It is a comparison of the current BMD to a normal young adult population of the same gender and is the preferred clinical guideline (DHHS, 2004a). Osteopenia (weakened bone mass as defined by T score between –1 and –2.5 and osteoporosis (T score greater than –2.5) occur in 10 million Americans, 8 million of which are women, and if a fracture occurs, 25% will die in a year from a complication (DHHS, 2004a). With declining levels of estrogen over time, osteoclastic-mediated bone loss increases (i.e., osteoclast cells breakdown bone tissue while osteoblasts form new bone tissue), and osteoblastic bone resorption decreases (Riley & Jan de Beur, 2008). Estrogen deficiency is also responsible for increased renal excretion of calcium and decreased calcium absorption in the intestines, thus elevating the parathyroid hormone levels, which in turn increase bone turnover (DHHS, 2004a). Risk factors for osteopenia and osteoporosis are outlined in Figure 14-8.

Women who develop iatrogenic menopause because of surgery, chemotherapy, radiation therapy, or hormone blockade have an increased propensity to undergo accelerated bone mineral loss, most prominently in the spine, within one to two years after becoming menopausal. Therefore, patients with gynecologic cancers are at increased risk for bone loss (Knobf, 2006). Treatment recommendations begin with assessment of risk factors, determination of baseline BMD, and education/counseling regarding bone loss and interventions to lessen it. Daily calcium intake (1,000–1,500 mg) is recommended (but in divided doses, as the intestine can only absorb 500 mg at a time), together with adequate vitamin D sources (e.g., sunlight, fortified products, egg yolks, fish, liver) or supplementation (800 IU–1,000 IU daily). Dietary management includes foods higher in calcium (see Figure 14-9 for list of specific food products). Exercise recommendations should include 30 minutes daily of regular weight-bearing and resistance exercise to preserve bone mass, prevent further loss, and build muscle to

Figure 14-8. Risk Factors for Osteoporosis

Nonmodifiable Risk Factors
- Increasing age
- Family history
- Personal history of a hip or vertebral fracture
- Celiac or Crohn disease

Modifiable Risk Factors
- Calcium intake
- Physical activity
- Smoking cessation
- Alcohol consumption
- Caffeine consumption
- Medications (e.g., glucocorticoids, aromatase inhibitors, immunosuppressive drugs, chemotherapy)
- Total body weight less than 127 pounds

Figure 14-9. Calcium-Rich Foods

- Sardines
- Dark, leafy greens
- Cheese and dairy products
- Lima beans
- Figs
- Almonds
- Oatmeal
- Broccoli

protect bone. Napoli, Thompson, Citivelli, and Armemento-Villareal (2007) suggest calcium from dietary sources in appropriate amounts provides for a better improvement in bone mineral density. Patient education is needed to help prevent falls that can lead to fractures. This education should include recommendations to clear floors of objects, keep areas well lit, add nightlights, install grab bars and extra handrails, and ensure that vision is checked and optimized with glasses, if necessary (DHHS, 2004a).

Prescription medications may be used, especially if the T score is greater than –1, for prevention and for treatment if the T score is greater than –2.5. The bisphosphonates (e.g., alendronate, risedronate, ibandronate) are used for both prevention and treatment as first-line pharmacologic interventions, one not being better than the other (Bruno & Feeney, 2007; Harvard Medical School, 2008). These are effective in preventing bone loss in premenopausal women with iatrogenic ovarian failure. The major side effect is gastrointestinal irritation. To avoid or lessen this effect, education is necessary on proper administration of the drug. If gastrointestinal problems persist or the woman is not a candidate for oral administration, IV zoledronic acid, which is another bisphosphonate, can be given once or twice yearly (Harvard Medical School, 2008). Other pharmacologic options may include the SERM raloxifene (Evista®, Eli Lilly) or calcitonin nasal spray. Parathyroid hormone, marketed as Forteo® (Eli Lilly) is an anabolic treatment that is self-injected daily. This is effective in stimulating new bone formation but is expensive, and the patient has to be taught to self-inject.

Ideally, a woman's bone health begins in childhood and continues through young adulthood with a calcium-rich diet, adequate vitamin D, and regular exercise. A woman begins losing bone mass in her mid-30s, so the emphasis on prevention begins long before a woman reaches perimenopause. For women with a gynecologic cancer, the issue of osteoporosis prevention and treatment is emphasized after treatments are completed during well-woman counseling. If the patient experiences recurrence, cancer treatment and control of treatment-related symptoms become paramount.

Summary

The issues of long-term survivorship are getting more attention in cancer care as treatments improve survival time (Houldin et al., 2006). However, research lacks prospective, longitudinal studies and RCTs that look at the specific issues of women with a gynecologic cancer who survive long-term. Evidence-based guidelines and further research, including nursing research, are needed for this population to guide clinical practice. In the interim, clinicians can use the available information to help improve symptom management and quality of life.

Special thanks to George Monemvasitis for his editorial assistance.

References

Abu-Rustum, N.R., Alektiar, K., Iasonos, A., Lev, G., Sonoda, Y., Aghajanian, C., et al. (2006). The incidence of lower extremity lymphedema following treatment of uterine corpus malignancies: A 12 year experience at Memorial Sloan-Kettering Cancer Center. *Gynecologic Oncology, 103*(2), 714–718.

Abu-Rustum, N.R., Gemignani, M.L., Moore, K., Sonoda, Y., Venkatraman, E., Brown, C., et al. (2003). Total laparoscopic radical hysterectomy with pelvic lymphadenectomy using the argon-beam coagulator: Pilot data and comparison to laparotomy. *Gynecologic Oncology, 91*(2), 402–409.

Alexander, I.M., & Andrist, L.C. (2005). Menopause. In K.D. Schuiling & F.E. Likis (Eds.), *Women's gynecologic health* (pp. 249–289). Sudbury, MA: Jones and Bartlett.

Almadrones, L., & Arcot, R. (1999). Patient guide to peripheral neuropathy. *Oncology Nursing Forum, 26*(8), 1359–1360.

Almadrones, L., Armstrong, T., Gilbert, M., & Schwartz, R. (2002). *Chemotherapy-induced neurotoxicity: Current trends in management. A multidisciplinary approach* [Monograph]. Philadelphia: Phillips Group Oncology Communications.

Almadrones, L., McGuire, D., Walzak, J., Florio, C., & Tian, C. (2004). Psychometric evaluation of two scales assessing functional status and peripheral neuropathy associated with chemotherapy for ovarian cancer: A Gynecologic Oncology Group study. *Oncology Nursing Forum, 31*(3), 615–623.

Altman, D., Granath, F., Cnattingius, S., & Falconer, C. (2007). Hysterectomy and risk of stress-urinary-incontinence surgery: Nationwide cohort study. *Lancet, 270*(9597), 1494–1499.

American College of Obstetricians and Gynecologists. (2007, June). *Hormone replacement therapy: Is it right for you?* Retrieved May 5, 2008, from http://www.acog.org/acog_districts/dist_notice.cfm?recno=1&bulletin=2321

Anderson, G.L., Judd, H.L., Kaunitz, A.M., Barad, D.H., Beresford, S.A., Pettinger M., et al., (2003). Effects of estrogen plus progestin on gynecologic cancers and associated diagnostic procedures: The Women's Health Initiative randomized trial. *JAMA, 290*(13), 1739–1748.

Antoine, C., Liebens, F., Carly, B., & Pastijn, A. (2007). Safety of alternative treatments for menopausal symptoms after breast cancer: A qualitative systematic review. *Climacteric, 10*(1), 23–26.

Armer, J.M., Radina, M.E., Porock, D., & Culbertson, S.D. (2003). Predicting breast cancer–related lymphedema using self-reported symptoms. *Nursing Research, 52*(6), 370–379.

Armer, J.M., & Porock, D. (2002). Self-management of fatigue among women with lymphedema. *Lymphology, 35*(Suppl.), 208–213.

Armstrong, D.K., Bundy, B., Wenzel, L., Huang, H.Q., Baergen, R., Lele, S., et al. (2006). Intraperitoneal cisplatin and paclitaxel in ovarian cancer. *New England Journal of Medicine, 354*(1), 34–43.

Armstrong, T., Almadrones, L., & Gilbert, M. (2005). Chemotherapy-induced peripheral neuropathy. *Oncology Nursing Forum, 32*(2), 305–311.

Auchincloss, S.S. (1995). After treatment: Psychosocial issues in gynecologic cancer survivorship. *Cancer, 76*(10), 2117–2124.

Barakat, R.R., Bundy, B.N., Spirtos, N.M., Bell, J., & Mannel, R.S. (2006). Randomized double-blind trial of estrogen replacement therapy versus placebo in stage I or II endometrial cancer: A Gynecologic Oncology Group study. *Journal of Clinical Oncology, 24*(4), 587–592.

Barton, D., & Loprinzi, C.L. (2004). Making sense of the evidence regarding nonhormonal treatments for hot flashes. *Clinical Journal of Oncology Nursing, 8*(1), 39–42.

Barton, D.L., Loprinzi, C.L., Quella, S.K., Sloan, J.A., Veeder, M.H, Egner, J.R., et al. (1998). Prospective evaluation of vitamin E for hot flashes in breast cancer survivors. *Journal of Clinical Oncology, 16*(2), 495–500.

Bennett, G.J., & Paice, J.A. (2007). Peripheral neuropathy: Experimental findings, clinical approaches. *Supportive Oncology, 5*(2), 61–63.

Bhoola, S., & Hoskins, W.J. (2006). Diagnosis and management of epithelial ovarian cancer. *Obstetrics and Gynecology 107*(6), 1399–1410.

Biglia, N., Mariani, L., Marneco, D., Robba, C., Peano, E., Kubatzki, F., et al. (2006). Hormonal replacement therapy after gynaecological cancer. *Gynäkologisch-geburtshilfliche Rundschau, 46*(4), 191–196.

Blumenthal, M., Goldberg, A., & Brinckmann, J. (2000). *Herbal medicine: Expanded commission E monographs*. Newton, MA: Integrative Medicine Communications.

Booth-LaForce, C., Thurston, R.C., & Taylor, M.R. (2007). A pilot study of a Hatha yoga treatment for menopausal symptoms. *Maturitas, 57*(3), 286–295.

Bordeleau, L., Pritchard, K., Goodwin, P., & Loprinzi, C. (2007). Therapeutic options for the management of hot flashes in breast cancer survivors: An evidence-based review. *Clinical Therapeutics, 29*(2), 230–241.

Brewer, V.H., Hahn, K.A., Rohrbach, B.W., & Baddour, L.M. (2000). Risk factor analysis for breast cellulitis complicating breast conservation therapy. *Clinical Infectious Diseases, 31*(3), 654–659.

Brown, J. (2004). A clinically useful method for evaluating lymphedema. *Clinical Journal of Oncology Nursing, 8*(1), 35–38.

Brown, J.K., Byers, T., Doyle, D., Coumeya, K.S., Denmark-Whanefried, W., Kushi, L.H., et al. (2003). Nutrition and physical activity during and after cancer treatment: An American Cancer Society guide for informed choices. *CA: A Cancer Journal for Clinicians, 53*(5), 268–291.

Bruno, D., & Feeney, K.J. (2006). Management of postmenopausal symptoms in breast cancer survivors. *Seminars in Oncology, 33*(6), 696–707.

Cadron, I., Van Gorp, T., Amant, F., Leunen, K., Neven, P., & Vergote, I. (2007). Chemotherapy for recurrent cervical cancer. *Gynecologic Oncology, 107*(1, Suppl. 1), S113–S118.

Cammu, H., Vany Nylen, M., & Amy, J.J. (2000). A 10-year follow-up after Kegel pelvic floor muscle exercises for genuine stress incontinence. *British Journal of Urology International, 85*(6), 655–688.

Carpenter, J.S., Storniolo, A.M., Johns, S., Monahan, P.O., Azzouz, F., Elam, J.L., et al. (2007). Randomized, double-blind, placebo-controlled crossover trials of venlafaxine for hot flashes after breast cancer. *Oncologist, 12*(1), 124–125.

Casley-Smith, J.R. (1997). *Grades of lymphodema: Information about lymphoedema for patients* (6th ed.). Malvern, Australia: Lymphoedema Association of Australia.

Cavaletti, G., & Zanna, C. (2002). Current status and future prospects for the treatment of chemotherapy-induced peripheral neurotoxicity. *European Journal of Cancer, 38*(14), 1832–1837.

Cerosimo, R.J. (1989). Cisplatin neurotoxicity. *Cancer Treatment Reviews, 16*(4), 195–211.

Chaudry, V., Rowinsky, E., Sartorius, S., Donehower, R., & Cornblath, D. (1994). Peripheral neuropathy for Taxol and cisplatin combination chemotherapy: Clinical and electrophysiological studies. *Annals of Neurology, 35*(3), 304–311.

Cheville, A.L. (2007). Current and future trends in lymphedema management: Implications for women's health. *Physical Medicine and Rehabilitation Clinics of North America, 18*(3), 539–553.

Cheville, A.L., McGarvey, C.L., Petrek, J.A., Russo, S.A., Taylor, M.E., & Thiadens, S.R. (2003). Lymphedema management. *Seminars in Radiation Oncology, 13*(3), 214–225.

Cohen, B.E., Kanaya, A.M., Macer, J.L., Shen, H., Chang, A.A., & Grady, D. (2007). Feasibility and acceptability of restorative yoga for treatment of hot flushes: A pilot trial. *Maturitas, 56*(2), 198–204.

Col, N.F., Kim J.A., & Chlebowski, R.T. (2005). Menopausal hormone therapy after breast cancer: A meta-analysis and critical appraisal of the evidence. *Breast Cancer Research, 7*(4), R535–R540.

Cramer, G., Xu, H., & Harlow, B.L. (1995). Family history as a predictor of early menopause. *Fertility and Sterility, 64*(4), 740–745.

Criscuolo, S., Auletta, C., Lippi, S., Brogi, F., & Brogi, A. (2004). Oxcarbazine (Trileptal®) monotherapy dramatically improves quality of life in two patients with postherpetic neuralgia refractory to carbamazepine and gabapentin. *Journal of Pain and Symptom Management, 28*(6), 535–536.

Elkind-Hirsch, K. (2001). Effect of dietary phytoestrogens on hot flushes: Can soy-based proteins substitute for traditional estrogen replacement therapy? *Menopause, 8*(3), 154–156.

England, J., Gronseth, G., Franklin, G., Miller, R., Asbury, A., Carter, G., et al. (2005). Distal symmetric polyneuropathy: A definition for clinical research: Report of the American Academy of Neurology, the American Association of Electrodiagnostic Medicine and the American Academy of Physical Medicine and Rehabilitation. *Neurology, 64*(2), 199–207.

Foeldi, M., Foeldi, E., & Dubik, S. (Eds.). (2003). *Textbook of lymphology for physicians and lymphedema therapists* [English printing of German 5th ed.] Munich, Germany: Urban and Fischer.

Foldi, E., (1998). The treatment of lymphedema. *Cancer, 83*(12, Suppl. American), 2833–2834.

Freedman, R.R. (2005). Hot flashes: Behavioral treatments, mechanisms, and relation to sleep. *American Journal of Medicine, 118*(Suppl. 12B), 124–180.

Freedman, R.R., & Woodward, S. (1992). Behavioral treatment of menopausal hot flushes: Evaluation by ambulatory monitoring. *American Journal of Obstetrics and Gynecology*, *167*(2), 436–439.

Gary, D.E. (2007). Lymphedema diagnosis and management. *Journal of the American Academy of Nurse Practitioners, 19*(2), 72–78.

Graf, M.C., & Geller, P.A. (2003). Treating hot flashes in breast cancer survivors: A review of alternative treatments to hormone replacement therapy. *Clinical Journal of Oncology Nursing, 7*(6), 637–640.

Germaine, L.M., & Freedman, R.R. (1984). Behavioral treatment of menopausal hot flashes: Evaluation by objective methods. *Journal of Consulting and Clinical Psychology, 52*(6), 1072–1079.

Gross, R.E. (2006). Evidence-based management of vasomotor symptoms in female cancer survivors. *Journal of Gynecologic Oncology Nursing, 16*(2), 18–24.

Guttoso, T., Jr., Kurlan, R., McDermott, M.P., & Kieburtz, K. (2003). Gabapentin's effects on hot flashes in postmenopausal women: A randomized controlled trial. *Obstetrics and Gynecology, 101*(2), 337–345.

Hamilton, A.B. (1999). Psychologocial aspects of ovarian cancer. *Cancer Investigator, 17*(5), 335–341.

Hammar, M., Berg, G., & Lindgren, R. (1990). Does physical exercise influence the frequency of postmenopausal hot flashes? *Acta Obstetricia et Gynecologica Scandinavica, 69*(5), 409–412.

Harvard Medical School. (2008). Eight for 2008: Eight things you should know about osteoporosis and fracture risk. *Harvard Women's Health Watch, 15*(5), 1–3.

Hausheer, F.H., Schilsky, R.L., Bain, S., Berghorn, E.J., & Lieberman, F. (2006). Diagnosis, management, and evaluation of chemotherapy-induced peripheral neuropathy. *Seminars in Oncology, 33*(1), 15–49.

Henningfield, J.E., Fant, R.V., Buchhalter, A.R., & Stitzer, M.L. (2005). Pharmacotherapy for nicotine dependence. *CA: A Cancer Journal for Clinicians, 55*(5), 281–299.

Hilkens, P.H., & ven den Bent, M.J. (1997). Chemotherapy-induced peripheral neuropathy. *Journal of the Peripheral Nervous System, 2*(4), 350–361.

Holmberg, L., Anderson, H., & HABITS Steering and Monitoring Committees. (2004). HABITS (hormonal replacement therapy after breast cancer—Is it safe?), a randomized comparison: Trial stopped. *Lancet, 363*(9407), 453–355.

Holmes, M.D., Chen, W.Y., Feskanich, D., Kroenke, C.H., & Colditz, G.A. (2005). Physical activity and survival after breast cancer diagnosis. *JAMA, 293*(20), 2479–2486.

Houldin, A., Curtiss, C.P., & Haylock, P.J. (2006). Executive summary: The state of science on nursing approaches to managing late and long-term sequelae of cancer and cancer treatment. *American Journal of Nursing, 106*(3), 54–59.

Hu, S.A. (2004). Risks and benefits of soy isoflavones for breast cancer survivors. *Oncology Nursing Forum, 31*(2), 249–263.

Hughes, R.A. (2002). Peripheral neuropathy. *BMJ (Clinical Research Edition), 324*(7335), 466–469.

International Society of Lymphology. (2003). The diagnosis and treatment of peripheral lymphedema: Consensus document of the International Society of Lymphology. *Lymphology, 36*(2), 84–91.

Irvin, J.H., Donnar, A.D., Clark, C., Zuttmeister, P.C., & Freidman, R. (1996). The effects of relaxation response training on menopausal symptoms. *Journal of Psychosomatic Obstetrics and Gynaecology, 17*(4), 202–207.

Jacobsen, J.S., Troxel, A.B., Evans, J., Klaus, L., Vahdat, L., Kinne, D., et al. (2001). Randomized trial of black cohosh for treatment of hot flashes among women with a history of breast cancer. *Journal of Clinical Oncology, 19*(10), 2739–2745.

Jemal, A., Siegel, R., Ward, E., Hao, H., Xu, J., Murray, T., et al. (2008) Cancer statistics, 2008. *CA: A Cancer Journal for Clinicians, 58*(2), 71–96.

Jin, Y., Desta, Z., Stearns, V., Ward, B., Ho, H., Lee, K.H., et al. (2005). CYP2D6 genotype, antidepressant use, and tamoxifen metabolism during adjuvant breast cancer treatment. *Journal of the National Cancer Institute, 97*(1), 30–39.

Knobf, M.T. (2006). Reproductive and hormonal sequelae of chemotherapy in women. *Cancer Nursing, 29*(Suppl. 2), 60–65.

Lerner, R. (1998). Complete decongestive physiotherapy and the Lerner Lymphedema Services. *Academy of Lymphatic Studies. Cancer, 83*(Suppl. 12), 2861–2863.

Leduc, O., Leduc, A., Bourgeois, P., & Belgrado, J.P. (1998). The physical treatment of upper arm limb edema. *Cancer, 83*(Suppl. 12), 2835–2839.

Li, C., Samioe, G., & Iosif, C. (1999a). Quality of life in endometrial cancer survivors. *Maturitas, 31*(3), 227–236.

Li, C., Samioe, G., & Iosif, C. (1999b). Quality of life in long-term survivors of cervical cancer. *Maturitas, 32*(2), 95–102.

Li, C., Samioe, G., Borgfeldt, C., Lidfeldt, J., Agardh, C.D., & Nerband, C. (2003). Menopause-related symptoms: What are the background factors? A prospective population-based cohort study of Swedish women. *American Journal of Obstetrics and Gynecology, 189*(6), 1646–1653.

Lockwood-Rayerman, S. (2007). Lymphedema in gynecologic cancer survivors: An area for exploration? *Cancer Nursing, 30*(4), E11–E18.

Loprinzi, C.L., Kugler, J.W., Sloan, J.A., Mailliard, J.A., LaVasseur, B.I., Barton, D.L., et al. (2000). Venlafaxine in management of hot flashes in survivors of breast cancer: A randomized controlled trial. *Lancet, 356*(9247), 2059–2063.

Loprinzi, C.L., Sloan, J.A., Perez, E.A., Quella, S.K., Mailliard, J.A., Halvard, M.Y., et al. (2002). Phase III evaluation of fluoxetine for treatment of hot flashes. *Journal of Clinical Oncology, 20*(6), 1578–1583.

Mariani, L., Quattrini, M., Atante, M., Galati, M., Barbati, A., & Giannarelli, D. (2005). Hot-flashes in breast cancer survivors: Effectiveness of low-dosage fluoxetine. A pilot study. *Journal of Expert Clinical Cancer Research, 24*(3), 373–378.

Marrs, J., & Newton, S. (2003). Updating your peripheral neuropathy "know-how." *Clinical Journal of Oncology Nursing, 7*(3), 299–303.

McMeekin, D.S., Alektiar, K.M., Sabbatini, P., & Zaino, R.J. (2009). Corpus: epithelial tumors. In R.R. Barakat, M. Markman, & M.E. Randall (Eds). *Principles and practice of gynecologic oncology* (5th ed.). Baltimore, MD: Lippincott Williams & Wilkins.

Meek, A.G. (1998). Breast radiotherapy and lymphedema. *Cancer, 83*(Suppl. American), 2788–2797.

Memorial Sloan-Kettering Cancer Center. (2008, October 20). *About herbs: Black cohosh.* Retrieved April 21, 2009, from http://www.mskcc.org/mskcc/html/69140.cfm

Miller, E.R., Pastor-Barriuso, R., Dalal, D., Reimersma, R.A., Appel, L.J., & Guallar, E. (2005). Meta-analysis: High dose vitamin E may increase all cause mortality. *Annals of Internal Medicine, 142*(1), 37–46.

Moffat, C.J., Franks, P.J., Doherty, D.C., Williams, A.F., Badger, C., Jeffs, E., et al., (2003). Lymphoedema: An underestimated health problem. *Quarterly Journal of Medicine, 96*(10), 731–738.

Mortimer, P.S. (1998). The pathophysiology of lymphedema. *Cancer, 83*(Suppl. 12), 2798–2802.

Musacari, E. (2004). Lymphedema: Responding to our patient's needs. *Oncology Nursing Forum, 31*(5), 905–912.

Napoli, N., Thompson, J., Citivelli, R., & Armamento-Villareal, R.C. (2007). Effects of dietary calcium compared with calcium supplements on estrogen metabolism and bone mineral density. *American Journal Clinical Nutrition, 85*(5), 1428–1433.

National Institutes of Health. (2005). *NIH consensus and state-of-the-science statements: Management of menopause-related symptoms.* Bethesda, MD: Author.

National Institutes of Health State-of-the-Science Panel. (2005). National Institutes of Health state-of-the-science conference statement: Management of menopause-related symptoms. *Annals of Internal Medicine, 142*(12, Pt. 1), 1003–1013.

National Lymphedema Network Medical Advisory Committee. (2008a). *Position statement of the National Lymphedema Network—Topic: Air travel.* Oakland, CA: National Lymphedema Network. Retrieved May 29, 2009, from http://www.lymphnet.org/pdfDocs/nlnairtravel.pdf

National Lymphedema Network Medical Advisory Committee. (2008b). *Position statement of the National Lymphedema Network—Topic: Lymphedema risk reduction practices.* Oakland, CA: National Lymphedema Network. Retrieved May 29, 2009, from http://www.lymphnet.org/pdfDocs/nlnriskreduction.pdf

Nelson, H.D., Vesco, K.K., Haney, E., Fu, R., Nedrow, A., Miller J., et al. (2006). Nonhormonal therapies for menopausal hot flashes: Systematic review and metanalysis. *JAMA, 295*(17), 2057–2071.

North American Menopause Society. (2004a). *Menopause practice: A clinician's guide.* Cleveland, OH: Author.

North American Menopause Society. (2004b). Treatment of menopause-associated vasomotor symptoms: Position statement of The North American Menopause Society. *Menopause, 11*(1), 11–33.

Ocean, A.J., & Vahdat, L.T. (2004). Chemotherapy-induced peripheral neuropathy: Pathogenesis and emerging therapies. *Supportive Care in Cancer, 12*(9), 619–625.

Pace, A., Savarese, A., Picardo, M., Maresca, V., Pacetti, U., Del Monte, G., et al. (2003). Neuroprotective effect of vitamin E supplementation in patient treated with cisplatin chemotherapy. *Journal of Clinical Oncology, 21*(5), 927–931.

Pandya, K.J., Morrow, G.R., Roscoe., J.A., Zhao, H., Hickok, J.T., Paion, E., et al. (2005). Gabapentin for hot flashes in 420 women with breast cancer: A randomized double-blind placebo-controlled trial. *Lancet, 366*(9488), 818–824.

Pandya, K.J., Thummala, A.R., Griggs, J.J., Rosenblatt, J.D., Sahasrabudhe, D.M., Guttoso, T.J., et al. (2004). Pilot study using gabapentin for tamoxifen-induced hot flashes in women with breast cancer. *Breast Cancer Research and Treatment 83*(1), 87–89.

Penson, R.T., Wenzel, L.B., Vernte, I., & Cella, D. (2006). Quality of life considerations in gynecologic cancer. FIGO 6th Annual Report on the Results of Treatment in Gynecologic Cancer. *International Journal of Gynaecology and Obstetrics, 95*(Suppl. 1), S247–S257.

Philip, H.A. (2003). Hot flashes—a review of literature on alternative and complementary treatment approaches. *Alternative Medicine Review, 8*(3), 284–302.

Pignata, S., Ballatori, E., Favalli G., & Scambia, G. (2001). Quality of life: Gynaecologic cancers. *Annals of Oncology, 12*(Suppl. 3), S37–S42.

Poncelet, A.N. (1998). An algorhythm for the evaluation of peripheral neuropathy. *American Family Physician, 57*(4), 755–764.

Quasthoff, S., & Hartung, H.P. (2002). Chemotherapy-induced peripheral neuropathy. *Journal of Neurology, 249*(1), 9–17.

Rees, M. (2006). Gynaecolgocial oncology perspective on management of menopause. *European Journal of Surgical Oncology, 32*(8), 892–897.

Ridner, S.H. (2002). Breast cancer lymphedema: Pathophysiology and risk reduction guidelines. *Oncology Nursing Forum, 29*(9), 1285–1293.

Riley, L.H., & Jan de Beur, S.M. (2008). *Back pain and osteoporosis*. Baltimore, MD: Johns Hopkins School of Medicine White Papers.

Rouzier, R., Haddad, B., Dubernard, G., Dubois, P., & Paniel, B.J. (2003). Inguinofemoral dissection for carcinoma of the vulva: Effect of modifications of extent and technique on morbidity and survival. *Journal of the American College of Surgeons, 196*(3), 442–450.

Ryan, M., Stainton, M.C., Slaytor, E.K., Jaconelli, C., Watts, S., & Mackenzie, P. (2003a). Aetiology and prevalence of lower limb lymphoedema following treatment for gynaecological cancer. *Australia and New Zealand Journal of Obstetrics and Gynaecology, 43*(2), 148–151.

Ryan, M., Stainton, M.C., Slaytor, E.K., Jaconelli, C., Watts, S., Mackenzie, P., et al. (2003b). The experience of lower limb lymphedema for women after treatment for gynecologic cancer. *Oncology Nursing Forum, 30*(3), 417–423.

Sandberg, M., Wijma, K., Wyon, Y., Nedstrand, E., & Hammar, M. (2002). Effects of electro-acupuncture on psychological distress in postmenopausal women. *Complementary Therapies in Medicine, 10*(3), 161–169.

Skouby, S. (2002). Consequences of HRT following HERSII and WHI reports. *Acta Obstetricia et Gynecologica Scandinavica, 81*, 793–798.

Smith, E., Beck, S., & Cohen, J. (2008). The total neuropathy score: A tool for measuring chemotherapy-induced peripheral neuropathy. *Oncology Nursing Forum, 35*(1), 96–102.

Stearns, V., Beebe, K.L., Iynengar, M., & Dube, E. (2003). Paroxetine controlled release in the treatment of menopausal hot flushes: A randomized controlled trial. *JAMA, 289*(21), 2827–2834.

Stearns, V., Isaacs, C., Rowland, J., Crawford, J., Ellis, M.J. Kramer, R., et al. (2000). A pilot trial assessing the efficacy of paroxetine hydrochloride (Paxil) in controlling hot flashes in breast cancer survivors. *Annals of Oncology, 11*(1), 17–22.

Stearns, V., Johnson, M.D., Rae, J., Morocho, A., Novielli, A., Bhargava, P., et al. (2003). Active tamoxifen metabolite plasma concentrations after coadministration of tamoxifen and the selective serotonin reuptake inhibitor paroxetine. *Journal of the National Cancer Institute, 95*(23), 1758–1764.

Szuba, A., Shin, W.S., Strauss, H.W., & Rockson, S. (2003). The third circulation: Radionuclide lymphscintigraphy in the evaluation of lymphedema. *Journal of Nuclear Medicine, 44*(1), 43–57.

Tabano, M., Condosta, D., & Coons, M. (2002). Symptoms affecting quality of life in women with gynecologic cancer. *Seminars in Oncology Nursing, 18*(3), 223–230.

U.S. Department of Health and Human Services. (2004a). *Bone health and osteoporosis: A report of the Surgeon General*. Rockville, MD: U.S. Department of Health and Human Services, Office of the Surgeon General.

U.S. Department of Health and Human Services. (2004b). *The health consequences of smoking, A report of the Surgeon General*. Washington, DC: U.S. Government Publishing Office.

Verstappen, C.C., Heimans, J.J., Hekman, K., & Postma, T.J. (2003). Neurotoxic complications, of chemotherapy in patients with cancer: Clinical signs and optimal management. *Drugs, 63*(15), 1549–1563.

Visovsky, C., Collins, M., Abbott, L., Aschenbrenner, J., & Hart, C. (2007). Putting evidence into practice: Evidence-based interventions for chemotherapy-induced peripheral neuropathy. *Clinical Journal of Oncology Nursing, 11*(6), 901–913.

Warnecke, G. (1985). Beeinflussung klimakterischer beschwerden durch ein Phytotherapeutikum: Erfolgreiche therapie mit *Cimicifuga*-Monoextrakt (Influence of phytotherapy on menopausal syndrome: Successful treatments with the monoextract of *Cimicifuga*). *Medizinische Welt, 36*, 871–874.

Wenzel, L., Dogan-Ates, A, Habbal, R., Berkowitz, R., Godstein, D.P, Bernstein, M., et al. (2005). Defining and measuring reproductive concerns of female cancer survivors. *Journal of the National Cancer Institute Monographs, 2005*(34), 94–98.

Werngren-Elgstrom, M., & Lidman, D. (1994). Lymphoedema of the lower extremities after surgery and radiotherapy for cancer of the cervix. *Scandinavian Journal of Plastic and Reconstructive Surgery and Hand Surgery, 28*(4), 289–293.

Whiteman, M.K., Staropoli, C.A., Lengenberg, P.W., McCarter, R.J., Kierulff, K.H., & Flaws, J.A. (2003). Smoking, body mass, and hot flashes in midlife women. *Obstetrics and Gynecology, 101*(2), 264–272.

Wickham, R. (2007). Chemotherapy-induced peripheral neuropathy: A review and implications for oncology nursing practice. *Clinical Journal of Oncology Nursing, 11*(3), 361–376.

Wilbur, J., Miller, A.M., McDevitt, J., Wang, E., & Miller, J. (2005). Menopausal status, moderate-intensity walking, and symptoms in midlife women. *Research and Theory in Nursing Practice, 19*(2), 163–180.

Willis, W.D. (2000). The nervous system. In R.M. Berne & M.N. Levy (Eds.), *Principles of physiology* (3rd ed., pp. 68–94). St. Louis, MO: Mosby.

Women's Health Initiative Steering Committee. (2004). Effects of conjugated equine estrogen in postmenopausal women with hysterectomy: The Women's Health Initiative randomized controlled trial. *JAMA, 291*(14), 1701–1712.

Writing Group for the Women's Health Initiative Investigators. (2002). Risks and benefits of estrogen plus progestin in health menopausal women: Principal results from the Women's Health Initiative randomized controlled trial. *JAMA, 288*(3), 321–333.

Wuttke, W., Seidlova-Wurttke, D., & Gorkow, C. (2003). The cimicifuga preparation BNO 1055 vs. conjugated estrogens in a double-blind placebo-controlled study: Effects on menopause symptoms and bone markers. *Maturitas, 44*(Suppl. 1), S67–S77.

Wyon, Y., Lindgren, R., Hammar, M., & Lundeberg, T. (1994). [Acupuncture against climacteric disorders? Lower number of symptoms after menopause]. *Lakartidningen, 91*(23), 2318–2322.

Wyon, Y., Wijma, K., Nedstrand, E., & Hammar, M. (2004). A comparison of acupuncture and oral estradiol treatment of vasomotor symptoms in postmenopausal women. *Climacteric, 7*(2), 153–164.

Zaborowska, E., Brynhildsen, J., Damberg, S., Fredriksson, M., Lindh-Astrand, L., Nedstrand, E., et al. (2007). Effects of acupuncture, applied relaxation, estrogens and placebo on hot flushes in postmenopausal women: An analysis of two prospective, parallel, randomized studies. *Climacteric, 10*(1), 38–45.

Zibecchi, L., Greendale, G.A., & Ganz, P.A. (2003). Comprehensive menopausal assessment: An approach to managing vasomotor symptoms and urogenital symptoms in breast cancer survivors. *Oncology Nursing Forum, 30*(3), 393–407.

APPENDIX

International Federation of Gynecology and Obstetrics Staging Classification for Gynecologic Cancer

Staging Classification by Site	
Vulva	
0	Carcinoma in situ; preinvasive carcinoma
I	Tumor confined to vulva or vulva and perineum; 2 cm or less in greatest dimension; nodes are negative
IA	Stromal invasion no greater than 1 mm
IB	Stromal invasion greater than 1 mm
II	Tumor confined to vulva or vulva and perineum; more than 2 cm in greatest dimension; nodes are negative
III	Tumor of any size with adjacent spread to the lower urethra, vagina, or the anus and/or with unilateral regional lymph node metastasis
IVA	Tumor invades any of the following: bladder mucosa, rectal mucosa, or upper urethral mucosa; or is fixed to bone and/or bilateral regional node metastases
IVB	Distant metastasis, including pelvic lymph nodes
Vagina	
0	Carcinoma in situ; intraepithelial neoplasia grade 3
I	The carcinoma is limited to the vaginal wall
II	The carcinoma involves subvaginal tissues but does not extend to the pelvic wall
III	The carcinoma extends to the pelvic wall
IV	The carcinoma extends beyond the true pelvis or involves the mucosa of the bladder or rectum; bullous edema as such does not permit a case to be allotted to Stage IV
IVA	Tumor invades bladder and/or rectal mucosa and/or extends beyond the true pelvis
IVB	Distant metastasis
Cervix Uteri	
0	Carcinoma in situ (preinvasive carcinoma)
I	Carcinoma confined to the cervix (extension to corpus should be disregarded)
IA	Invasive carcinoma diagnosed only by microscopy (all macroscopically visible lesions—even with superficial invasion—are Stage IB)
IA1	Stromal invasion no greater than 3 mm in depth and 7 mm or less in horizontal spread

(Continued on next page)

Staging Classification by Site *(Continued)*	
IA2	Stromal invasion more than 3 mm and not more than 5 mm in depth, with a horizontal spread of 7 mm or less
IB	Clinically visible lesion confined to the cervix or microscopic lesion greater than IA2
IB1	Clinically visible lesion 4 cm or less in greatest dimension
IB2	Clinically visible lesion more than 4 cm in greatest dimension
II	Tumor invades beyond the uterus but not to pelvic wall or to lower third of the vagina
IIA	Without parametrial invasion
IIB	With parametrial invasion
III	Tumor extends to pelvic wall and/or involves the lower third of the vagina and/or causes hydronephrosis or nonfunctioning kidney
IIIA	Tumor involves lower third of vagina; no extension to pelvic wall
IIIB	Tumor extends to pelvic wall and/or causes hydronephrosis or nonfunctioning kidney
IV	Carcinoma has extended beyond the true pelvis or has clinically involved the mucosa of the bladder or rectum
IVA	Tumor invades mucosa of bladder or rectum and/or extends beyond true pelvis
IVB	Distant metastasis
Corpus Uteri	
I	Tumor confined to corpus uteri
IA	Tumor limited to endometrium
IB	Tumor invades up to or less than one half of the myometrium
IC	Tumor invades more than one half of the myometrium
II	Tumor invades cervix but does not extend beyond uterus
IIA	Endocervical glandular involvement only
IIB	Cervical stromal invasion
III	Local and/or regional spread
IIIA	Tumor involves serosa and/or adnexa (direct extension or metastasis) and/or cancer cells in ascites or peritoneal washings
IIIB	Vaginal involvement (direct extension or metastasis)
IIIC	Metastasis to pelvic and/or paraaortic lymph nodes
IVA	Tumor invades bladder mucosa and/or bowel mucosa
IVB	Distant metastasis (excluding metastasis to vagina, pelvic serosa, or adnexa, and including metastasis to intraabdominal and/or inguinal lymph nodes)
Fallopian Tube	
0	Carcinoma in situ (preinvasive carcinoma)
I	Tumor confined to fallopian tube(s)
IA	Tumor limited to one tube, without penetrating the serosal surface; no ascites
IB	Tumor limited to both tubes, without penetrating the serosal surface; no ascites

(Continued on next page)

Staging Classification by Site *(Continued)*	
IC	Tumor limited to one or both tube(s), with extension onto or through the tubal serosa; or with positive malignant cells in the ascites or positive peritoneal washings
II	Tumor involves one or both fallopian tube(s) with pelvic extension
IIA	Extension and/or metastases to uterus and/or ovaries
IIB	Extension to other pelvic structures
IIC	Pelvic extension with positive malignant cells in the ascites or positive peritoneal washings
III	Tumor involves one or both fallopian tube(s) with peritoneal implants outside the pelvis and/or positive retroperitoneal or inguinal nodes
IIIA	Microscopic peritoneal metastasis outside the pelvis
IIIB	Macroscopic peritoneal metastasis outside the pelvis 2 cm or less in greatest dimension
IIIC	Peritoneal metastasis more than 2 cm in greatest dimension and/or positive retroperitoneal or inguinal lymph nodes
IV	Distant metastasis beyond the peritoneal cavity
Ovary	
I	Tumor confined to the ovaries
IA	Tumor limited to one ovary; capsule intact, no tumor on ovarian surface; no malignant cells in ascites or peritoneal washings
IB	Tumor limited to both ovaries; capsule intact, no tumor on ovarian surface; no malignant cells in ascites or peritoneal washings
IC	Tumor limited to one or both ovaries, with any of the following: capsule ruptured, tumor on ovarian surface; positive malignant cells in the ascites or positive peritoneal washings
II	Tumor involves one or both ovaries with pelvic extension
IIA	Extension and/or implants in uterus and/or tube(s); no malignant cells in the ascites or peritoneal washings
IIB	Extension to other pelvic organs; no malignant cells in the ascites or peritoneal washings
IIC	Pelvic extension with any of the following: capsule ruptured, tumor on ovarian surface; malignant cells in ascites or peritoneal washings
III	Tumor involves one or both ovaries with microscopically confirmed peritoneal metastasis outside the pelvis and/or retroperitoneal or inguinal lymph node metastasis
IIIA	Microscopic peritoneal metastasis beyond the pelvis
IIIB	Macroscopic peritoneal metastasis beyond the pelvis 2 cm or less in greatest dimension
IIIC	Peritoneal metastasis beyond pelvis more than 2 cm in greatest dimension and/or positive retroperitoneal or inguinal lymph nodes
IV	Distant metastasis beyond the peritoneal cavity
Gestational Trophoblastic Disease	
I	Disease strictly confined to the uterine corpus
II	Disease extends to the adnexa or to the vagina, but limited to the genital structures
III	Disease extends to the lungs, with or without known genital tract involvement
IV	All other metastatic sites

Note. From *Staging Classifications and Clinical Practice Guidelines for Gynaecological Cancers* (3rd ed., pp. 7, 26, 39, 64, 85, 97, & 129), by S. Pecorelli, H.Y.S. Ngan, and N.F. Hacker (Eds.), 2006, London, UK: International Federation of Gynecology and Obstetrics (FIGO).

World Health Organization Risk Factor Scoring With FIGO Staging for Gestational Trophoblastic Disease

	Score			
Prognostic Factor	**0**	**1**	**2**	**4**
Age (years)	< 40	≥ 40	–	–
Antecedent pregnancy	Hydatidiform mole	Abortion	Term	–
Interval from index pregnancy (months)	< 4	4–6	7–12	> 12
Pretreatment hCG (Milli mIU/ml)	$< 10^3$	10^3–10^4	10^4–10^5	$> 10^5$
Largest tumor, including uterus	–	3–4 cm	≥ 5 cm	–
Sites of metastases, including uterus	Lung	Spleen, kidney	Gastrointestinal tract	Brain, liver
Number of metastases identified	–	1–4	5–8	> 8
Previous failed chemotherapy	–	–	Single drug	Two or more drugs

The identification of an individual patient's stage and risk score will be expressed by allotting a Roman numeral to the stage and an Arabic numeral to the risk score, separated by a colon. Total score is interpreted as follows: low risk, 0–4; intermediate risk, 5–7; high risk, ≥ 8.

Note. From *Staging Classifications and Clinical Practice Guidelines for Gynaecological Cancers* (3rd ed., p. 130), by S. Pecorelli, H.Y.S. Ngan, and N.F. Hacker (Eds.), 2006, London, UK: International Federation of Gynecology and Obstetrics (FIGO).

Index

The letter f *after a page number indicates that relevant content appears in a figure; the letter* t, *in a table.*

A

abdominal distention/pain, management of, 159*t*
ablation, for preinvasive cervical disease, 42
acetic acid, and vaginal cancer, 132–133
actinomycin-D
  for gestational trophoblastic neoplasia, 119, 119*t*–121*t*
  for ovarian germ cell tumors, 94, 96
acupuncture, for menopausal symptoms, 173
ADC. *See* adenosquamous carcinoma
adenocarcinoma
  of cervix, 47, 50*t*
  of vagina, 132
adenocarcinoma in situ (AIS), 38
  management of, 41*t*
adenoid cystic carcinoma, of cervix, 50*t*
adenoma malignum, of cervix, 50*t*
adenosquamous carcinoma (ADC)
  of cervix, 50*t*
  HPV and, 19
adventitia, 8
African American women
  and cervical cancer, 18
  and endometrial cancer, 28, 63, 65
  and epithelial ovarian cancer, 75
  and ovarian germ cell tumors, 92
  and trophoblastic disease, 114
AGC. *See* atypical glandular cells
age, and ovarian cancer, 24
air travel, and lymphedema, 169
AIS. *See* adenocarcinoma in situ
AJCC. *See* American Joint Committee on Cancer
alendronate, for osteoporosis, 176
alfa interferon, and peripheral neuropathy, 164*t*
alkylating agents, side effects of, 153*t*
alopecia, management of, 156*t*
alpha-fetoprotein, with ovarian germ cell tumors, 92, 93*t*
alpha-tocopherol, for peripheral neuropathy, 165
altretamine, for epithelial ovarian cancer, 84*f*
amenorrhea, 13–14
American Indian women, and epithelial ovarian cancer, 75
American Joint Committee on Cancer (AJCC), on staging of cervical cancer, 51
amiodarone, and peripheral neuropathy, 164*t*
amitriptyline, and peripheral neuropathy, 164*t*–165*t*
ampulla, 7
anastrozole, for epithelial ovarian cancer, 84*f*
androgens, 4
anemia, management of, 154*t*
anesthetics, local, for peripheral neuropathy, 165*t*
anorexia, management of, 156*t*
anterior pelvic exenteration, 140, 141*f*
anthracycline, for gynecologic sarcomas, 108
antibiotics
  for alteration in vaginal mucous membranes, 160*t*
  for infection, 154*t*
  for lymphedema, 169
  side effects of, 153*t*
anti-CA-125 monoclonal antibody, for epithelial ovarian cancer, 83
anticonvulsant drugs, for peripheral neuropathy, 165, 165*t*
antidepressants
  for menopausal symptoms, 174
  for peripheral neuropathy, 165*t*
antimetabolite agents, side effects of, 153*t*
anxiety, management of, 149, 150*t*
apoptosis, 117
appendix, epithelial ovarian cancer and, 80
areola, 11
aromatase inhibitors
  for endometrial cancer, 69
  for epithelial ovarian cancer, 84*f*
arometase inhibitor, side effects of, 153*t*
arzoxifene, and endometrial cancer, 64
ASC-H. *See* atypical squamous cells—cannot rule out high grade lesion
ASCUS. *See* atypical squamous cells of undetermined significance
Ashkenazi Jewish women, and ovarian cancer, 24, 77
Asian women
  and ovarian germ cell tumors, 92
  and trophoblastic disease, 114
aspirin, contraindications to, 154*t*
Astroglide®, for menopausal symptoms, 174
atypical glandular cells (AGC), 38
  excision of, 41
  management of, 41*t*, 42
atypical squamous cells—cannot rule out high grade lesion (ASC-H), 38, 38*t*
  management of, 41*t*
atypical squamous cells of undetermined significance (ASCUS), 37–38, 38*t*
  management of, 41*t*
autonomic nerves, 163

B

Bartholin glands, 9
Bartholinitis, 10
Bassett-Way operation, 129
benign, term, 1
BEP protocol
  for gestational trophoblastic neoplasia, 120, 121*t*
  for ovarian germ cell tumors, 94, 95*t*
  for sex cord stromal tumors, 98

Bethesda system (TBS), 37–38, 38*t*
bevacizumab (Avastin®)
  for cervical cancer, 58
  emetic risk potential of, 158*t*
  for endometrial cancer, 71
  for epithelial ovarian cancer, 84, 84*f*
  side effects of, 153*t*
bilateral salpingo-oophorectomy (BSO)
  for hereditary EOC, 77
  for ovarian germ cell tumors, 93
  in pelvic exenteration, 140
  for sex cord stromal tumors, 97
biopsy
  in diagnosis of cervical cancer, 50
  in diagnosis of preinvasive cervical disease, 41
  in diagnosis of vaginal cancer, 132–133
  in diagnosis of vulvar cancer, 129
  endometrial, 66–67, 67*f*
bisphosphonates
  for osteoporosis, 176
  side effects of, 176
black cohosh, for menopausal symptoms, 173
black women. *See* African American women
bladder dysfunction, radical hysterectomy and, 52
bleeding
  dysfunctional uterine, 13
  management of, 152*t,* 154*t*
  vaginal, 66, 107
bleomycin
  emetic risk potential of, 158*t*
  for gestational trophoblastic neoplasia, 120, 121*t*
  for ovarian germ cell tumors, 94, 95*t,* 96
  for sex cord stromal tumors, 98
  side effects of, 153*t*
  for vulvar cancer, 131
blood-brain barrier, 163
body image alteration, nursing care for, 151*t*
bortezomib, and peripheral neuropathy, 163
bowel alterations, management of, 150*t*–151*t*
bowel obstruction, management of, 160*t*
Bowen disease, 127–128
  incidence of, 127–128
  risk factors for, 128
brachytherapy
  for cervical cancer, 53, 55–56
  for endometrial cancer, 70
  nursing care for, 161*t*
  for vaginal cancer, 134–135
  for VAIN, 133
BRCA1 gene, and ovarian cancer, 24, 75–77, 76*t*
BRCA2 gene, and ovarian cancer, 24, 75–77, 76*t*
breast-feeding, and ovarian cancer, 25
breast-ovarian syndrome, hereditary, 24, 24*f*
breasts, 11, 12*f*
  abcess, 11
  benign pathophysiology of, 11
breathing techniques
  for lymphedema, 169
  for menopausal symptoms, 172–173
BSO. *See* bilateral salpingo-oophorectomy
bupropion, for smoking cessation, 172

C

CA-125, 27
  and epithelial ovarian cancer, 78–79, 85
  and ovarian germ cell tumors, 92
calcitonin, for osteoporosis, 176
calcium
  foods rich in, 175*f*
  for osteoporosis, 175–176
capecitabine, for epithelial ovarian cancer, 84*f*
carbamazepine, for peripheral neuropathy, 165*t*
carboplatin
  emetic risk potential of, 158*t*
  for endometrial cancer, 71
  for epithelial ovarian cancer, 80–81
  for gynecologic sarcomas, 108
  for ovarian germ cell tumors, 94
  and peripheral neuropathy, 163
  for sex cord stromal tumors, 98
  side effects of, 153*t*
carcinoma in situ (CIS), 38*t*
  vaginal, 133
carcinosarcoma, 106
  survival rates with, 105*t,* 106
cardiac toxicity, management of, 157*t*
CD10, and endometrial stromal sarcoma, 105
CDT. *See* complete decongestive therapy
cervical cancer
  barriers to screening for, 42
  bulky, treatment of, 55–56
  challenges with, 21
  diagnosis of, 50
  diagnostic tests for, 38–39
  education on, 20–21
  follow-up for, 57
  future directions in, 58
  histology of, 47, 50*t*
  incidence of, 17, 47, 48*f*
  invasive, 47–61
  metastasis of, 51, 56
  microinvasive, treatment of, 53
  mortality rates with, 17, 37, 47, 49*f*
  palliative care for, 57–58
  pathophysiology of, 17
  and pregnancy, 57
  preinvasive, 37–45
  prevention and early detection of, 17–23
  recurrent, 56–57
  risk factors for, 17–18, 18*f*
  screening for, 22–23, 38, 47
  signs and symptoms of, 47–50
  staging of, 51, 181–182
  treatment of, 51–57
  types of, 47
cervical cone biopsy, 41
cervical intraepithelial neoplasia (CIN), 17, 37
  management of, 40–41
cervical sampling, additional, rationale for, 39, 40*f*
cervical sarcomas, 106–107
  incidence of, 103
cervix, 7–8, 17
  benign pathophysiology of, 8
  evaluation of, 37–38
chemotherapy, 149–158, 153*t*–157*t*
  for cervical cancer, 52, 55–56
  and emetic risk potential, 158*t*
  for endometrial cancer, 70–71
  for EOC, 82–83, 82*t*
  for epithelial ovarian cancer, 79–83
  for gestational trophoblastic neoplasia, 118–120, 119*t,* 120*f,* 120*t*–121*t*
  for gynecologic sarcomas, 107–108
  nursing care for, 159*t*
  oral, 85
  for ovarian germ cell tumors, 94, 95*t*
  for placental site trophoblastic tumor, 122
  in pregnancy, 57
  for recurrent epithelial ovarian cancer, 84, 84*f*
  for sex cord stromal tumors, 98
  side effects of, 82–83, 85, 136, 149
  for vaginal cancer, 131, 135–136
  for vulvar cancer, 130–131
chemotherapy-induced peripheral neuropathy (CIPN), 163–166
  diagnosis of, 164
  incidence of, 164
  symptoms of, 164
chlamydia, 12–13
Chlamydia trachomatis, 13
choriocarcinoma, 113, 118
  incidence of, 114
chorionic villi, in trophoblastic disease, 115–116
cigarette smoking
  and cervical cancer, 18
  and endometrial cancer, 65–66
  and menopausal symptoms, 172
  and vulvar intraepithelial neoplasia, 40
cilia, 7
cimetadine, and peripheral neuropathy, 164*t*
Cimicifuga racemosa, for menopausal symptoms, 173
CIN. *See* cervical intraepithelial neoplasia
CIPN. *See* chemotherapy-induced peripheral neuropathy
CIS. *See* carcinoma in situ
cisplatin
  for cervical cancer, 56–58
  emetic risk potential of, 158*t*
  for endometrial cancer, 70
  for epithelial ovarian cancer, 81–82
  for gestational trophoblastic neoplasia, 120, 121*t*
  for gynecologic sarcomas, 108
  for ovarian germ cell tumors, 94, 95*t,* 96
  and peripheral neuropathy, 163–164
  for sex cord stromal tumors, 98
  side effects of, 153*t*
  for vaginal cancer, 136
  for vulvar cancer, 131
cisterna chyli, 166
citalopram, for peripheral neuropathy, 165*t*
citrovorum factor, for gestational trophoblastic neoplasia, 119*t*
CKC. *See* cold knife conization
clear cell adenocarcinoma
  of cervix, 50*t*
  of vagina, 134*t*

clitoris, 9, 10*f*
clomipramine, for peripheral neuropathy, 165*t*
clonidine, for peripheral neuropathy, 165*t*
coasting, 164
colchicine, and peripheral neuropathy, 164*t*
cold knife conization (CKC), 50
colostomy
  care of, 148*f*
  pelvic exenteration and, 147, 147*f*
colposcopy, 39–40, 50, 129
  abnormal findings in, 39*t*
  follow-up for, 42
complete decongestive therapy (CDT), 168
compression devices, for lymphedema, 168, 168*t*, 169
computed tomography (CT)
  and epithelial ovarian cancer, 78
  and staging of cervical cancer, 51, 58
  and trophoblastic disease, 117
condyloma acuminatum. *See* warts
cone biopsy, 41
conization, 41
  cold knife, 50
constipation, management of, 150*t*
continent urostomy, care of, 148*f*
cortex, 3, 5
corticosteroids
  for alteration in vaginal mucous membranes, 160*t*
  for peripheral neuropathy, 165*t*
cryotherapy
  for mucositis, 155*t*
  for preinvasive cervical disease, 42
CT. *See* computed tomography
cyclophosphamide
  emetic risk potential of, 158*t*
  for epithelial ovarian cancer, 84*f*
  for gestational trophoblastic neoplasia, 119, 120*t*
  for ovarian germ cell tumors, 94, 96
  for sex cord stromal tumors, 98
  side effects of, 153*t*
cystectomy, total, in pelvic exenteration, 140
cystitis, management of, 159*t*
cysts
  breast, 11
  ovarian, 6

D

dapsone, and peripheral neuropathy, 164*t*
darbepoetin alfa, for fatigue, 150*t*
deep vein thrombosis (DVT)
  in lymphedema, 167
  pelvic exenteration and, 143, 146
desipramine, for peripheral neuropathy, 165*t*
dexamethasone, for peripheral neuropathy, 165*t*
DEXA scan, 175
diabetes
  and endometrial cancer, 65
  and peripheral neuropathy, 165
diarrhea, management of, 151*t*
diet
  and endometrial cancer, 29, 66
  and ovarian cancer, 24–25
diphenhydramine, for gestational trophoblastic neoplasia, 121*t*
docetaxel
  emetic risk potential of, 158*t*
  for epithelial ovarian cancer, 81, 84*f*
  for gynecologic sarcomas, 108
  and peripheral neuropathy, 163
  side effects of, 153*t*
doxepin, for peripheral neuropathy, 165*t*
doxorubicin
  emetic risk potential of, 158*t*
  for endometrial cancer, 70
  for epithelial ovarian cancer, 84*f*
  for gynecologic sarcomas, 108
  for sex cord stromal tumors, 98
  side effects of, 153*t*
  for vaginal cancer, 136
DVT. *See* deep vein thrombosis
dysfunctional uterine bleeding (DUB), 13
dysgerminoma, 91
  chemotherapy for, 94
dysmenorrhea, 13
dysplasia, term, 37
dyspnea, management of, 159*t*

E

EBRT. *See* external beam radiation therapy
ECC. *See* endocervical curettage
edema, pelvic exenteration and, 146
education. *See* patient education
EGFRs. *See* epidermal growth factor receptors
EIN. *See* endometrial intraepithelial neoplasia
electrolyte alterations, management of, 156*t*
EMA-CO protocol
  for gestational trophoblastic neoplasia, 119–120, 120*f*, 120*t*
  for placental site trophoblastic tumor, 122
embolism, pulmonary, with surgery, prevention/management of, 152*t*
emotional issues, 1
endocervical curettage (ECC), 39, 50, 67, 67*f*
endometrial biopsy, 66–67
  instruments used in, 67*f*
endometrial cancer, 63–73
  clinical presentation of, 66
  comorbidity with, 65
  diagnostic evaluation of, 66–67
  epidemiology of, 63–64
  etiology of, 63
  future trends in, 71
  incidence of, 63
  mortality rates with, 64
  occult, 68
  prevention and early detection of, 28–31
  prognosis in, 68*f*
  recurrent, 71
  risk factors for, 28–30, 64–65, 66*t*, 68*f*
  risk reduction and protective effects, 65–67
  screening for, 30–31, 66
  staging of, 67
  treatment of, 67–71
endometrial hyperplasia, 30
  classification of, 66, 66*t*
endometrial intraepithelial neoplasia (EIN), 66
endometrial sampling, 31
endometrial stromal nodule, 105–106
endometrial stromal sarcoma (ESS)
  etiology and epidemiology of, 105–106
  mortality rates with, 105
  recurrent, 105
  survival rates with, 105, 105*t*
  types of, 105
endometriosis, 7–8
  and epithelial ovarian cancer, 76
endometrium, 7, 63, 66
environmental factors
  and epithelial ovarian cancer, 76
  and ovarian cancer, 24–25
EOC. *See* epithelial ovarian cancer
EP-EMA protocol
  for gestational trophoblastic neoplasia, 121*t*
  for placental site trophoblastic tumor, 122
epidermal growth factor receptors (EGFRs), in trophoblastic disease, 118
epipodophyllotoxin group, side effects of, 153*t*
epirubicin
  emetic risk potential of, 158*t*
  side effects of, 153*t*
epithelial ovarian cancer (EOC), 75–89
  advanced-stage, treatment of, 81, 82*t*
  consolidation therapy for, 83
  diagnostic testing for, 78
  early-stage, 80–81, 81*f*
  epidemiology of, 75–76
  future outlook for, 85–86
  maintenance therapy for, 83
  metastasis of, 79
  pathology classifications of, 80, 80*t*
  prognosis in, 80
  protective factors for, 75, 76*f*
  recurrent, 84–85, 84*f*
  risk factors for, 75–76, 76*f*
  staging surgery for, 79–80
  surveillance for, 83–84
  survival rates with, 75
  symptoms of, 77–78, 78*f*
  treatment of, 80–85, 84*f*
epoetin alfa, for fatigue, 150*t*
EP protocol, for sex cord stromal tumors, 98
erlotinib
  for cervical cancer, 58
  for epithelial ovarian cancer, 84*f*
ERT. *See* estrogen replacement therapy
ESS. *See* endometrial stromal sarcoma
estradiol, 4, 14
Estring®, for menopausal symptoms, 174
estrogen, 3–4
  for alteration in vaginal mucous membranes, 160*t*
  and epithelial ovarian cancer, 75
  and gynecologic sarcomas, 104
  for menopausal symptoms, 174
  obesity and, 64
  for premalignant vaginal lesions, 42

estrogen replacement therapy (ERT), 171
and endometrial cancer, 29, 64
and gynecologic sarcomas, 106
and ovarian cancer, 25
ethnicity
and epithelial ovarian cancer, 77
See also race
etoposide
emetic risk potential of, 158*t*
for epithelial ovarian cancer, 84*f*
for gestational trophoblastic neoplasia, 119–120, 120*t*–121*t*
for ovarian germ cell tumors, 94, 95*t*, 96
and peripheral neuropathy, 163
for sex cord stromal tumors, 98
side effects of, 153*t*
evidence-based practice, and trophoblastic disease, 122
excision
in diagnosis of cervical cancer, 50
for preinvasive cervical disease, 41
exemestane, for epithelial ovarian cancer, 84*f*
exenteration. *See* pelvic exenteration
exercise
and endometrial cancer, 31
for lymphedema, 168*t*, 169
for menopausal symptoms, 172
for osteoporosis, 175
and sexual health, 175
external beam radiation therapy (EBRT)
nursing care for, 159*t*–160*t*
for vaginal cancer, 134–135
external os, 8
extracellular fluid, 166

F

fallopian tube, 5*f*, 6–7
benign pathophysiology of, 7
carcinoma of, 75
staging of cancer of, 182–183
falls, prevention of, 176
family education, and pelvic exenteration, 146
fatigue
lymphedema and, 169
management of, 149, 150*t*
female reproductive system, 1
external, 9–10, 10*f*
internal, 3–9, 4*f*
lymphatic drainage of, 10
nursing care and, 14
female sexuality, 11–12
See also sexual function
fentanyl, for peripheral neuropathy, 165*t*
fertility-sparing treatment
for cervical cancer, 53–54
for endometrial cancer, 69
for epithelial ovarian cancer, 79
for gynecologic sarcomas, 107
for ovarian germ cell tumor, 93–94
fertilization, 7
fibroadenoma, 11
fibromas, characteristics and treatment of, 99*t*
field effect, 131
FIGO. *See* International Federation of Gynecology and Obstetrics
filgrastim, 120*t*–121*t*
for infection, 154*t*
fimbriae, 7
fistula, vaginal, 9
flap, in pelvic exenteration
care of, 147
gracilis, 141–142, 145*f*
modified Singapore, 141–142, 144*f*
pudendal thigh, 141–142, 144*f*
rectus abdominis myocutaneous, 141–142, 144*f*
fluid retention, management of, 157*t*
5-fluorouracil (5-FU)
emetic risk potential of, 158*t*
management of side effects of, 155*t*
for premalignant vaginal/vulvar lesions, 42
side effects of, 153*t*
for vaginal cancer, 136
for VAIN, 133
for vulvar cancer, 131
fluoxetine (Prozac®)
contraindications to, 174
for menopausal symptoms, 174
for peripheral neuropathy, 165*t*
folinic acid, for gestational trophoblastic neoplasia, 120
follicles, 3, 5–6
follicle-stimulating hormone (FSH), 4
follicular/proliferative phase, 4–5, 6*f*
fornix, 8
5-FU. *See* 5-fluorouracil

G

gabapentin
for menopausal symptoms, 174
for peripheral neuropathy, 165, 165*t*
side effects of, 174
galactocele, 11
gastrointestinal complications, pelvic exenteration and, 146–147
gemcitabine
emetic risk potential of, 158*t*
for epithelial ovarian cancer, 84*f*
for gynecologic sarcomas, 108
side effects of, 153*t*
genetic factors
and endometrial cancer, 29–30, 64–65
and epithelial ovarian cancer, 76–77, 76*t*
and gestational trophoblastic disease, 114
and ovarian cancer, 24
testing for, 76*t*, 77
gestational trophoblastic disease (GTD), 113–117
chromosomal characteristics of, 114
clinical presentation of, 114–115
diagnostic evaluation of, 115–116
etiology of, 114
incidence of, 113–114
management of, 116–117
risk factors for, 184
staging of, 183–184
gestational trophoblastic neoplasia (GTN), 113, 117–120
classification of, 118
follow-up for, 120
incidence of, 114
management of, 118–120, 119*t*, 120*f*, 120*t*–121*t*
risk factors for, 114*f*
staging of, 118, 119*t*
survival rates with, 119
gonadotropin-releasing hormone agonists, for endometrial cancer, 69
gonadotropin-releasing hormone (GnRH), 4
gonorrhea, 12
gracilis flap, 141–142, 145*f*
granisetron, for gestational trophoblastic neoplasia, 121*t*
granulosa stromal cell tumors, 96
GTD. *See* gestational trophoblastic disease
GTN. *See* gestational trophoblastic neoplasia
gynandroblastoma, characteristics and treatment of, 99*t*
gynecologic cancers, 1–2
acute symptom management for, 149–162, 150*t*–151*t*
long-term symptom management for, 163–180
prevention and early detection of, 17–36
resources on, 158*f*
staging of, 181–184
gynecologic oncologists, 1
and epithelial ovarian cancer, 79–80
and ovarian germ cell tumors, 93–94
and pelvic exenteration, 140
and vaginal cancer, 132
and vulvar cancer, 127
gynecologic sarcomas, 103–111
etiology and epidemiology of, 103–107
incidence of, 103
recurrent, 108
risk factors for, 103
staging of, 107
treatment of, 107–108

H

HCG. *See* human chorionic gonadotropin
HDR. *See* high-dose brachytherapy
hereditary nonpolyposis colorectal cancer (HNPCC), 24, 24*f*, 64–65, 76*t*, 77
hereditary syndromes, and ovarian cancer, 24, 24*f*
HER2/neu gene, and epithelial ovarian cancer, 80
herpes, genital, 12–13
high-dose brachytherapy (HDR), for cervical cancer, 53
high-grade endometrial stromal sarcoma, 105
high-grade squamous intraepithelial lesion (HSIL), 37–38, 38*t*
management of, 41*t*
Hispanic American women
and cervical cancer, 18
and epithelial ovarian cancer, 75
HIV. *See* human immunodeficiency virus
HNPCC. *See* hereditary nonpolyposis colorectal cancer

hormonal factors
and endometrial cancer, 29
and ovarian cancer, 25
hormone replacement therapy (HRT), 171
and endometrial cancer, 29
and ovarian cancer, 25
hormone therapy, for endometrial cancer, 69
hot flashes, 171–172
management of, 171–174, 172*f*
HPV. *See* human papillomavirus
HPV DNA testing, in management of preinvasive cervical disease, 40–41
HRT. *See* hormone replacement therapy
HSIL. *See* high-grade squamous intraepithelial lesion
human chorionic gonadotropin (HCG)
with ovarian germ cell tumors, 92, 93*t*
in trophoblastic disease, 116–118
human immunodeficiency virus (HIV), 13
and HPV, and preinvasive cervical disease, 42
human papillomavirus (HPV), 8, 13
and cervical cancer, 17–18, 18*f*, 37
controversies on, 21
epidemiology of, 18–20
and HIV, and preinvasive cervical disease, 42
persistent, 19
testing for, 39
transmission of, 20
types associated with genital lesions, 20*t*
vaccination for, 13, 20, 20*f*
and vulvar intraepithelial neoplasia, 39, 127
Hybrid Capture 2 test, 22
hydralazine, and peripheral neuropathy, 164*t*
hydromorphone, for peripheral neuropathy, 165*t*
hyperemesis gravidarium, in trophoblastic disease, 115
hypersensitivity reactions, management of, 157*t*
hypertension, and endometrial cancer, 65
hyperthyroidism, in trophoblastic disease, 115
hysterectomy
for cervical cancer, 52–53
for endometrial hyperplasia, 30
for gestational trophoblastic neoplasia, 119
and incontinence, 175
for ovarian germ cell tumors, 93
for placental site trophoblastic tumor, 122
and sexual function, 53
for trophoblastic disease, 116

I

ibandronate, for osteoporosis, 176
ifosfamide
emetic risk potential of, 158*t*
for epithelial ovarian cancer, 84*f*
for gynecologic sarcomas, 108
for ovarian germ cell tumors, 96
side effects of, 153*t*
ileal conduit, care of, 148*f*
imipramine, for peripheral neuropathy, 165*t*
imiquimod, for premalignant vaginal/vulvar lesions, 42
immunohistochemical staining
and endometrial stromal sarcoma, 105
and trophoblastic disease, 115–116
immunomarkers, and epithelial ovarian cancer, 80
immunosuppression, and cervical cancer, 18
infection, management of, 152*t*, 154*t*
infertility, and epithelial ovarian cancer, 76
infundibulum, 7
inhibin, and sex cord stromal tumors, 97
insomnia, lymphedema and, 169
internal os, 8
International Federation of Gynecology and Obstetrics (FIGO), on staging of cervical cancer, 51
International Union Against Cancer, on staging of cervical cancer, 51
intraperitoneal chemotherapy
for EOC, 82–83, 82*t*
nursing care for, 159*t*
side effects of, 82–83
intrauterine device (IUD)
and endometrial cancer, 65
progestin-secreting, for endometrial cancer, 69
and trophoblastic disease, 117
intravaginal radiation therapy (IVRT)
effects of, 70
for endometrial cancer, 70
invasive cervical cancer, 47–61
invasive mole, 118
incidence of, 114
IP chromic phosphate, for epithelial ovarian cancer, 83
irinotecan
emetic risk potential of, 158*t*
side effects of, 153*t*
irregular uterine bleeding, 13
isoflavones
and endometrial cancer, 66
for menopausal symptoms, 173
isoniazid, and peripheral neuropathy, 164*t*
IUD. *See* intrauterine device
IVRT. *See* intravaginal radiation therapy
ixabepilone, for epithelial ovarian cancer, 84*f*

J

Japan, gestational trophoblastic disease in, 114
juvenile granulosa cell tumors, characteristics and treatment of, 99*t*

K

kaempferol, 25
Kegel exercises, 175
keratinizing squamous cell carcinoma, of cervix, 50*t*
knowledge deficit. *See* patient education
koilocytosis, 37
K-Y®, for menopausal symptoms, 174

L

labia majora, 9, 10*f*
labia minora, 9, 10*f*
lactate dehydrogenase (LDH), with ovarian germ cell tumors, 92, 93*t*
Lactobacillus acidophilus, 8
laparoscopically assisted vaginal hysterectomy (LAVH), for endometrial cancer, 67
laparoscopic-assisted radical hysterectomy, 54–55
laparoscopy
for endometrial cancer, 67–68
for epithelial ovarian cancer, 79
laser therapy, for preinvasive cervical disease, 42
laser vaporization, 133
Latinas. *See* Hispanic American women
LAVH. *See* laparoscopically assisted vaginal hysterectomy
laxatives, for constipation, 150*t*
LDH. *See* lactate dehydrogenase
LDR. *See* low-dose brachytherapy
LEEP. *See* loop electro excision procedure
leiomyoma, differential diagnosis of, 105
leiomyosarcoma (LMS), 103
etiology and epidemiology of, 104–105
survival rates with, 104, 105*t*
Leser-Trélat syndrome, 77
letrozole
for epithelial ovarian cancer, 84*f*
side effects of, 153*t*
leucovorin, for gestational trophoblastic neoplasia, 120*t*–121*t*
LH. *See* luteinizing hormone
Lhermitte sign, 164
lichen sclerosis, 127–128
lidocaine
for alteration in vaginal mucous membranes, 160*t*
for peripheral neuropathy, 165*t*
lifestyle modifications, for menopausal symptoms, 172, 172*f*
lignans, and endometrial cancer, 66
lipoid cell tumors, ovarian, 98
liposomal doxorubicin
emetic risk potential of, 158*t*
side effects of, 153*t*
liquid-based Pap test, 22
lithium, and peripheral neuropathy, 164*t*
LMP. *See* low malignant potential
LMS. *See* leiomyosarcoma
loop electro excision procedure (LEEP), 41, 50
low-dose brachytherapy (LDR), for cervical cancer, 53
lower extremity lymphedema, 166–170, 167*f*
low-grade endometrial stromal sarcoma, 105
low-grade squamous intraepithelial lesion (LSIL), 37–38, 38*t*
ablation of, 42
HPV and, 20
management of, 40, 41*t*

low malignant potential (LMP), ovarian tumors of, 80
LSIL. *See* low-grade squamous intraepithelial lesion
Lubrin®, for menopausal symptoms, 174
luteal/secretory phase, 4–5, 6*f*
luteinizing hormone (LH), 4
LVSI. *See* lymphovascular space invasion
lymphadenectomy, for gynecologic sarcomas, 107
lymphatic drainage
  of breasts, 11, 12*f*
  of female genital tract, 10
lymphatic system, 166
lymphedema, 166–170, 167*f*
  diagnosis of, 167–168
  etiology of, 166
  incidence of, 166
  and quality of life, 169–170
  resources on, 168
  risk factors for, 166–167
  risk reduction recommendations for, 168–169, 169*t*
  stages of, 167*f*, 167*t*
  symptoms of, 167
  treatment of, 168, 168*t*
lymph nodes, 166
  dissection of, in pelvic exenteration, 140
  in vulvar cancer, 129–130
lymphoscintigraphy, 168
lymphovascular space invasion (LVSI), 51, 130
Lynch syndrome, 64–65, 76*t*, 77
  II, 24, 29–30

M

magnetic resonance imaging (MRI)
  and epithelial ovarian cancer, 78
  in pregnancy, 57
  and staging of cervical cancer, 51
  and trophoblastic disease, 117
manual lymph drainage (MLD), 168, 168*t*
mastalgia, 11
matrix-associated laser desorption ionization time-of-flight (MALDI-TOF) technology, and epithelial ovarian cancer, 79
MCL-1 gene, and trophoblastic disease, 117
MDM2 gene, and trophoblastic disease, 118
medroxyprogesterone acetate, for endometrial cancer, 69
medulla, 3
megestrol acetate, for endometrial cancer, 69
melanoma, vaginal, 132, 134*t*
melphalan, for sex cord stromal tumors, 98
menopause, 3, 14
  definition of, 170
  management of, 170–176
  symptoms of, 170
menstruation, 4–5, 6*f*
  issues affecting, 13–14
metaplasia, 47
methadone, for peripheral neuropathy, 165*t*
methotrexate
  for gestational trophoblastic neoplasia, 119, 119*t*, 120, 120*t*–121*t*
  for ovarian germ cell tumors, 96
  side effects of, 153*t*
  for vaginal cancer, 136
  for vulvar cancer, 131
metronidazole, and peripheral neuropathy, 164*t*
metrorrhagia, and cervical cancer, 50
mexiletine, for peripheral neuropathy, 165*t*
microinvasive disease, cervical, treatment of, 53
mifepristone, contraindications to, 116
minimally invasive surgery
  for cervical cancer, 54–55
  for endometrial cancer, 67–68
MIS. *See* Müllerian inhibitory substance
mitomycin
  emetic risk potential of, 158*t*
  side effects of, 153*t*
mitomycin C, for vaginal cancer, 136
mixed mesodermal sarcoma, 103–104
MLD. *See* manual lymph drainage
MLH1 gene, and endometrial cancer, 30, 65
MLH2 gene, and endometrial cancer, 65
modified Singapore flap, 141–142, 144*f*
molar pregnancy. *See* gestational trophoblastic disease
mons pubis, 9
mood, menopause and, 172
morphine, for peripheral neuropathy, 165*t*
motor nerves, 163
MRI. *See* magnetic resonance imaging
MSH2 gene, and endometrial cancer, 30
mTOR inhibitors, for endometrial cancer, 71
mucositis, management of, 155*t*
mucus plug, 8
Müllerian adenosarcoma, 106
  survival rates with, 105*t*
Müllerian inhibitory substance (MIS), and sex cord stromal tumors, 97
multiple papilloma, 11
myometrium, 7

N

Native American women, and epithelial ovarian cancer, 75
nausea
  management of, 155*t*–156*t*
  risk factors for, 158
Neisseria gonorrhoeae, 13
nerves, types of, functions of, 163
neuroendocrine carcinoma, of cervix, 50*t*
neuropathic pain, 164
  mechanism of, 165
neutropenia, management of, 154*t*
nicotine replacement, for smoking cessation, 172
night sweats, 171
  See also vasomotor symptoms
nipple discharge, 11
nondysgerminomatous tumors, 91
  chemotherapy for, 94, 95*t*
nonepithelial ovarian cancer, 91–101
nonkeratinizing squamous cell carcinoma, of cervix, 50*t*
nortriptyline, for peripheral neuropathy, 165*t*
nursing care, 158
  with brachytherapy, 161*t*
  with chemotherapy, 154*t*–157*t*, 159*t*
  with EBRT, 159*t*–160*t*
  and female reproductive system, 14
  with intraperitoneal chemotherapy, 159*t*
  with menopause, 171
  with pelvic exenteration, 144–147
  with peripheral neuropathy, 166
  with trophoblastic disease, 123

O

obesity
  and endometrial cancer, 28–29, 63–64
  and menopausal symptoms, 172
  and ovarian cancer, 24–25
OGCT. *See* ovarian germ cell tumors
oocyte, 3
oophorectomy, for cervical cancer, 53
opioids, for peripheral neuropathy, 165, 165*t*
oral contraceptives
  and cervical cancer, 18
  and endometrial cancer, 29, 31, 65
  and epithelial ovarian cancer, 75
  and gynecologic sarcomas, 104
  and ovarian cancer, 25
  and trophoblastic disease, 113, 114*f*, 117
os, 8, 17
osteopenia, definition of, 175
osteoporosis, 175–176
  definition of, 175
  risk factors for, 175*f*
ostomy care, 148*f*
ova, 3, 6
ovarian cancer, 23–28
  early signs and symptoms of, 25, 25*f*
  epithelial, 75–89
  incidence of, 75
  mortality rates with, 75
  multimodal screening for, 27–28
  nonepithelial, 91–101
  research initiatives on, 28
  screening for, 77
  staging of, 183
  treatment of, 23, 23*f*
  types of, 91, 91*f*
ovarian cycle, 4–5, 6*f*
ovarian cysts, 6
ovarian germ cell tumors (OGCT), 91–96
  circulating tumor marker substances with, 92, 93*t*
  clinical presentation of, 92
  diagnostic evaluation of, 92
  epidemiology of, 91–92
  etiology of, 91–92
  histologic typing of, 92*f*
  incidence of, 91
  long-term sequelae in, 94–95
  recurrent, 95–96
  staging of, 92–93
  treatment of, 93–94
ovarian sarcomas, 98–99, 106
  incidence of, 103
ovarian tumors
  benign, 6
  of low malignant potential, 80
ovaries, 3–6, 5*f*

benign pathophysiology of, 6
ovulation, 4–5, 6*f*
oxycodone, for peripheral neuropathy, 165*t*
oxygen therapy, for hypersensitivity reaction, 157*t*
oxytocin
contraindications to, 116
for trophoblastic disease, 116

P

p21 gene, in trophoblastic disease, 118
^{32}P, for epithelial ovarian cancer, 83
p57, in trophoblastic disease, 116
paced respirations, for menopausal symptoms, 172–173
paclitaxel
emetic risk potential of, 158*t*
for endometrial cancer, 70–71
for epithelial ovarian cancer, 80–83, 84*f*
for gynecologic sarcomas, 108
for ovarian germ cell tumors, 96
and peripheral neuropathy, 163
for sex cord stromal tumors, 98
side effects of, 153*t*
PAC protocol, for sex cord stromal tumors, 98
pain, with surgery, prevention/management of, 152*t*
palliative care, for cervical cancer, 57–58
pancytopenia, 136
papillary serous type endometrial cancer, treatment of, 71
Pap test, 22–23, 23*f,* 47, 50
Bethesda system and, 37–38, 38*t*
education on, 20–21, 42
endocervical, 22, 23*f*
liquid-based, 22
and management of preinvasive cervical disease, 41
and vaginal cancer, 132
parathyroid hormone (Forteo®), for osteoporosis, 176
paroxetine (Paxil®)
contraindications to, 174
for menopausal symptoms, 174
for peripheral neuropathy, 165*t*
patient education
on brachytherapy, 161*t*
on cervical cancer, 20–21
on chemotherapy, 154*t,* 159*t*
on external beam radiation, 159*t*–160*t*
on intraperitoneal chemotherapy, 159*t*
on lymphedema, 169*f*
on pelvic exenteration, 146
on peripheral neuropathy, 165
on radiation therapy, 158, 159*t*–160*t*
on surgery, 151*t*
on symptom management, 149, 150*t*–151*t*
pegfilgrastim, for infection, 154*t*
pelvic examination, 22, 22*f*
and epithelial ovarian cancer, 78
and ovarian cancer, 25, 26*f*
and trophoblastic disease, 117
and vaginal cancer, 132
pelvic exenteration, 139–148
anterior, 140, 141*f*
complications of, 142–143, 146*f*
contraindications to, 139, 139*f*
indications for, 139*f*
mortality rates with, 139
patient selection for, 139
posterior, 140, 142*f*
postoperative care, 146–147, 147*f*
preoperative care, 144–146, 146*f*
survival rates with, 139
for vaginal cancer, 134
pelvic inflammatory disease (PID), 12–13
pelvic lymphadenectomy, for cervical cancer, 52
pelvic lymph nodes, in endometrial cancer treatment, 69–70
pelvic pain, 13
pelvic reconstruction, 139–148
complications of, 142–143, 146*f*
pelvic support, disorders of, 9
perimenopause, definition of, 170
peripheral neuropathy (PN), 163–166
definition of, 163
etiologies of, 164*t*
treatment of, 165–166, 165*t*
PET. *See* positron emission tomography
phenoxodiol, for epithelial ovarian cancer, 84*f*
phenytoin, and peripheral neuropathy, 164*t*–165*t*
PHLDA2, in trophoblastic disease, 116
physical activity, and endometrial cancer, 31, 66
phytoestrogens, and endometrial cancer, 66
PID. *See* pelvic inflammatory disease
Pipelle®, 66–67, 67*f*
placental site trophoblastic tumor (PSTT), 113, 121–122
clinical presentation of, 121
diagnostic evaluation of, 121–122
management of, 122
plant alkaloids
and peripheral neuropathy, 163
side effects of, 153*t*
platinum
for epithelial ovarian cancer, 81
for gestational trophoblastic neoplasia, 120, 121*t*
and peripheral neuropathy, 163
PMS. *See* premenstrual syndrome
PN. *See* peripheral neuropathy
poly(ADP-ribose) polymerases, for epithelial ovarian cancer, 84
polycystic ovarian syndrome, 6
and endometrial cancer, 65
POMB-ACE protocol, for ovarian germ cell tumors, 96
positron emission tomography (PET)
and epithelial ovarian cancer, 78
and staging of cervical cancer, 51, 58
posterior pelvic exenteration, 140, 142*f*
prednisone, for peripheral neuropathy, 165*t*
preeclampsia, in trophoblastic disease, 115
pregnancy
and cervical cancer, 57
and endometrial cancer, 65
and ovarian cancer, 25, 94
trophoblastic disease and, 113–125
preinvasive cervical disease, 37–45
diagnostic tests for, 38–39
management of, 40–41, 41*t*
special considerations in, 42–43
premalignant lesions, vaginal/vulvar, 42
premature ovarian failure, 6
premenstrual syndrome (PMS), 13
primary peritoneal carcinoma, 75
prochlorperazine, for gestational trophoblastic neoplasia, 121*t*
procidentia, 7
progesterone, 3–4, 171
progesterone challenge, 30
progestin
and endometrial cancer, 65, 69
for endometrial hyperplasia, 30
for gynecologic sarcomas, 108
prostaglandin, contraindications to, 116
proteomic screening, for ovarian cancer, 28, 79
PSTT. *See* placental site trophoblastic tumor
psychosocial impact
of pelvic exenteration, 140, 143–144
of trophoblastic disease, 122–123
of vulvar cancer, 129
PTEN tumor suppressor gene, and endometrial cancer, 31
pudendal thigh flap, 141–142, 144*f*
pulmonary embolism, with surgery, prevention/management of, 152*t*
pyridoxine, and peripheral neuropathy, 164*t*

R

race
and cervical cancer, 18
and endometrial cancer, 28, 63, 65
and epithelial ovarian cancer, 75
and ovarian cancer, 23
and ovarian germ cell tumors, 92
and trophoblastic disease, 114
and uterine sarcomas, 103–104
radiation therapy (RT), 158
for cervical cancer, 52, 55–56
for endometrial cancer, 69–70
for epithelial ovarian cancer, 83
for gestational trophoblastic neoplasia, 120
for gynecologic sarcomas, 108
for ovarian germ cell tumors, 95
for sex cord stromal tumors, 98

side effects of, 52–53, 158
for vaginal cancer, 131, 134–135, 136*t*
for vulvar cancer, 130–131
radical hysterectomy
for cervical cancer, 52–53
classes of, 52
complications of, 52
laparoscopic-assisted, 54–55
in pelvic exenteration, 140
and sexual function, 53
radical trachelectomy
for cervical cancer, 53–54
selection criteria for, 54*f*
RALH. *See* robotic-assisted laparoscopic hysterectomy
raloxifene (Evista®)
and endometrial cancer, 29, 64
for epithelial ovarian cancer, 84*f*
for osteoporosis, 176
RB gene, in trophoblastic disease, 118
reconstruction. *See* pelvic reconstruction; vaginal reconstruction
rectus abdominis myocutaneous (RAM) flap, 141–142, 144*f*
relaxin, 4
Remifemin®, for menopausal symptoms, 173
renal transplants, and cervical cancer, 18
Replens®, for menopausal symptoms, 174
reproductive factors, and endometrial cancer, 29
reproductive function, pelvic exenteration and, 143
respiratory complications, pelvic exenteration and, 146
risendronate, for osteoporosis, 176
risk-reducing salpingo-oophorectomy (RRSO), 25–26
robotic-assisted laparoscopic hysterectomy (RALH), for endometrial cancer, 67
RT. *See* radiation therapy
rugae, 8

S

salpingo-oophorectomy
for ovarian germ cell tumors, 95*t*
risk-reducing, 25–26
See also bilateral salpingo-oophorectomy
sampling
cervical, additional, rationale for, 39, 40*f*
endometrial, 31
sarcomas
cervical, 103, 106–107
endometrial stromal, 105–106, 105*t*
gynecologic, 103–111
mixed mesodermal, 103–104
ovarian, 98–99, 103, 106
uterine, 103–108
vaginal, 132, 134*t*
vulvar-vaginal, 103, 107
sargramostim, for infection, 154*t*
SCC. *See* squamous cell carcinoma
SCJ. *See* squamocolumnar junction
screening
barriers to, 42
for cervical cancer, 22–23, 38, 42, 47
for endometrial cancer, 30–31, 66
for ovarian cancer, 27–28, 77
sedentary lifestyle, and menopausal symptoms, 172
SELDI-TOF technology, 79
selective estrogen-receptor response modulators (SERMs)
and endometrial cancer, 64
for epithelial ovarian cancer, 84*f*
side effects of, 153*t*
selective serotonin reuptake inhibitors (SSRIs)
for menopausal symptoms, 174
for peripheral neuropathy, 165*t*
sensory nerves, 163
sentinel lymph node mapping, in vulvar cancer, 130
SERMs. *See* selective estrogen-receptor response modulators
serosa, 7
serotonin norepinephrine reuptake inhibitor (SNRI), for menopausal symptoms, 174
Sertoli-Leydig tumors, characteristics and treatment of, 99*t*
sertraline, for peripheral neuropathy, 165*t*
sex cord stromal tumors, 96–98
classification of, 96*f*
clinical presentation of, 96–97
diagnostic evaluation of, 97
epidemiology of, 96
etiology of, 96
prognosis in, 97*t*
recurrent, 98
staging of, 97
treatment of, 97–98, 99*t*
sexual function, 11–12
cervical cancer treatment and, 53
menopausal symptoms and, 174–175
nursing care for, 151*t*–152*t*
ovarian cancer treatment and, 94
pelvic exenteration and, 143
vulvar cancer and, 127
sexually transmitted diseases (STDs), 12–13
See also human papillomavirus
SIL. *See* squamous intraepithelial lesions
site-specific familial ovarian cancer syndrome, 24, 24*f*
Skene glands, 9
skin care
for lymphedema, 168, 168*t*, 169
for radiation therapy, 160*t*
skip lesions, 133
small bowel obstruction, management of, 160*t*
small cell carcinoma
of cervix, 50*t*
ovarian, 98
smoking. *See* cigarette smoking
SNRI. *See* serotonin norepinephrine reuptake inhibitor
Society of Gynecologic Nurse Oncologists (SGNO), 1
sorafenib, for epithelial ovarian cancer, 84*f*
soy, for menopausal symptoms, 173
spiritual issues, 1
squamocolumnar junction (SCJ), 17, 47
squamous cell carcinoma (SCC), 38*t*
cervical, 47, 50*t*
HPV and, 19
vaginal, 132–133, 134*t*
vulvar, 127, 128*t*
squamous intraepithelial lesions (SIL), 38
SSRIs. *See* selective serotonin reuptake inhibitors
STDs. *See* sexually transmitted diseases
stratum basalis, 7
stratum functionalis, 7
streptococci, and PID, 13
suction curettage, for trophoblastic disease, 116
surface-enhanced laser desorption ionization time-of-flight (SELDI-TOF) technology, and epithelial ovarian cancer, 79
surgery, 149
for cervical cancer, 52, 54–55
completion, for cervical cancer, 56
for endometrial cancer, 67–68, 69*f*
exenterative, 140–144, 141*f*
for gestational trophoblastic neoplasia, 120
for gynecologic sarcomas, 107
for hereditary EOC, 77
minimally invasive, 54–55, 67–68
nursing care for, 151*t*–152*t*
for ovarian germ cell tumors, 93–94
second-look, for epithelial ovarian cancer, 83
for sex cord stromal tumors, 97–98
staging, for epithelial ovarian cancer, 79–80
for vaginal cancer, 133–134, 135*t*–136*t*
for vulvar cancer, 129
syphilis, 12

T

TAH. *See* total abdominal hysterectomy
tamoxifen
and endometrial cancer, 29, 64, 69
for epithelial ovarian cancer, 84*f*
and gynecologic sarcomas, 104, 106
side effects of, 153*t*
SSRIs and, 174
taxane
for epithelial ovarian cancer, 81, 84*f*
and peripheral neuropathy, 163
side effects of, 153*t*
TBS. *See* Bethesda system
temozolomide, for gynecologic sarcomas, 108
tenaculum, 67, 67*f*
testosterone, menopause and, 174
theca cells, 5
theca lutein cysts, in trophoblastic disease, 115–116
thecomas, characteristics and treatment of, 99*t*
ThinPrep, 22, 39
thrombocytopenia, management of, 154*t*

thyroid storm, 115
TNM system, 51, 129
tocainide, for peripheral neuropathy, 165*t*
topoisomerase-1 inhibitor, side effects of, 153*t*
topotecan
  for cervcial cancer, 57
  for epithelial ovarian cancer, 84*f*
  side effects of, 153*t*
total abdominal hysterectomy (TAH)
  for ovarian germ cell tumors, 93
  for sex cord stromal tumors, 97
TP53 gene, in trophoblastic disease, 118
trachelectomy, radical
  for cervical cancer, 53–54
  selection criteria for, 54*f*
transformation zone (TZ), 17, 37–38
transvaginal ultrasound (TVUS)
  and endometrial cancer, 30–31
  and ovarian cancer, 25–26
trastuzumab (Herceptin®)
  for endometrial cancer, 71
  and epithelial ovarian cancer, 80
trichomoniasis, 13
  vaginal, 12
tricyclic antidepressants, for peripheral neuropathy, 165, 165*t*
trophoblastic disease, 113–125
  definition of, 113
  epidemiology of, 113–114
  evidence-based practice and, 122
  psychosocial impact of, 122–123
  resources on, 123
  variants of, 113*f*
Trousseau syndrome, 77
tubercules of Montgomery, 11
tumor, node, metastasis (TNM) system, 51, 129
TVUS. *See* transvaginal ultrasound
TZ. *See* transformation zone

U

ultrasound
  and endometrial cancer, 30–31
  and epithelial ovarian cancer, 78
  and ovarian cancer, 25–26
  and trophoblastic disease, 115–117
undifferentiated endometrial sarcoma, 105
urinary alteration, management of, 152*t*, 159*t*
urinary diversions, pelvic exenteration and, 147, 147*f*
urogenital symptoms, of menopause, 170, 172
  management of, 174–175
urostomy, continent, care of, 148*f*
uterine bleeding, irregular, 13
uterine cancer, staging of, 182
uterine sarcomas
  clinical presentation of, 107
  diagnostic evaluation of, 107
  etiology and epidemiology of, 103–106, 104*t*
  histology of, 104, 105*t*
  incidence of, 103, 104*t*
  metastasis of, 104
  recurrent, 104
  staging of, 107
  survival rates with, 105*t*
  treatment of, 107–108
uterine sound, 67, 67*f*
uterine tumors resembling ovarian sex-cord tumors (UTROSCT), 106
uterus, 5*f*, 7–8
  benign pathophysiology of, 7–8
  examination of, 68, 70*f*
  prolapse of, 7
  See also endometrial cancer
UTROSCT. *See* uterine tumors resembling ovarian sex-cord tumors

V

VAC protocol, for sex cord stromal tumors, 98
Vagifem®, for menopausal symptoms, 174
vagina, 8–9, 140
  anatomy and natural history of, 132
  atrophy of, 174
  benign pathophysiology of, 8–9
  infection of, 9
  pH of, 8
  prolapse of, 9
vaginal bleeding
  in endometrial cancer, 66
  in uterine sarcomas, 107
vaginal cancer, 131–136
  clinical presentation of, 132
  diagnosis of, 132–133
  histology of, 133, 134*t*
  incidence of, 132
  recurrent, 136
  risk factors for, 132
  staging of, 133, 181
  survival rates with, 133
  treatment of, 133–136
vaginal defects, classification of, 141, 143*f*
vaginal discharge, 9
vaginal fistula, 9
vaginal intraepithelial neoplasia (VAIN), 40, 131, 133
  risk factors for, 40, 132
  treatment of, 133–134, 135*t*
vaginal mucous membranes, alteration in, management of, 160*t*
vaginal reconstruction, 140–142
  complications of, 142–143, 146*f*
vaginitis, 9, 12
VAIN. *See* vaginal intraepithelial neoplasia
valproic acid, for peripheral neuropathy, 165*t*
vasomotor symptoms, of menopause, 170
  management of, 171–174, 172*f*
  risk factors for, 171, 172*f*
VBP protocol, 94
venlafaxine (Effexor®)
  for menopausal symptoms, 174
  side effects of, 174
verrucous carcinoma, of cervix, 50*t*
VIN. *See* vulvar intraepithelial neoplasia
vinblastine
  for ovarian germ cell tumors, 94, 96
  for vaginal cancer, 136
vincristine (Oncovin®)
  for gestational trophoblastic neoplasia, 119, 120*t*
  for ovarian germ cell tumors, 94, 96
  and peripheral neuropathy, 163
vinorelbine
  emetic risk potential of, 158*t*
  for epithelial ovarian cancer, 84*f*
  side effects of, 153*t*
vitamin D, for osteoporosis, 175
vitamin E
  for menopausal symptoms, 173
  for peripheral neuropathy, 165
VNNED. *See* vulvar non-neoplastic epithelial disorder
vomiting
  management of, 155*t*–156*t*
  risk factors for, 158
vulva, 9–10, 10*f*
  benign pathophysiology of, 9–10
vulvar cancer, 127–131
  clinical presentation of, 128–129
  diagnosis of, 127, 129, 129*t*
  etiology and epidemiology of, 127–128, 128*t*
  metastasis in, 129
  prevalence of, 127
  prognosis in, 129
  recurrent, 131
  staging of, 127, 129, 181
  treatment of, 127, 129–130
vulvar intraepithelial neoplasia (VIN), 39–40, 127
  presentation of, 128
  risk factors for, 40
vulvar non-neoplastic epithelial disorder (VNNED), 127
  presentation of, 128
vulvar-vaginal sarcomas
  etiology and epidemiology of, 107
  incidence of, 103
vulvitis, 10

W

WAI. *See* whole abdominal irradiation
warts, genital, 12
  ablation of, 42
  and cervical cancer, 50*t*
  HPV and, 20, 20*t*, 37
  incidence of, 20
  and vulvar intraepithelial neoplasia, 39
weight control, for menopausal symptoms, 172
whole abdominal irradiation (WAI), for endometrial cancer, 70
Williams, John, 37

X

Xylotax®, for epithelial ovarian cancer, 83

Z

zoledronic acid, for osteoporosis, 176